Socioemotional Development
in Cultural Context

**SOCIAL, EMOTIONAL, AND PERSONALITY
DEVELOPMENT IN CONTEXT**
Kenneth H. Rubin, *Series Editor*

Handbook of Peer Interactions, Relationships, and Groups
*Edited by Kenneth H. Rubin, William M. Bukowski,
and Brett Laursen*

The Development of Shyness and Social Withdrawal
Edited by Kenneth H. Rubin and Robert J. Coplan

Socioemotional Development in Cultural Context
Edited by Xinyin Chen and Kenneth H. Rubin

SOCIOEMOTIONAL DEVELOPMENT IN CULTURAL CONTEXT

Edited by

Xinyin Chen
Kenneth H. Rubin

THE GUILFORD PRESS
New York   London

© 2011 The Guilford Press
A Division of Guilford Publications, Inc.
72 Spring Street, New York, NY 10012
www.guilford.com

Printed in the United States of America

This book is printed on acid-free paper.

Last digit is print number: 9 8 7 6 5 4 3 2 1

The authors have checked with sources believed to be reliable in their efforts to
provide information that is complete and generally in accord with the standards
of practice that are accepted at the time of publication. However, in view of the
possibility of human error or changes in behavioral, mental health, or medical
sciences, neither the authors, nor the editor and publisher, nor any other party
who has been involved in the preparation or publication of this work warrants
that the information contained herein is in every respect accurate or complete,
and they are not responsible for any errors or omissions or the results obtained
from the use of such information. Readers are encouraged to confirm the
information contained in this book with other sources.

Library of Congress Cataloging-in-Publication Data

Socioemotional development in cultural context / edited by Xinyin Chen and
Kenneth H. Rubin.
    p. cm. — (Social, emotional, and personality development in context)
    Includes bibliographical references and index.
    ISBN 978-1-60918-186-4 (cloth: alk. paper)
    1. Child psychology. 2. Child development. 3. Emotions in children.
4. Culture—Psychological aspects. I. Chen, Xinyin. II. Rubin, Kenneth H.
    BF721.S5737 2011
    155.4—dc22

                                                                   2011001077

About the Editors

Xinyin Chen, PhD, is Professor of Psychology in the Applied Psychology–Human Development Division, Graduate School of Education, at the University of Pennsylvania in Philadelphia. He is a Fellow of the American Psychological Association and the Association for Psychological Science and a member of the Executive Committee of the International Society for the Study of Behavioral Development. Dr. Chen has received a William T. Grant Scholars Award, a Shanghai Eastern Scholars Award, and several other academic awards. His primary research interest is children's and adolescents' socioemotional functioning (e.g., shyness–inhibition, social competence, and affect) and social relationships from a cultural–contextual perspective. He has coedited the books *Peer Relationships in Cultural Context* (2006) and *Social Change and Human Development: Concepts and Results* (2010), and published a number of articles in major journals such as *Child Development, Developmental Psychology*, and *Annual Review of Psychology* and book chapters concerning culture, children's social behaviors and peer relationships, and parental socialization practices.

Kenneth H. Rubin, PhD, is Professor of Human Development and Director of the Center for Children, Relationships, and Culture at the University of Maryland in College Park. He is a Fellow of the Canadian Psychological Association, the American Psychological Association, and the Association for Psychological Science. In 2008, Dr. Rubin received the award for Distinguished Contributions to the International Advancement of Research and Theory in Behavioral Development from the International Society for the Study of Behavioral Development. In 2010, he received the Developmental Psychology Mentor Award from the American Psychological Association.

Dr. Rubin has twice served as Associate Editor of *Child Development* and is currently on several editorial boards. From 1998 to 2002, he was President of the International Society for the Study of Behavioral Development, and he is currently a member of the Governing Council of the Society for Research in Child Development.

Dr. Rubin's publications include 19 books and over 270 peer-reviewed chapters and journal articles on such topics as social competence, social cognition, play, aggression, social anxiety and withdrawal, and children's peer and family relationships. He is currently Principal Investigator for research projects on friendship and psychosocial adjustment in middle childhood and adolescence and a multimethod early intervention program for socially reticent, inhibited preschoolers, both funded by the National Institute of Mental Health.

Contributors

Alaina Brenick, PhD, Human Behaviour in Social and Economic Change Program, University of Jena, Jena, Germany

Xinyin Chen, PhD, Applied Psychology–Human Development Division, Graduate School of Education, University of Pennsylvania, Philadelphia, Pennsylvania

Michiko Otsuki Clutter, PhD, Department of Psychology, University of South Florida, St. Petersburg, Florida

Pamela M. Cole, PhD, Department of Psychology, The Pennsylvania State University, University Park, Pennsylvania

Madeleine Currie, EdM, Graduate School of Education, Harvard University, Cambridge, Massachusetts

Sara Douglass, MA, Department of Applied Developmental Psychology, Fordham University, Bronx, New York

Katie Ellison, BA, Department of Human Development, University of Maryland, College Park, Maryland

Doran C. French, PhD, Child Development and Family Studies Department, Purdue University, West Lafayette, Indiana

Nancy G. Guerra, PhD, Department of Psychology, University of California, Riverside, California

Amber J. Hammons, PhD, Family Resiliency Center, University of Illinois at Urbana–Champaign, Urbana, Illinois

Sara Harkness, PhD, Center for the Study of Culture, Health, and Development, University of Connecticut, Storrs, Connecticut

Heidi Keller, PhD, Faculty of Human Sciences, University of Osnabrueck, Osnabrueck, Germany

Melanie Killen, PhD, Department of Human Development, University of Maryland, College Park, Maryland

Caroline Johnston Mavridis, MA, Center for the Study of Culture, Health, and Development, University of Connecticut, Storrs, Connecticut

Melissa Menzer, BA, Department of Human Development, University of Maryland, College Park, Maryland

Wonjung Oh, PhD, Department of Psychology, University of Michigan, Ann Arbor, Michigan

Hiltrud Otto, PhD, Faculty of Human Sciences, University of Osnabrueck, Osnabrueck, Germany

Fred Rothbaum, PhD, Eliot–Pearson Department of Child Development, Tufts University, Medford, Massachusetts

Kenneth H. Rubin, PhD, Center for Children, Relationships, and Culture, University of Maryland, College Park, Maryland

Natalie Rusk, EdM, Eliot–Pearson Department of Child Development, Tufts University, Medford, Massachusetts

Rainer K. Silbereisen, PhD, Department of Developmental Psychology, University of Jena, Jena, Germany

Joan Stevenson-Hinde, ScD, Sub-Department of Animal Behaviour, Department of Zoology, University of Cambridge, Cambridge, United Kingdom

Charles M. Super, PhD, Department of Human Development and Family Studies, University of Connecticut, Storrs, Connecticut

Martin J. Tomasik, PhD, Center for Applied Developmental Science, University of Jena, Jena, Germany

Gisela Trommsdorff, PhD, Department of Psychology, University of Konstanz, Konstanz, Germany

Tiffany Yip, PhD, Department of Psychology, Fordham University, Bronx, New York

Hirokazu Yoshikawa, PhD, Graduate School of Education, Harvard University, Cambridge, Massachusetts

Contents

III. SOCIOEMOTIONAL PROCESSES

IV. ADAPTIVE AND MALADAPTIVE SOCIAL FUNCTIONING

Culture and Socioemotional Development
An Introduction

XINYIN CHEN *and* KENNETH H. RUBIN

C hildren across cultures generally differ in observed socioemotional characteristics. For example, Asian children are less expressive of positive emotions (e.g., smiling and laughing) than their Western counterparts (e.g., Camras et al., 1998; Gartstein et al., 2006; Knyazev, Zupancic, & Slobodskaya, 2008). Young children in many non-Western societies, particularly in such group-oriented societies as Mayan (Gaskins, 2000), Bedouin Arab (Ariel & Sever, 1980), and Kenyan, Mexican, and Indian societies (Edwards, 2000), tend to engage in less sociodramatic play than Western children. Relatedly, the themes of social pretense vary across cultural and ethnic groups; Farver, Kim, and Lee (1995) found that the sociodramatic play of Korean-American children involved more thematic, daily-life activities (e.g., family role play) and fewer fantasy themes (e.g., actions related to legend or fairy tale characters) than Anglo-American children.

In general, children in traditional societies in which extended families live together and children are required to assume family responsibilities tend to display more prosocial–cooperative behaviors than children in economically complex societies with class structures and occupational divisions of labor (Edwards, 2000). Moreover, as a society increases in urbanization, children's cooperative behavior seems to decline (e.g., Graves &

1

Graves, 1983). There is also evidence that children in China, India, Korea, and some South American countries are more cooperative in their social interactions than children in North American countries (e.g., Farver et al., 1995; Kagan & Knight, 1981; Orlick, Zhou, & Partington, 1990). Relative to their North American counterparts, children in Australia, in some Asian countries such as China, Korea, and Thailand, and in some European nations such as Sweden and the Netherlands appear to exhibit less aggressive and oppositional behaviors (e.g., Bergeron & Schneider, 2005; Russell, Hart, Robinson, & Olsen, 2003; Weisz et al., 1988). Zahn-Waxler, Friedman, Cole, Mizuta, and Hiruma (1996) found that Japanese children showed less anger than U.S. children in their responses to hypothetical situations involving conflict and distress. Considerable variability also exists in children's social attitudes and behaviors within a society. Cole, Tamang, and Shrestha (2006), for example, found that Brahman children are more likely to endorse aggressive behavior than Tamang children in Nepal. Brahman children react to difficult social situations such as peer conflict with anger and other negative emotions more often than Tamang children do.

Finally, Asian and Western children have been found to differ in their reactivity to stressful situations. Rubin et al. (2006) found that Korean and Chinese toddlers exhibited more fearful and anxious reactivity in unfamiliar laboratory situations than Italian and Australian toddlers. In a comprehensive analysis of children's inhibited behavior in laboratory situations, Chen et al. (1998) found that, compared with Canadian toddlers, Chinese toddlers were more vigilant and reactive in novel situations. Chinese toddlers stayed closer to their mothers and were less likely to explore the environment. Also, Chinese toddlers displayed more anxious behaviors, as reflected in their greater latency to approach unfamiliar adults and objects.

Given this brief background, it would appear essential to ask the following questions:

1. What specific social-contextual factors are responsible for cultural variability in children's socioemotional functioning?
2. How do distinct patterns of socioemotional functioning emerge in particular societies or communities?
3. Do cultural factors affect the developmental outcomes of a specific socioemotional characteristic or behavior? If so, what processes can explain these outcomes?

To answer these questions, it is important to understand the meaning of socioemotional functioning within given cultures. Cultural norms and values serve as a framework for interpreting and evaluating socioemotional characteristics (Benedict, 1934; Chen & French, 2008). As a result, children who display specific behaviors may evoke predictable responses from others in their social milieus (e.g., acceptance, rejection); in turn, these responses may serve to guide children's maintenance or inhibition of these behaviors during the course of their development.

Theoretical Perspectives

Traditionally, theorists have attempted to explain the relations between culture and human development from either socioecological (Bronfenbrenner & Morris, 2006; Super & Harkness, 1986) or sociocultural perspectives (Rogoff, 2003; Vygotsky, 1978). According to socioecological theory, the beliefs and practices that are endorsed within a cultural group play an important role as a part of the socioecological environment in shaping children's social and cognitive development. In addition to its direct effects, culture may regulate development through organizing various social settings such as community services, schools, and daycare facilities. Sociocultural theory, on the other hand, focuses primarily on the internalization of external symbolic systems such as language and symbols, along with their cultural meanings, from the interpersonal level to the intrapersonal level. Collaborative or guided learning in which more experienced peers or adults assist the child in understanding and solving problems represents the primary mechanism for development (e.g., Rogoff, 2003).

In this edited compendium, both Joan Stevenson-Hinde and Xinyin Chen discuss culture and socioemotional development from the perspective of social interactions and relationships. Drawing from a conceptual model proposed by Hinde (1987), Stevenson-Hinde and Chen argue that there are multiple dynamic social processes linking the individual and culture. While constrained by underlying biological processes, individuals are embedded in networks of social relationships and groups. According to Stevenson-Hinde (Chapter 1, this volume), each level of social complexity has its emergent properties. For example, although the quality of given relationships may be a product of a history of interactions between individuals, relationships are actually more complex than the simple sum of interactions. Moreover, each level of complexity affects, and is affected by, other levels. At the same time, individuals—and their interactions and relationships—influence and are influenced by cultural beliefs, values, and norms. In his contextual–developmental model, Chen (Chapter 2, this volume) emphasizes such interaction processes as social evaluations and responses as primary mediators of cultural influence on individual behavior and development. He argues that children, who carry biologically based dispositional tendencies, play an active role in their development through participating in culturally directed social interactions. Therefore, the processes of social development are bidirectional and transactional. Through these processes, personal characteristics, socialization, and cultural factors collectively shape children's socioemotional functioning and its developmental patterns.

Methodological Issues

Cross-cultural researchers often compare two or more cultures on a given phenomenon of interest. In the case of socioemotional development, this approach is useful in revealing cultural variations in children's attitudes, emotions, and behaviors. Despite many methodological difficulties in this approach (e.g., selecting representative cultural groups; controlling for confounding factors such as socioeconomic status; establishing equivalence in measurement; and making culturally appropriate interpretations of the data; Schneider, French, & Chen, 2006), in the past 20 years, cross-cultural research has amassed valuable information about the role of cultural contexts in children's socioemotional functioning.

Common methods for studying socioemotional development include teacher, parent, and self reports; peer evaluations; observations; qualitative interviews; and, to a lesser extent, physiological assessments. Each of these methods has its noticeable strengths and weaknesses. Self-report data are most commonly used in cross-cultural studies because they are relatively easy and inexpensive to obtain. However, there are obvious limitations in the use of self-report data; these limitations include culturally specific response biases, the "reference group" effect, and differences in participants' understanding of the items and their willingness to reveal personal information to others. Each of these limitations can undermine the validity of data (e.g., Peng, Nisbett, & Wong, 1997; Schneider et al., 2006). This is dramatically illustrated by the findings of Weisz, Chaiyasit, Weiss, Eastman, and Jackson (1995) who discovered that, although Thai teachers provided higher behavior problem ratings to students than did American teachers, trained observers found that Thai students displayed fewer behavioral problems than their American counterparts. Peer evaluation (e.g., the Revised Class Play; Masten, Morison, & Pellegrini, 1985), another common technique in assessing children's socioemotional functioning, is particularly useful for cross-cultural research because it taps insiders' perspectives about child behavior and reputation. However, peer evaluation can be used only with children who are old enough to understand the methodological process (perhaps from beyond the age of 7 years). Moreover, it does not permit direct cross-cultural comparisons on group mean scores, because peer nomination or rating data often need to be standardized within a classroom or grade. Behavioral observation, either in controlled laboratory or naturalistic settings, provides relatively objective information about social behaviors. However, it is a challenge to maintain equivalent conditions in different observation settings, develop culturally sensitive coding systems, and train coders to reliably code observational data from different cultures. Given the strengths and weakness of each method, it is necessary to consider a multimethod approach, which can likely reduce potential biases and errors in the data from a single source. Through integrative analysis, data from multiple sources allow for the detection of general and convergent patterns, rather than specific variables or scores (see Keller & Otto, Chapter 7; Killen & Brenick, Chapter 10, this volume).

An important goal of the cross-cultural study of socioemotional functioning is understanding its meaning in a cultural context. This goal may be achieved in a variety of ways. Consistent with the contextual–developmental perspective (Chen, Chapter 2, this volume), researchers may examine (1) how a specific behavior is associated with the quality of children's social interactions and relationships and (2) how the behavior develops (e.g., how it is associated with other culturally relevant variables and what developmental outcomes it leads to) in the culture. An exploration of a given behavior in the context of social interactions and relationships helps the researcher to comprehend the functional meaning that the culture ascribes to the behavior. Longitudinal research may tap into the developmental significance and processes of the behavior.

The Organization of the Book

Despite prevailing arguments on the importance of the cultural context for human development (e.g., Hinde, 1987; Vygotsky, 1978), the role of culture in children's and adolescents' socioemotional functioning has traditionally received inadequate attention from developmental scientists. As a result, the understanding of socioemotional development has been largely limited to Western, particularly North American cultures. In the past two decades, interest in cultural involvement in socioemotional development in childhood and adolescence has burgeoned and expanded exponentially in many regions of the world, particularly in Asia, Europe, and South America. A number of research programs have been developed in different cultural contexts; the findings have consistently supported the view that children's socioemotional functioning may vary in its prevalence, interpretation, causes, and consequences across cultures.

This book responds to the need for a comprehensive discussion of the relationship between culture and socioemotional development. Leading scholars in the field who are committed to understanding cultural issues in children's socioemotional functioning address issues such as the impact of social circumstances and cultural values on socioemotional functioning; culturally prescribed socialization processes in socioemotional development; the cultural definitions and interpretations of children's socioemotional experience, expression, and regulation; and maladaptive socioemotional functioning from a cultural perspective. The paired roles of culture and development are emphasized in each chapter. The authors incorporate into their discussions findings from research programs that have used (1) multiple methodologies, including both qualitative (e.g., interviewing and observational) and quantitative (e.g., large-scale surveys, standardized questionnaires) approaches and (2) a wide range of ages (from early childhood to the teen years) of individuals growing up in cultures from East to West and from South to North (including Asia, South America, the Middle East, Eastern Europe) and ethnic groups in the United States.

Part I focuses on theoretical issues and the policy implications of studying culture and socioemotional development. The first two chapters provide general frameworks for a discussion of the processes of cultural involvement in development from the perspectives of attachment/fearfulness (Stevenson-Hinde, Chapter 1) and peer interaction (Chen, Chapter 2). Yoshikawa and Currie (Chapter 3) analyze the impact of public policies, such as those pertaining to immigration, on socialization beliefs and goals.

Part II discusses parental belief systems and socialization practices in a cultural context. Harkness, Super, and Mavridis (Chapter 4) argue that, to a large extent, culture determines parental beliefs, values, and practices at both the general (e.g., images of children, models of good parenting) and specific (e.g., particular parenting styles, views of emotion expression and suppression) levels. Cultural scripts of socialization practices, in turn, shape children's socioemotional development in various areas. Rothbaum and Rusk (Chapter 5) further discuss how socialization goals, strategies, and cultural circumstances mesh with one another, which has implications for individual development.

Part III explores the role culture plays in major socioemotional processes including emotion and emotion regulation (Trommsdorff and Cole, Chapter 6), autonomy (Keller and Otto, Chapter 7), self-identity (Yip and Douglass, Chapter 8), and dyadic relationships (Rubin, Oh, Menzer, and Ellison, Chapter 9). Through its influence on social relationships, culture may serve to regulate the development of individual characteristics including autonomy, self-regulatory ability, and self-image. In addition, as shown by Rubin and colleagues, cultural norms and values may affect the structure, function, and nature of dyadic relationships between parents and their children and between friends.

The chapters in Part IV tap into relatively wide ranges of adaptive and maladaptive social functioning such as morality and social exclusion (Killen and Brenick, Chapter 10), conflict management (French, Chapter 11), and aggression (Guerra, Hammons, and Clutter, Chapter 12). These chapters emphasize that adaptive and maladaptive socioemotional functioning is often defined by cultural norms and, thus, an understanding of the developmental patterns of adaptive and maladaptive behaviors must take cultural factors into account. Moreover, as described by Silbereisen and Tomasik (Chapter 13), social, political, economic, and cultural contexts are constantly changing. As a result, it is increasingly common for children to live in an environment with mixed values and lifestyles and for children with diverse backgrounds to interact with one another. Research on children's and adolescents' socioemotional functioning in changing circumstances is important in developmental science.

This book is unique in many ways. To begin with, it emphasizes social and cultural contexts, perspectives from multidisciplinary backgrounds, and the presentation of recent research findings based on qualitative and quantitative approaches. It comprises not only reviews of existing studies, but also serves as a guide in transcending the assumptions of middle-class Western culture about socioemotional development. The material in the book is likely to fill a significant gap in the literature on basic developmental processes as well as context for human development.

References

Ariel, S., & Sever, I. (1980). Play in the desert and play in the town: On play activities of Bedouin Arab children. In H.B. Schwartzman (Ed.), *Play and culture* (pp. 164-175). West Point, NY: Leisure Press.

Benedict, R. (1934). Anthropology and the abnormal. *Journal of General Psychology, 10,* 59–82.

Bergeron, N., & Schneider, B.H. (2005). Explaining cross-national differences in peer-directed aggression: A quantitative synthesis. *Aggressive Behavior, 31,* 116–137.

Bronfenbrenner, U., & Morris, P. A. (2006). The bioecological model of human development. In W. Damon (Series Ed.) & R. M. Lerner (Vol. Ed.), *Handbook of child psychology: Vol 1. Theoretical models of human development* (pp. 793–828). New York: Wiley.

Camras, L. A., Oster, H., Campos, J., Campos, R., Ujiie, T., Miyake, K., Wang, L., et al. (1998). Production of emotional facial expressions in European American, Japanese, and Chinese infants. *Developmental Psychology, 34,* 616–628.

Chen, X. & French, D. (2008). Children's social competence in cultural context. *Annual Review of Psychology, 59,* 591-616.

Chen, X., Hastings, P., Rubin, K. H., Chen, H., Cen, G., & Stewart, S. L. (1998). Childrearing attitudes and behavioral inhibition in Chinese and Canadian toddlers: A cross-cultural study. *Developmental Psychology, 34,* 677–686.

Cole, P. M., Tamang, B. L., & Shrestha, S. (2006). Cultural variations in the socialization of young children's anger and shame. *Child Development, 77,* 1237–1251.

Edwards, C. P. (2000). Children's play in cross-cultural perspective: A new look at the Six Culture Study. *Cross-Cultural Research, 34,* 318–338.

Farver, J. M., Kim, Y. K., & Lee, Y. (1995). Cultural differences in Korean- and Anglo-American preschoolers' social interaction and play behaviors. *Child Development, 66,* 1088–1099.

Gartstein, M. A., Gonzalez, C., Carranza, J. A., Ahadi, S. A., Ye, R., Rothbart, M. K., et al.. (2006). Studying cross-cultural differences in the development of infant temperament: People's Republic of China, the United States of America, and Spain. *Child Psychiatry & Human Development, 37,* 145–161.

Gaskins, S. (2000). Children's daily activities in a Mayan village: A culturally grounded description. *Cross-Cultural Research, 34,* 375–389.

Graves, N. B., & Graves, T. D. (1983). The cultural context of prosocial development: An ecological model. In D.L. Bridgeman (Ed.), *The nature of prosocial development* (pp. 795–824). San Diego, CA: Academic Press.

Hinde, R. A. (1987). *Individuals, relationships and culture.* Cambridge: Cambridge University Press.

Kagan, S., & Knight, G. P. (1981). Social motives among Anglo-American and Mexican-American children: Experimental and projective measures. *Journal of Research in Personality, 15,* 93–106.

Knyazev, G. G., Zupancic, G. G., & Slobodskaya, H. R. (2008). Child personality in Slovenia and Russia: Structure and mean level of traits in parent and self-ratings. *Journal of Cross-Cultural Psychology, 39,* 317–334.

Masten, A., Morison, P., & Pellegrini, D. (1985). A revised class play method of peer assessment. *Developmental Psychology, 21* 523–533.

Orlick, T., Zhou, Q. Y., & Partington, J. (1990). Co-operation and conflict within Chinese and Canadian kindergarten settings. *Canadian Journal of Behavioral Science, 22,* 20–25.

Peng, K., Nisbett, R. E., & Wong, N. Y. (1997). Validity problems comparing values across cultures and possible solutions. *Psychological Methods, 2,* 329–344.

Rogoff, B. (2003). *The cultural nature of human development.* New York, Oxford University Press.

Rubin, K. H., Hemphill, S. A., Chen, X., Hastings, P., Sanson, A., LoCoco, A. et al. (2006b). A cross-cultural study of behavioral inhibition in toddlers: East-west-north-south. *International Journal of Behavioral Development, 30,* 219–226.

Russell, A., Hart, C. H., Robinson, C. C., & Olsen, S. F. (2003). Children's sociable and aggressive behavior with peers: A comparison of the US and Australia, and contributions of temperament and parenting styles. *International Journal of Behavioral Development, 27,* 74–86.

Schneider, B., French, D., & Chen, X. (2006). Peer relationships in cultural perspective: Methodological reflections. In X. Chen, D. French, & B. Schneider (Eds.), *Peer relationships in cultural context* (pp. 489–500). New York: Cambridge University Press.

Super, C. M., & Harkness, S. (1986). The developmental niche: A conceptualization at the interface of child and culture. *International Journal of Behavioral Development, 9,* 545–569.

Vygotsky, L. S. (1978). In M. Cole, V. John-Steiner, S. Scribner & E. Souberman (Eds.), *Mind in society: The development of higher psychological processes.* Cambridge, MA: Harvard University Press.

Weisz, J. R., Chaiyasit, W., Weiss, B., Eastman, K. L., & Jackson, E. E. (1995). A multimethod study of problem behavior among Thai and American children in school: Teacher reports versus direct observations. *Child Development, 66,* 402–415.

Weisz, J. R., Suwanlert, S., Chaiyasit, W., Weiss, B., Walter, B. R., & Anderson, W. W. (1988). Thai and American perspectives on over-and undercontrolled child behavior problems: Exploring the threshold model among parents, teachers, and psychologists. *Journal of Consulting and Clinical Psychology, 56,* 601–609.

Zahn-Waxler, C., Friedman, R. J., Cole, P. M., Mizuta, I., & Hiruma, N. (1996). Japanese and United States preschool children's responses to conflict and distress. *Child Development, 67,* 2462–2477.

PART I

THEORETICAL PERSPECTIVES AND POLICY IMPLICATIONS

CHAPTER 1

Culture and Socioemotional Development, with a Focus on Fearfulness and Attachment

JOAN STEVENSON-HINDE

As implied by its title—*Socioemotional Development in Cultural Context*—this book covers a broad canvas, ranging from underlying physiological mechanisms to cultural values. Therefore, it may be helpful to view the chapters within the overall framework developed by Hinde (1979, 1987), which emphasizes the dialectical relations among various levels of analysis, from internal physiological and psychological processes, to individual behavior, interactions, relationships, groups, and society (see Figure 1.1). Additionally, each level influences and is influenced by the sociocultural context, with its shared values and conventions, as well as by the socioeconomic context. The latter may involve the availability of resources such as education, work, and social mobility. Both types of context are reflected in Super and Harkness's (1986) term *developmental niche*, namely, "(1) the physical and social settings in which the child lives; (2) culturally regulated customs of child care and child rearing; and (3) the psychology of the caretakers. . . . The three components of the developmental niche form the cultural context of child development" (p. 552).

But before moving on, it is worth noting that the framework developed by Hinde owes its origins not to the study of humans, but rather to research with rhesus monkeys, and before that to ethology and the development of John Bowlby's attachment theory. In seeking to understand why mater-

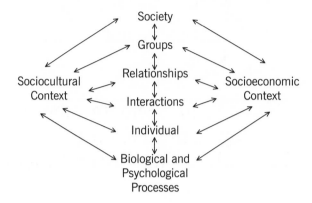

FIGURE 1.1. A framework indicating dialectical relations among successive levels of social complexity. Each level influences and is influenced by other levels, operating within cultural and socioeconomic contexts. Not illustrated is a "diachronic perspective," that involves continuous creation and change over time through the dialectical influences within and among the levels. Based on Hinde (1987, 2009).

nal separation should have long-lasting negative effects on young children, Bowlby came across ethology. Here he found the focus was not on the unconscious fantasies of his psychoanalytic training, but rather on behavioral observations in naturally occurring contexts. Such observations gave rise to relevant concepts such as "imprinting" (Lorenz, 1935) and underlying "behavior systems" (Baerends, 1976; see also Hinde, 2005, Stevenson-Hinde, 2007). In discussions with Hinde, Bowlby suggested setting up a rhesus monkey colony where separation effects could be observed under controlled conditions. Infants were born into any one of six groups, each consisting of several females, their offspring, and an adult male. Separation effects were indeed found, with their severity depending upon the mother's responsiveness to her infant upon reunion (Hinde, 1977; Hinde & McGinnis, 1977).

In addition to permitting planned separations, the research with monkeys illustrated what might have been more difficult to appreciate in humans. That is, detailed observations could be made routinely from before birth onward; the interactions and relationship with the mother were highlighted since a rhesus mother is virtually the only caregiver; and the influence of the social group was clear since interactions with other group members could be readily observed. Concerning the overall development of the mother–infant relationship, Hinde concluded that, although particular *interactions* change with age, the nature of the *relationship* transcends any particular set of interactions and indeed may be said to exist even during separation.

Additionally, mother–infant interactions and relationships were influenced by other members of the group. This perception led to the framework (e.g., Hinde & Stevenson-Hinde, 1976) that informed later research.

Returning to the framework developed for humans (see Figure 1.1), each level has emergent properties not relevant to the level below. For example, although relationships are built upon antecedent behavioral interactions, relationships are more than the simple sum of interactions, with inferred qualities such as sensitivity or warmth. Additionally, "each level is affected by other levels: the nature of a personal relationship is affected not only by its constituent interactions, but also by the group in which it is embedded. . . . Furthermore, each of the levels of complexity affects, and is affected by, the sociocultural structure of the ideology, beliefs, values, norms, institutions and so on, more or less shared by the individuals in the group or society." Finally, "Each level must thus be treated not as an entity but as involving processes of continuous creation, change or degradation through the dialectical influences within and between levels" (Hinde, 1999, pp. 19–20; see also Hinde, 2009).

Thus, Figure 1.1 represents a dynamic framework with bidirectional influences. This basic conception is not unlike that of family systems theorists, who stress continuous cycles of interactions within a system that involves both stability and change (e.g., Minuchin, 1985). Transactional models and dynamic systems theory, involving a continuous process of change with innovative outcomes, are particularly relevant to childrearing. As stated by Kuczynski (2003) in his review of bidirectional frameworks, "The task of parenting is to rear a rapidly changing organism; therefore, adaptation to change rather than stability is an essential element of successful parenting" (p. 7).

Two Major Developmental Constructs

Central to socioemotional development are two major constructs, fearfulness and attachment. In terms of our dialectical framework (Figure 1.1), we may identify underlying processes that interact with an individual's fearful behavior or attachment behavior, which in turn influence and are influenced by interactions and relationships. Furthermore, cultural beliefs and norms "help interpret the acceptability of individual characteristics and the types and ranges of interactions and relationships that are likely or permissible" (Rubin, 1998, p. 611).

Appreciating cultural influences is not incompatible with Bowlby's proposition concerning *origins*, namely that both fearful behavior and attachment behavior are universal and share a common evolutionary function, protection from harm (Bowlby, 1969/1982). Bowlby's argument is that, unlike other individuals, those individuals who exhibited *appropriate* (neither too little nor too much) fear of the unfamiliar would have been more apt to survive and leave offspring who, in turn, successfully reproduce. In a similar way, attachment behavior[1] (defined as behavior that increases proximity to an attachment figure in times of stress) and its complement, caregiving behavior, must have been selected for during the course of evolution (for an excellent overview of attachment, see Cassidy, 2008). "Therefore a core element of attachment theory is the idea of the universality of this bias in infants to become attached, regardless of their specific cultural niche" (van IJzendoorn & Sagi, 2008, p. 881). Fearfulness and attachment will now be considered in turn.

Fearfulness

All the major theories of childhood temperament contain a dimension related to fearfulness (reviewed in Goldsmith et al., 1987; see also Vaughn, Bost, & van IJzendoorn, 2008), a trait that has been recognized over the centuries (e.g., Kagan, 1994). Furthermore, consistent individual differences in fearfulness appear to be universal across a broad range of species, from fish to primates (e.g., Gosling & John, 1999; Stevenson-Hinde & C.A. Hinde, in press), and underlying biological processes have been identified. With humans, fearful behavior in unfamiliar and challenging situations (behavioral inhibition) has been associated with a high and steady heart rate, elevated cortisol levels, and right frontal (vs. left frontal) EEG asymmetry. Models based on research with both animals and humans focus on variation in the excitability of neural circuits in the limbic system, with the amygdala playing a central role (reviewed in Davidson & Rickman, 1999; Fox, Henderson, Marshall, Nichols, & Ghera, 2005; Marshall & Stevenson-Hinde, 2001—see their fig. 1).

Behavior genetic studies of twins and adoptees have indicated that individual differences in fearfulness are heritable, with genetic factors accounting for around 40–60% of the variance. Of current interest is a molecular genetic approach aimed at identifying particular genes that code for the regulation and transportation of neurotransmitters and then relating them to complex human traits (reviewed in Plomin & Rutter, 1998; Schmidt, Polak, & Spooner, 2001). For example, dopamine receptor (*DRD4*) polymorphisms (long alleles) have been associated with novelty seeking and related behavior. Since short alleles code for a receptor apparently more efficient in binding dopamine, "The theory is that individuals with the long-repeat *DRD4* allele are dopamine deficient and seek novelty to increase dopamine release" (Plomin & Caspi, 1998, p. 393). However, a meta-analysis concluded that the mean association between the DRD4 long allele and novelty seeking, on the basis of data aggregated over almost 4000 individuals, is negligible and statistically not significant. . . . Thus the pattern of results suggests, contrary to initial reports, and consistent with recent reviews that there is no *simple* association between DRD4 polymorphism and novelty seeking. (Kluger, Siegfried, & Ebstein, 2002, pp. 714–715)

The story is similar with anxiety-related traits, where a polymorphism in the promoter region of the serotonin transporter gene (*5-HTTLPR*) gene was identified (e.g., Lesch et al., 1996). The short allele is associated with diminished *5-HTT* transcription, lower transporter levels, and reduced serotonin uptake. Without the regulating effects of serotonin, the amygdala and hypothalamic–pituitary–adrenal (HPA) system becomes overactive, leading to the physiological profile of a fearful or anxious individual. However, consistent with the above *DRD4* meta-analysis, a review of studies relating the *5-HTT* gene to childhood fearfulness produced mixed results (Fox, Nichols, et al., 2005). This is not surprising, since a *single* gene will account for only a very small proportion of the variance in a complex trait, with many unidentified genes and interactions between genes involved in outcome. Thus, it is becoming clear that any simple association between a single genetic polymorphism and a behavioral trait will tend to lose its significance with increasing population size.

Instead, there is increasing evidence for gene–environment *interactions*. Of relevance to the trait of fearfulness is the Fox, Nichols, et al. study (2005) showing that children with the short *5-HTT* allele *in combination with* low family social support as perceived by mothers were at risk for high observed behavioral inhibition as well as shyness as reported by mothers. How genes are expressed in development depends upon past environmental influences, particularly behavioral interactions with parents, other caregivers, and peers (see Fox, Henderson, et al., 2005), all of which are influenced by the cultural context (see Figure 1.1).

Such an interactionist view of development is not new. What is new is the further proposition that a genetic predisposition may indicate children who are particularly susceptible to positive *and* negative rearing effects, "for better and for worse" (Belsky, Bakermans-Kranenburg, & van IJzendoorn, 2007). For example, the presence or absence of the long 7-repeat *DRD4* allele and mothers' state of mind with respect to loss or trauma (i.e., "unresolved" or "not unresolved") was associated with the level of attachment disorganization shown by infants upon reunion with mother in the Ainsworth strange situation. That is, the double risk of a long *DRD4* allele and mothers with unresolved loss was significantly associated with the *highest* levels of infant disorganization. Moreover, the long *DRD4* allele infants of mothers with no unresolved loss had the *lowest* levels of disorganization. Disorganization levels of infants *without* the long allele were in between these extremes and showed no significant effect of mothers' status (Bakermans-Kranenburg & van IJzendoorn, 2007; van IJzendoorn & Bakermans-Kranenburg, 2006). Further evidence that dopamine-related genes are associated with differential susceptibility to the rearing environment is reviewed in Bakermans-Kranenburg & van IJzendoorn (2010).

Following on from this, could it be that children with fearful dispositions are particularly sensitive to their environments, whether supportive or negative? If so, cultural influences could be augmented, for better (e.g., in China, where shyness is valued) or for worse (e.g., in North America, where it is discouraged). In traditional Chinese society, with its concern for social order and harmony, caution and self-restraint are valued, whereas assertiveness and self-expression are much more valued in the West. Chen's research group has shown that, compared with North American children, Chinese children tend to display more shy, inhibited behavior in a variety of novel situations (reviewed in Chen, Wang, & DeSouza, 2006). Unlike the situation in North America, Chinese mothers were accepting and approving of shyness, and peers were supportive and cooperative. Such positive associations with shyness continued into middle and later childhood. A longitudinal study of a Chinese sample showed that shyness in early childhood predicted later sociometric status, social and academic competence, and indices of psychological well-being. This pattern contrasts with the negative associations in the West, where shyness is associated with such characteristics as negative mood and problem behavior with peers (e.g., Stevenson-Hinde & Glover, 1996) and where toddlers' high behavioral inhibition carries a two- to four-fold risk for later anxiety disorders (reviewed in Pine, 2007).

Importantly, Chen's research also documents changes and differences *within* China by means of "natural experiments." First, while the cited positive associations with shyness occurred in an urban setting in 1990, they decreased in 1998 and even reversed themselves by 2002, when shyness had become associated with peer rejection, school problems, and depression. Such changes over time were associated with economic reform toward a capitalist system and a competitive environment that valued assertiveness over shyness (Chen, Cen, Li, & He, 2005). Second, differences at a particular time occurred within an urban context. Whereas shyness was associated with indices of psychological well-being and social competence in children whose families had migrated to Beijing from rural areas (rural migrant children), the opposite held for children of strictly urban families who did not maintain traditional socialization beliefs and practices (Chen, Wang, & Wang, 2009). This distinction neatly illustrates the importance of carefully describing the cultural context in order to make clear links with behavioral development (see also Chen, Chapter 2, this volume).

Thus, we have seen the influence of changes in cultural context on the development and correlates of shyness, and it is highly unlikely that these changing contexts are creating genetic polymorphisms. But the stability of these changes across populations and across time does not rule out a developmental change in the availability of genes to be expressed. Recent advances in chromatin biology (DNA and its enveloping histone proteins) offer a conceptual framework for understanding long-lasting changes in gene expression that are not heritable but constitute the basis for epigenetics (see Keverne & Curley, 2008). "Influences that determine the expression of DNA without altering the sequence of DNA are referred to as epigenetic, meaning 'in addition to genetic'" (Champagne & Mashoodh, 2009, p. 128). Thus, even monozygotic twins reveal increasing discordance in behavioral, physiological, and disease susceptibility phenotypes that cannot be explained by Mendelian inheritance but is consistent with epigenetic chromatin modifications. Furthermore, epigenetic mechanisms may mediate the long-term effects of maternal care on development (reviewed in Champagne & Curley, 2009), something to bear in mind in the following section. Of particular importance to development, epigenesis enables genetic and environmental information to stably construct a program of gene expression, to be erased and available for reprogramming in subsequent generations.

Attachment

Since attachment theory is increasingly being applied beyond its original limits, it may be constructive here to review empirical support for its basic tenets. In keeping with Bowlby's formulation of attachment theory, attachment behavior and the subsequent development of an enduring attachment relationship with a caregiver may be regarded as universal, including an infant's ability to form multiple attachments (see e.g., Cassidy, 2008; Howes & Spieker, 2008). Indeed, it was in a non-Western culture (Uganda) that an infant's use of mother as a "secure base" within a network of multiple caregivers was first fully appreciated and documented over 9 months, along with caregiving practices (Ainsworth, 1967; see also Ainsworth, 1977). Mary Ainsworth's second observational study of attachment behavior was conducted in Baltimore, with extensive home visits over the first year followed by a standardized laboratory procedure in which attachment behavior was elicited by two brief separations. The *organization* of attachment behavior and emotions toward the mother upon reunion provided the basis for assessing aspects of the *attachment relationship*, such as the degree of security (rated from 1 to 9) or the pattern of attachment (Ainsworth, Blehar, Waters, & Wall, 1978). Thus, Ainsworth's original research showed how infant–caregiver interactions over the first year of life lead to the development of an attachment relationship with its own emergent properties.

The nature of this relationship is significantly dependent upon antecedent infant–caregiver interactions rather than genetic influences. Neither a behavior genetic study of two samples of twins in London and Leiden (Bokhurst et al., 2003) nor a molecular genetic study with a reasonably large sample size (N = 132; Bakermans-Kranenburg & van IJzendoorn, 2004) found any significant genetic influence on patterns of attachment. Although, as we have seen, the *DRD4* 7-repeat allele did *interact* with maternal style (lack of resolution of mourning) to increase levels of disorganized attachment, no direct link between this allele and disorganization was found, even with an analysis of six samples (N = 542; Bakermans-Kranenburg & van IJzendoorn, 2007).

Thus, both theory and research indicate that the key influence on patterns of attachment is maternal (or caregiver) styles of interaction, including emotional communication. In Bowlby's (1991) words, "What is happening during these early years is that the pattern of communication that a child adopts towards his mother comes to match the pattern of communication that she has been adopting towards him" (pp. 295–296). Thanks to Mary Ainsworth, the style of "sensitive responsiveness," which she defined as reading signals accurately and responding appropriately, has been related to security of attachment in cultures ranging from Baltimore (Ainsworth et al., 1978) to Indonesia (Zevalkink, 1997). Indeed, a meta-analysis over many studies, including non-Western cultures with various caregiving arrangements, has shown significant associations between sensitivity and security (DeWolff & van IJzendoorn, 1997). Furthermore, intervention studies indicate the causal influence of maternal sensitivity in promoting security (Bakermans-Kranenburg, van IJzendoorn, & Juffer, 2003). In a review chapter van IJzendoorn & Bakermans-Kranenburg (2004) conclude that correlational, experimental, and cross-cultural studies have replicated the association between sensitivity and attachment numerous times. Thus, the main tenets of attachment theory appear to be universal: (1) the phenomenon of an infant showing attachment behavior from birth, leading to (2) the formation of an attachment bond with one or more specific caregivers and (3) the security of that attachment bond being dependent on antecedent caregiver responsiveness to the infant's signals.

Consistent with Bowlby's emphasis on universals, the occurrence of particular items of behavior is *not* the focus of attachment theory. That is, *attachment behavior* is defined in terms of context and outcome rather than content (attaining proximity to caregiver when stressed, regardless of exactly how that outcome is achieved), caregiver *sensitive responsiveness* is defined in terms of context-appropriate communication within the dyad, and *attachment* is assessed in terms of how attachment behavior is organized toward the caregiver. Accordingly, infants may show culture-specific attachment behavior to express their emotions about separations and reunions, and at the same time the organization of that behavior may produce patterns of attachment that are distributed similarly across very different cultures, including the Gusii of Kenya (in van IJzendoorn & Sagi, 2008). Thus, measures typically of interest in cross-cultural research concerning specific practices, attitudes, and values (e.g., valuing relatedness vs. autonomy) lie outside the focus of attachment theory.

However, that observation does not imply that attachment-related practices such as sleeping arrangements are irrelevant to the development of security. Indeed, insecurity was associated with the former practice in many Israeli kibbutzim of collective sleeping arrangements away from parents, starting from a few months after birth. In our evolutionary past, darkness carried particular dangers, and to this day children show nighttime fears, when they may need an attachment figure most. This kibbutzim practice of sleeping away contrasts sharply with the practice of infants sleeping with their mothers and feeding on demand, such as with the !Kung San of northwestern Botswana or the Efé of northeastern Zambia (reviewed in van IJzendoorn & Sagi, 2008).

Such cross-cultural differences enhance our understanding of attachment relationships and the diversity of caregiving practices underlying them (see, e.g., Morelli & Rothbaum, 2007; Rothbaum & Rusk, Chapter 5, this volume). Accordingly, van IJzendoorn & Sagi (2008) point to an insufficient number of attachment studies within vast countries such as China, with over 56 nationalities, and a lack of attachment studies in India and most Islamic countries. Nevertheless, the three basic attachment patterns identified in Ainsworth's original Strange Situation (Ainsworth et al., 1978)—secure, insecure–avoidant and insecure–ambivalent—have been found in every culture studied thus far. When a mother returns after a brief separation, a child who expresses emotions appropriately and is readily comforted by her will be classified as "secure"; a child who keeps emotions closed and maintains a polite neutrality is "avoidant"; and a child who overexpresses emotions, showing ambivalence and anger, is "ambivalent" (for a recent review and interpretation of individual differences in attachment, see Weinfield, Sroufe, Egeland, & Carlson, 2008).

Although the three main patterns tend to be distributed similarly across cultures, with the secure pattern as the norm, peculiar distributions of patterns have been found. One often quoted Japanese study (Miyake, Chen, & Campos, 1985) reported a higher-than-expected proportion of children classified as insecure–ambivalent" (28%). However, rather than the recommended procedure of curtailing a 3-minute separation episode very soon after distress occurs (e.g., Ainsworth et al., 1978), as routinely done even in Western samples, Miyake et al. (1985) curtailed an episode after only 2 minutes of distress. With such prolonged distress, most 12-month-olds, in any culture, would be so upset that they would be difficult to soothe upon reunion and therefore would appear to fit an "ambivalent" classification. Such a modification of the Strange Situation as well as the low N of 25 render the findings questionable (for further details, see van IJzendoorn & Sagi, 2008). In Israel, where the Strange Situation was used properly, the ambivalent pattern was overrepresented, even in a study without any overnight sleeping arrangements away from parents. Finally, within Germany the Grossmanns found that an avoidant pattern was the norm in the industrialized northern city of Bielefeld, whereas in the Bavarian city of Regensburg a secure pattern predominated (Grossmann, Fremer-Bombik, Rudolph, & Grossmann, 1988).

In an attempt to understand how different distributions of attachment patterns might come to characterize different societies, Hinde and Stevenson-Hinde (1991) identified three "desiderata": biological, cultural, and psychological. Although interrelated, and perhaps even more so in our distant past, the desiderata may now be more distinct, especially in modern industrialized societies. A pattern required for the "biological desiderata" of increasing inclusive fitness need not be the same as a pattern fitting "cultural desiderata," particularly in those cultures where procreation is increasingly seen as a threat to survival rather than a goal. Even though an avoidant pattern might be most common and presumably "fits" a highly pressured society as in Bielefeld, it may not be optimal for psychological development. As a practicing psychiatrist, Bowlby focused on "psychological desiderata," and he argued that "psychological well-being" should be desirable in any culture, as is the case with "physical well-being" (cited in Stevenson-Hinde, 2007).

Bowlby postulated that experiences within early close relationships lead to an "internal working model" of the self in relation to others that guides future interactions. With a secure working model comes the expectation of gaining support when it's needed, along with feeling worthy of such support. Empirical studies have related security to particular developmental outcomes, including resilience, empathy, and social competence (reviewed in Weinfield et al., 2008; see also Thompson, 2008, for an overview of past research as well as current conceptual and empirical issues). A classic study—the Minnesota Longitudinal Study of Risk and Adaptation from Birth to Adulthood—involved a variety of assessments in multiple contexts of 180 children born into poverty. Security in infancy was a predictor of adaptation in play group, which along with security was an additional predictor of social competence in middle childhood. The Minnesota study illustrates how early close relationships may set the stage for later ones, which along with changing circumstances may affect outcome, in a probabilistic way. Finally, with its range of assessments and outcomes over time, the Minnesota study supports the view that attachment status should not and does not predict every aspect of development: "One of the emergent themes in our work is that the predictive power of variables depends on the particular outcome in question" (Sroufe, Egeland, Carlson, & Collins, 2005, p. 197).

Evidence relating security to developmental outcomes in non-Western cultures is understandably scarce, given the challenges of such longitudinal studies, as indicated above. In addition, cross-cultural studies have highlighted the need to take a child's network of attachment relationships into account in predicting outcome (for a thorough review, see van IJzendoorn & Sagi, 2008). A further challenge involves defining and assessing attachment-related outcomes in culturally appropriate ways (see, e.g., Chen, Chapter 2, this volume, for identifying cultural differences in outcomes of close friendships). Finally, developmental outcomes may be best characterized not by "simple frequencies of behaviors but [by] the organization of behavior within and across situations" (Sroufe et al., 2005, p. 147).

The Interplay between Fearfulness and the Ambivalent Pattern of Attachment: Cultural Considerations

In both the United States and Europe, the insecure–ambivalent pattern of attachment has been associated with significantly high behavioral inhibition (BI) (e.g., Stevenson-Hinde & Marshall, 1999; reviewed in Stevenson-Hinde, 2005). Nevertheless, over 50% of children with high BI have been classified as secure (Stevenson-Hinde, Shouldice, & Chicot, in press). As we have seen, insecurity is associated with insensitive maternal responsiveness to infants' signals, and mothers of insecure ambivalent children are observed to be both insensitive and unpredictable. Thus, their infants "live with the constant fear of being left vulnerable and alone . . . the anxiety associated with this fear of separation lasts beyond infancy" (Weinfield et al., 2008, p. 87). With regard to Figure 1.1, it appears that the *individual* characteristic of fearfulness may make a child particularly vulnerable to insensitive and unpredictable maternal *interactions* to promote an insecure–ambivalent *relationship* (Stevenson-Hinde et al., in press). Now, would this hold in spite of differing cultural norms for fearfulness? The answer is probably "yes," provided the cultural norm is used as an anchor for defining fearfulness levels. Within North America or Europe, one may expect the top 15% or so of an unselected "normal" sample to show "high" behavioral inhibition (e.g., Kagan, Reznick, & Snidman, 1987), and this might provide a meaningful cutoff in any culture.

Furthermore, one might predict that the cultural *norm* for behavioral inhibition, whatever it may be, should be associated with a secure pattern of attachment, since secure children do not tend to be "extreme in either the inhibited or uninhibited direction" (Calkins & Fox, 1992, p. 1469; Stevenson-Hinde & Marshall, 1999). Thus, in spite of a higher norm for behavioral inhibition in China as compared with North America, the distribution of attachment patterns should be similar. Indeed, Strange Situation assessments carried out in Beijing (Hu & Meng, 1996) produced distributions remarkably similar to the global ones: 68% secure infant–mother dyads, 16% insecure–avoidant, and 16% insecure–ambivalent. Typically for China, all the subjects (16 boys, 15 girls) were only children, and all but one family lived with grandparents. Thus, China could provide a fertile area for research not only for cross-cultural issues but also for comparison of attachment to mother with attachment to a grandmother who shares in caregiving.

Summary

We have seen how the cultural context may illuminate the development of two exemplars of an individual's emotional development, namely, fearful behavior and attachment behavior. Both are presumed to have evolved with the function of protection from harm. Thus, these behaviors were crucial for survival and are pancultural.

Levels of behavioral inhibition differ across cultures and across time within a culture, according to cultural attitudes and values. Thus, with reference to Figure 1.1, a key dialectic occurs between levels of behavioral inhibition and the *sociocultural context*. However, distributions of patterns of attachment are remarkably similar across cultures, and with a few exceptions the secure pattern is the norm. Why should this be so? First, caregivers from the United States to China perceive the "ideal child" as a securely attached child (via Attachment Q-Sorts; reviewed in van IJzendoorn & Sagi, 2008). Second, an individual's pattern of attachment is crucially dependent upon those caregivers, with "sensitive responsiveness" fostering security. Third, security is associated with positive outcomes such as a sense of competence and self-worth (Thompson, 2008), and it is a protective factor in adversity (Weinfield et al., 2008). It is tempting to conclude that Bowlby's focus on "psychological well-being" is of value in all cultures.

Conclusion

The framework discussed here (Figure 1.1), with a hierarchy of levels ranging from the individual to the cultural context, may serve at least two purposes for chapters in the present volume. One is to locate which levels any particular chapter is addressing and the dynamics between them. The other is to make one aware of levels *not* considered, with potential between-level dynamics overlooked, and possible ensuing weaknesses in predictive power. This perspective reflects the recent plea from the president of the Society for Research in Child Development (SRCD) to incorporate interdisciplinary perspectives in order to "do a much better job of understanding and predicting human development" (Sameroff, 2009, p. 3). Mirroring Hinde's framework, Sameroff (2009) points out that individuals are constrained by underlying biological processes and are embedded in networks of relationships. Groups and social institutions provide roles that children come to fill, and cultures provide meaning systems. Furthermore, individuals are limited by the availability of economically related resources, which determine whether or not they can realize their potential.

Finally, our dialectical framework suggests in a diagrammatic way what we already know but often conveniently overlook, namely, the ramifications for individuals, relationships, and social institutions when a culture and essential resources are actually destroyed. Yet, we all carry ultimate responsibility for such destruction, such as the clearfelling of life-supporting forests, mining operations in vulnerable villages, or "natural" disasters due to human-made climate change. Climate change has already impacted on agriculture in parts of sub-Saharan Africa, leading to an increase in malnutrition among children. Children are usually among the hardest hit by a disaster, despite being the ones least responsible for it. They may be denied their rights to life, nutrition, health care, education, family care, and protection. By the end of 2010, 106 million children younger than 15 years old were projected to have lost one or both parents. Such issues, including emergencies and special reports, appear on the UNICEF (United Nations International Children's Emergency Fund) website, as well as in relevant publications (e.g., Bhutta, et al., 2010).

Furthermore, nations continue to manufacture and export weapons and to support military aggression, however benignly described (e.g., "occupation" or "targeting terrorist strongholds"), with devastating effects on civilians. In the war in Afghanistan, concerted attacks by Coalition Forces in northwest Pakistan have sent thousands of families fleeing from their traditional villages to makeshift camps, with only tents to live in during the harsh winters. Latest news and individuals' stories may be found on the UNHCR (United Nations High Commission for Refugees) website, as well as global statistics. For example, at the end of 2009 there were 43.3 million forcibly displaced people worldwide, including 15.2 million refugees. Some were long-term refugees—4.8 million Palestinians—and some refugees were more recent—2.9 million from Afghanistan and 1.8 million from Iraq (UNHCR, 2010). Such grim facts, together with the world's precarious economic situation, require us all to be concerned with global issues if we are to truly foster socioemotional development in children.

Acknowledgments

I would like to thank Robert Hinde, Barry Keverne, and Marinus van IJzendoorn for their constructive suggestions.

Note

1. Borrowing from ethology, Bowlby (1969/1982) postulated an underlying "attachment behavior system" that exists in its own right, distinct from other motivational systems such as "exploration" or "fear." Activation of the fear behavior system leads to activation of the attachment behavior system and deactivation of the exploratory behavior system. Only when the attachment behavior system is deactivated (by gaining proximity with an attachment figure) is the infant then psychologically "free to explore." How much a culture encourages exploration of different kinds at different ages is a separate issue.

References

Ainsworth, M. D. S. (1967). *Infancy in Uganda: Infant care and the growth of love*. Baltimore, MD: Johns Hopkins University Press.

Ainsworth, M. D. S. (1977). Infant development and mother–infant interaction among Ganda and American families. In P. H. Leiderman, S. R. Tulkin, & A. Rosenfeld (Eds.), *Culture and infancy: Variations in the human experience* (pp. 119–149). New York: Academic Press.

Ainsworth, M. D. S., Blehar, M. C., Waters, E., & Wall, S. (1978). *Patterns of attachment*. Hillsdale, NJ: Erlbaum.

Baerends, G. P. (1976). The functional organization of behaviour. *Animal Behaviour, 24*, 726–738.

Bakermans-Kranenburg, M. J., & van IJzendoorn, M. H. (2004). No association of the dopamine D4 receptor (DRD4) and -521 C/T promoter polymorphisms with infant attachment disorganization. *Attachment and Human Development, 6*, 211–218.

Bakermans-Kranenburg, M. J., & van IJzendoorn, M. H. (2007). Research review: Genetic vulnerability or differential susceptibility in child development: The case of attachment. *Journal of Child Psychology and Psychiatry, 48*, 1160–1173.

Bakermans-Kranenburg, M. J., & van IJzendoorn, M. H. (2010). Parenting matters: Family science in the genomic era. *Family Science, 1*, 26–36.

Bakermans-Kranenburg, M. J., van IJzendoorn, M. H., & Juffer, F. (2003). Less is more: Meta-analyses of sensitivity and attachment interventions in early childhood. *Psychological Bulletin, 129*, 195–215.

Belsky, J., Bakermans-Kranenburg, M. J., & van IJzendoorn, M. H. (2007). For better *and* for worse: Differential susceptibility to environmental influences. *Current Directions in Psychological Science, 16*, 300–304.

Bhutta, Z. A., Chopra, M., Axelson, H., Berman, P., Boerma, T., Bryce, J., et al.,

(2010). Countdown to 2015 decade report (2000–10): Taking stock of maternal, newborn, and child survival. *Lancet, 375,* 2032–2044.

Bokhorst, C. L., Bakermans-Kranenburg, M. J., Fearon, R. M. P., van IJzendoorn, M. H., Fonagy, P., & Schuengel, C. (2003). The importance of shared environment in mother–infant attachment security: A behavioral genetic study. *Child Development, 74,* 1769–1782.

Bowlby, J. (1969/1982). *Attachment and loss: Vol. I. Attachment.* London: Hogarth Press.

Bowlby, J. (1991). Postscript. In C. M. Parkes, J. Stevenson-Hinde, & P. Marris (Eds.), *Attachment across the life cycle* (pp. 293–297). London: Routledge.

Calkins, S. D., & Fox, N. A. (1992). The relations among infant temperament, security of attachment, and behavioral inhibition at twenty-four months. *Child Development, 63,* 1456–1472.

Cassidy, J. (2008). The nature of the child's ties. In J. Cassidy & P. R. Shaver (Eds.), *Handbook of attachment: Theory, research, and clinical applications* (2nd ed., pp. 3–22). New York: Guilford Press.

Champagne, F. A., & Curley, J. (2009). Epigenetic mechanisms mediating the long-term effects of maternal care on development. *Neuroscience and Biobehavioral Reviews, 33,* 593–600.

Champagne, F. A., & Mashoodh, R. (2009). Gene–environment interplay and the origins of individual differences in behavior. *Current Directions in Psychological Science, 18,* 127–131.

Chen, X., Cen, G., Li, D., & He, Y. (2005). Social functioning and adjustment in Chinese children: The imprint of historical time. *Child Development, 76,* 182–195.

Chen, X., Wang, L., & DeSouza, A. (2006). Temperament, socioemotional functioning, and peer relationships in Chinese and North American children. In X. Chen, D. C. French, & B. H. Schneider (Eds.), *Peer relationships in cultural context* (pp. 123–147). Cambridge, UK: Cambridge University Press.

Chen, X., Wang, L., & Wang, Z. (2009). Shyness-sensitivity and social, school, and psychological adjustment in rural migrant and urban children in China. *Child Development, 80,* 1499–1513.

Davidson, R. J., & Rickman, M. (1999). Behavioral inhibition and the emotional circuitry of the brain. In L. A. Schmidt & J. Schulkin (Eds.), *Extreme fear, shyness, and social phobia* (pp. 67–87). Oxford, UK: Oxford University Press.

DeWolff, M. S., & van IJzendoorn, M. H. (1997). Sensitivity and attachment: A meta-analysis on parental antecedents of infant attachment. *Child Development, 68,* 571–591.

Fox, N. A., Henderson, H. A., Marshall, P. J., Nichols, K. E., & Ghera, M. M. (2005). Behavioral inhibition: Linking biology and behavior within a developmental framework. *Annual Review of Psychology, 56,* 235–262.

Fox, N. A., Nichols, K. E., Henderson, H. A., Rubin, K., Schmidt, L., Hamer, D., et al. (2005). Evidence for a gene–environment interaction in predicting behavioral inhibition in middle childhood. *Psychological Science, 16,* 921–926.

Goldsmith, H. H., Buss, A. H., Plomin, R., Rothbart, M. K., Thomas, A., Chess, S., et al. (1987). Roundtable: What is temperament? *Child Development, 58,* 505–529.

Gosling, S. D., & John, O. P. (1999). Personality dimensions in nonhuman animals: A cross-species review. *Current Directions in Psychological Science, 8,* 69–75.

Grossmann, K., Fremer-Bombik, E., Rudolph, J., & Grossmann, K. E. (1988). Maternal attachment representation as related to patterns of infant–mother attachment and maternal care during the first year. In R. A. Hinde & J. Stevenson-Hinde (Eds.), *Relationships within families* (pp. 241–262). Oxford, UK: Clarendon Press.

Hinde, R. A. (1977). Mother–infant separation and the nature of inter-individual relationships: Experiments with rhesus monkeys. *Proceedings of the Royal Society, 196,* 29–50.

Hinde, R. A. (1979). *Towards understanding relationships.* London: Academic Press.

Hinde, R. A. (1987). *Individuals, relationships, and culture.* Cambridge, UK: Cambridge University Press.

Hinde, R. A. (1999). *Why gods persist: A scientific approach to religion.* London: Routledge.

Hinde, R. A. (2005). Ethology and attachment theory. In K. E. Grossmann, K. Grossmann & E. Waters (Eds.), *Attachment from infancy to adulthood: The major longitudinal studies.* (pp. 1–12). New York: Guilford Press.

Hinde, R. A. (2009). *Why gods persist: A scientific approach to religion* (2nd ed.). London: Routledge.

Hinde, R. A., & McGinnis, L. (1977). Some factors influencing the effects of temporary mother–infant separation—some experiments with rhesus monkeys. *Psychological Medicine, 7,* 197–222.

Hinde, R. A., & Stevenson-Hinde, J. (1976). Towards understanding relationships: Dynamic stability. In P. P. G. Bateson & R. A. Hinde (Eds.), *Growing points in ethology* (pp. 451–479). Cambridge, UK: Cambridge University Press.

Hinde, R. A., & Stevenson-Hinde, J. (1991). Perspectives on attachment. In C. M. Parkes, J. Stevenson-Hinde, & P. Marris (Eds.), *Attachment across the life cycle* (pp. 52–65). London: Routledge.

Howes, C., & Spieker, S. (2008). Attachment relationships in the context of multiple caregivers. In J. Cassidy & P. R. Shaver (Eds.), *Handbook of attachment: Theory, research, and clinical applications* (2nd ed., pp. 317–332). New York: Guilford Press.

Hu, P., & Meng, Z. (1996). An examination of infant–mother attachment in China. Poster presented at the meeting of the International Society for the Study of Behavioral Development, Québec City, Québec, Canada.

Kagan, J. (1994). *Galen's prophecy.* New York: Basic Books.

Kagan, J., Reznick, J. S., & Snidman, N. (1987). The physiology and psychology of behavioral inhibition in children. *Child Development, 58,* 1459–1473.

Keverne, E. B., & Curley, J. P. (2008). Epigenetics, brain evolution and behaviour. *Frontiers in Neuroendocrinology, 29,* 398–412.

Kluger, A. N., Siegfried, Z., & Ebstein, R. P. (2002). A meta-analysis of the association between DRD4 polymorphism and novelty seeking. *Molecular Psychiatry, 7,* 712–717.

Kuczynski, L. (2003). Beyond Bidirectionality: Bilateral conceptual frameworks for understanding dynamics in parent–child relations. In L. Kuczynski (Ed.), *Handbook of dynamics in parent–child relations* (pp. 3–24). London: Sage.

Lesch, K. P., Bengel, D., Heils, A., Sabol, S. Z., Greenberg, B. D., Petri, S., et al. (1996). Association of anxiety-related traits with a polymorphism in the serotonin transporter gene regulatory region. *Science, 274,* 1527–1531.

Lorenz, K. (1935). Der Kumpan in der Umwelt des Vogels. *Journal für Ornithologie, 83,* 137–213.

Marshall, P. J., & Stevenson-Hinde, J. (2001). Behavioral inhibition: Physiological correlates. In W. R. Crozier & L. E. Alden (Eds.), *International handbook of social anxiety* (pp. 53–76). Chichester, UK: Wiley.

Minuchin, P. (1985). Families and individual development: Provocations from the field of family therapy. *Child Development, 56,* 289–302.

Miyake, K., Chen, S. J., & Campos, J. J. (1985). Infant temperament, mother's mode of interactions, and attachment in Japan: An interim report. In I. Bretherton & E. Waters (Eds.), Growing points of attachment theory and research. *Monographs of the Society for Research in Child Development, 50*(1–2, Serial No. 209), 276–297.

Morelli, G. A., & Rothbaum, R. (2007). Situating the child in context: Attachment relationships and self-regulation in different cultures. In S. Kitayama & D. Cohen (Eds.), *Handbook of cultural psychology* (pp. 500–527). New York: Guilford Press.

Pine, D. S. (2007). Research review: A neuroscience framework for pediatric anxiety disorders. *Journal of Child Psychology and Psychiatry, 48,* 631–648.

Plomin, R., & Caspi, A. (1998). DNA and personality. *European Journal of Personality, 12,* 387–407.

Plomin, R., & Rutter, M. (1998). Child development, molecular genetics, and what to do with genes once they are found. *Child Development, 69,* 1223–1242.

Rubin, K. H. (1998). Social and emotional development from a cultural perspective. *Developmental Psychology, 34,* 611–615.

Sameroff, A. (2009). How to become a developmental scientist. *SRCD Developments, 52,* 3.

Schmidt, L., Polak, C. P., & Spooner, A. L. (2001). Biological and environmental contributions to childhood shyness: A diathesis–stress model. In W. R. Crozier & L. E. Alden (Eds.), *International handbook of social anxiety* (pp. 29–51). Chichester, UK: Wiley.

Sroufe, L. A., Egeland, B., Carlson, E. A., & Collins, W. A. (2005). *The development of the person: The Minnesota study of risk and adaptation from birth to adulthood.* New York: Guilford Press.

Stevenson-Hinde, J. (2005). On the interplay between attachment, temperament, and maternal style: A Madingley perspective. In K. E. Grossmann, K. Grossmann, & E. Waters (Eds.). *Attachment from infancy to adulthood: The major longitudinal studies* (pp. 198–222). New York: Guilford Press.

Stevenson-Hinde, J. (2007). Attachment theory and John Bowlby: Some reflections. *Attachment and Human Development, 9,* 337–342.

Stevenson-Hinde, J., & Glover, A. (1996). Shy girls and boys: A new look. *Journal of Child Psychology and Psychiatry, 37,* 181–187.

Stevenson-Hinde, J., & Hinde, C. A. (in press). Individual characteristics—weaving psychological and ethological approaches. In A. Weiss, J. King, & L. Murray (Eds.), *Personality and temperament in nonhuman primates*. New York: Springer.

Stevenson-Hinde, J., & Marshall, P. J. (1999). Behavioral inhibition, heart period, and respiratory sinus arrhythmia: An attachment perspective. *Child Development, 70*, 805–816.

Stevenson-Hinde, J., Shouldice, A., & Chicot, R. (in press). Maternal anxiety, behavioral inhibition, and attachment. *Attachment and Human Development, 13*.

Super, C. M., & Harkness, S. (1986). The developmental niche: A conceptualization at the interface of child and culture. *International Journal of Behavioral Development, 9*, 545–569.

Thompson, R. A. (2008). Early attachment and later development: Familiar questions, new answers. In J. Cassidy & P. R. Shaver (Eds.), *Handbook of attachment: Theory, research, and clinical applications* (2nd ed., pp. 348–365). New York: Guilford Press.

UNHCR (2010). 2009 global trends: Refugees, asylum-seekers, returnees, and internally displaced and stateless persons. Geneva, Switzerland: UNHCR.

van IJzendoorn, M. H., & Bakermans-Kranenburg, M. J. (2004). Maternal sensitivity and infant temperament in the formation of attachment (pp. 233–258). In G. Bremner & A. Slater (Eds.), *Theories of Infant Development*. London: Blackwell.

van IJzendoorn, M. H., & Bakermans-Kranenburg, M. J. (2006). DRD4 7-repeat polymorphism moderates the association between material unresolved loss or trauma and infant disorganization. *Attachment and Human Development, 8*, 291–307.

van IJzendoorn, M. H., & Sagi-Schwartz, A. (2008). Cross-cultural patterns of attachment: Universal and contextual dimensions. In J. Cassidy & P. R. Shaver (Eds.), *Handbook of attachment: Theory, research, and clinical applications* (2nd ed., pp. 880–905). New York: Guilford Press.

Vaughn, B. E., Bost, K. K., & van IJzendoorn, M. H. (2008). Attachment and temperament: Additive and interactive influences on behavior, affect, and cognition during infancy and childhood. In J. Cassidy & P. R. Shaver (Eds.), *Handbook of attachment: Theory, research, and clinical applications* (2nd ed., pp. 192–216). New York: Guilford Press.

Weinfield, N. S., Sroufe, L. A., Egeland, B., & Carlson, E. A. (2008). Individual differences in infant–caregiver attachment: Conceptual and empirical aspects of security. In J. Cassidy & P. R. Shaver (Eds.), *Handbook of attachment: Theory, research, and clinical applications* (2nd ed., pp. 78–101). New York: Guilford Press.

Zevalkink, J. (1997). *Attachment in Indonesia: The mother–child relationship in context*. Doctoral dissertation, University of Nijmegen, Nijmegen, The Netherlands.

CHAPTER 2

Culture and Children's Socioemotional Functioning

A Contextual–Developmental Perspective

XINYIN CHEN

D evelopmental theorists have long been interested in social interactions and relationships as an organizing context for individual development (Hartup, 1992; Piaget, 1932; Vygotsky, 1978). Social interactions provide opportunities for children to learn from one another such problem-solving skills as negotiation and cooperation. The experience of social interactions is helpful for children in understanding the rules and standards for appropriate behaviors in various settings. Moreover, social affiliations established through interactions are an important source of the feelings of security and belongingness, which in turn constitute a basis for the development of psychological well-being (e.g., Bowlby, 1969; Sullivan, 1953). Consistent with these perceptions, empirical evidence indicates that social interactions and relationships are associated with children's adaptive and maladaptive behaviors and various adjustment outcomes (Coie, Terry, Lenox, Lochman, & Hyman, 1995; Coplan, Prakash, O'Neil, & Armer, 2004; DeRosier, Kupersmidt, & Patterson, 1994; Dodge, Greenberg, Malone, & Conduct Problems Prevention Research Group, 2008; Dodge, Petit, McClaskey, & Brown, 1986; Ladd & Troop-Gordon, 2003; Rubin, Bukowski, & Parker, 2006).

Social interactions and relationships are likely to be shaped by cultural norms and values in the society or community (Chen & French, 2008; Edwards, Guzman, Brown, & Kumru, 2006). According to Hinde (1987), diverse levels of social experiences are embedded within an all-encompassing cultural system. Similarly, Schneider, Smith, Posson, and Kwan (1997) point out that cultural background may affect many aspects of peer interactions and relationships. Indeed, research has indicated that culture plays an important role in determining the quality and function of children and adolescents' social interactions and relationships, such as parent–child attachment, friendship, and social networks (e.g., DeRosier & Kupersmidt, 1991; Farver, Kim, & Lee, 1995; French, Pidada, & Victor, 2005; Rothbaum, Weisz, Pott, Miyake, & Morelli, 2000).

Therefore, it seems reasonable to argue that social interactions and relationships serve as a mediator of cultural influence on individual development (see Stevenson-Hinde, Chapter 1, this volume). The significance of social relationships for development is generally recognized in the cross-cultural and developmental field. However, theorists and researchers in the field have traditionally focused on the socialization role of adults, especially parents and educators, in transmitting cultural values to the younger generation (e.g., Goodnow, 1997; LeVine et al., 1994; Parke & Buriel, 2006; Super & Harkness, 1986). Cultural influence on development is often conceptualized as a vertical process of interactions between adults and children, although the latter may be active participants in the socialization (Edwards et al., 2006; Rogoff, 2003). The sociocultural theory (Vygotsky, 1978), for example, emphasizes children's internalization of external symbolic systems such as language and symbols, along with their cultural meanings, from the interpersonal level to the intrapersonal level. According to this theory, an important mechanism of internalization is collaborative or guided learning in which adults or experienced members of the society act as skilled tutors and representatives of the culture and assist children in understanding and solving problems. The assistance and guidance of more knowledgeable members in children's activities are believed to be critical to the development of correct thought and behavior (e.g., Cole, 1996; Goodnow, 1997; Leontiev, 1981; Rogoff, 2003; Vygotsky, 1978).

The sociocultural theory and other vertical socialization perspectives indicate the importance of culture and culturally directed socialization practices for human development. However, the processes of cultural influence on individual development, particularly in socioemotional areas, are more complicated than internalization of cultural systems or learning from senior members of the society. A major issue, for example, is what motivates children to learn, accept, and follow cultural expectations during socioemotional development. Unlike symbolic systems or tools for solving cognitive tasks, many of the cultural norms and values endorsed in the society such as those that serve to maintain social harmony and group functioning (e.g., self-control in resource-limited situations, helping others when they need it) may not have inherent benefit per se and thus may not be readily appreciated by children. Maintaining behaviors according to cultural standards may even require personal sacrifice. Moreover, although the guidance and support of parents, teachers, and other adults help children understand rules and learn appropriate behaviors, adult influence becomes more indirect and perhaps inadequate as children develop greater autonomy and as children engage in more activities outside the home and classroom. Therefore, it is necessary to look into more context-relevant social processes that are involved in cultural influence on socioemotional development.

Based on the literature (e.g., Hinde, 1987; Stevenson-Hinde, Chapter 1, this volume) and the recent cross-cultural research on peer relationships, I have proposed a contextual–developmental perspective focusing on the role of social interaction *in the peer context* in bridging culture and socioemotional development (e.g., Chen, Chung, & Hsiao, 2009). According to this perspective, social interaction in dyadic, group, and larger settings is an important context that mediates cultural influence on individual development. The social evaluation and regulation processes in interaction play a crucial role in building and facilitating links between cultural norms and values, on the one hand, and the development of various behaviors and characteristics, on the other. Specifically, during social interaction, peers evaluate individual behaviors in a manner that is consistent with the norms and values that are endorsed in the peer world. Moreover, peers may react to these behaviors and express particular attitudes such as acceptance or rejection toward children who display the behaviors according to the norms and values. Social evaluations and reactions, in turn, may regulate children's behaviors and developmental patterns.

Culturally Based Social Evaluations in Peer Interaction

Children's social behaviors such as autonomy, cooperation, and emotion expression and regulation may be valued differently in different cultures (e.g., Rothbaum & Trommsdorff, 2006). The cultural values of social behaviors provide a basis for social evaluations and reactions in peer interaction. Consistent with the literature (e.g., Greenfield, Suzuki, & Rothstein-Fisch, 2006; Triandis, 1995), I focus on two major dimensions of socioemotional functioning, namely, social initiative and self-control (Chen & French, 2008). Social initiative, which refers to the tendency to initiate and maintain social participation (as often indicated by reactivity in challenging situations), is relatively more emphasized in Western self-oriented societies, whereas self-control, the ability to modulate behavioral and emotional reactivity in social interactions, is more valued in collectivist or group-oriented societies. Cultural values with regard to these two dimensions may be reflected in such behaviors as prosocial–cooperative behavior (active social participation with effective control), aggression–disruption (high social initiative and low self-control), and shyness (low social initiative and adequate control to constrain behaviors and emotions toward self).

Findings from a number of research programs have indicated evident cultural variations in children and adolescents' judgments and evaluations of social behaviors. According to Miller (1994), for example, while individuals in Western societies attempt to maintain a balance between prosocial concerns and individual freedom of choice, individuals in group-oriented societies regard responsiveness to the needs of others as a fundamental commitment. Similarly, Eisenberg, Fabes, and Spinrad (2006) and Greenfield et al. (2006) argue that while prosocial–cooperative behavior is often seen as a personal decision in Western societies, children view this behavior as more obligatory in societies that value group harmony. Consistent with these arguments, relative to their American counterparts, youths in some Asian and Latino societies tend to hold a higher standard of social responsibility and are more concerned about prosocial–cooperative behaviors in social interaction (e.g., Azmitia & Cooper, 2004; Chen, Li, Li, Li, & Liu, 2000; Greenfield et al., 2006; Miller, Bersoff, & Harwood, 1990; Schneider, Fonzi, Tomada, & Tani, 2000).

Cultural differences have also been found in children's attitudes toward aggressive behavior. Cole and her colleagues (Cole, Bruschi, & Tamang, 2002; Cole, Tamang, & Shrestha, 2006), for example, have noticed in rural Nepal that Brahmans are high-caste Hindus who value hierarchy and dominance in the caste, whereas Tamangs, with a background of Tibetan Buddhism, value social equality, compassion, modesty, and nonviolence. Accordingly, Brahman children are more likely to endorse anger and aggressive behaviors than Tamang children. Killen and Brenick (Chapter 10, this volume) have found that Korean children view aggression as more negative and peer exclusion of aggressive children as more legitimate than do U.S. children. In North America, although aggression is generally discouraged, aggressive behavior may be associated with social support and approval in certain peer groups (e.g., Rodkin, Farmer, Pearl, & van Acker, 2000). In cultures of the Yanoamo Indians, where aggressive and violent behaviors are considered socially acceptable or even desirable, aggressive children, especially boys, may be regarded as "stars" by their peers (Chagnon, 1983). In some central and southern Italian communities, owing to social and historical circumstances, aggressive and defiant behaviors may be perceived by children as reflecting social assertiveness and competence (Casiglia, Lo Coco, & Zappulla, 1998; Schneider & Fonzi, 1996). As a result, aggressive behavior is associated with fewer negative peer evaluations in these cultures than in cultures that strictly prohibit aggression (Chen, He, et al., 2004).

In the Western literature (see Coplan & Armer, 2007; Rubin, Coplan, & Bowker, 2009), the manifestation of shy-inhibited behavior is thought to derive from internal anxiety in challenging social situations; socially wary and restrained behavior is assumed to reflect fearfulness and a lack of confidence. Children who display shy-inhibited behavior are believed to be socially incompetent and maladaptive in cultures that value assertiveness, expressiveness, and competitiveness (Rubin et al., 2009; Triandis, 1995). Shyness appears to be viewed as less problematic in some Asian and European societies such as China, Indonesia, Korea, and Sweden (Eisenberg, Pidada, & Liew, 2001; Farver et al., 1995; Kerr, Lambert, & Bem, 1996) than in North America. In traditional Chinese culture, for example, shy-inhibited behavior is considered an indication of social maturity; shy, wary, and inhibited children are perceived as well behaved and understanding (e.g., Chen, 2010).

In a cross-cultural study of peer interaction based on laboratory observations, Chen, DeSouza, Chen, and Wang (2006) demonstrated different peer attitudes toward children who display shy and inhibited behaviors in China and Canada. When shy children in Canada displayed a social initiation, peers were likely to make negative responses such as overt refusal, disagreement, and intentional ignoring of an initiation (e.g., "No!," "I won't do it"). However, peers responded in a more positive manner in China by controlling their negative actions and by showing approval, cooperation, and support (e.g., "I really like your drawing!"). The wary and low-power behaviors displayed by shy children were perceived by others as incompetent in Canada but as appropriate or even desirable in China, indicating cautiousness, courteousness, and a signal of looking for social engagement (Chen et al., 2006). There were also differences between the samples in peer voluntary initiations to shy children. In Canada, relative to initiations made to non-shy children, initiations made to shy children were more likely to be coercive (e.g., a direct demand such as "Gimme that," or verbal teasing) and less likely to be cooperative (e.g., "Can I play with you?"). This was not the case within the Chinese sample, where peer voluntary initiations to shy and non-shy children did not differ. The results suggest that whereas peers are generally antagonistic, forceful, and unreceptive in their interactions with children who display shy behavior in Canada, peers appear more supportive and cooperative toward shy children in China.

Culturally based social evaluations are also reflected in more general peer attitudes such as acceptance and rejection of children who display certain behavioral characteristics. The existing evidence indicates that shy children seem to experience fewer problems in peer acceptance in societies where assertiveness and autonomy are not valued or encouraged. Eisenberg et al. (2001), for example, found that shyness in Indonesian children was negatively associated with peer nominations of dislike. Chen and his colleagues found that shyness was associated with peer rejection in Canadian children but with peer acceptance in Chinese children during the early 1990s (e.g., Chen, Rubin, & Li, 1995; Chen, Chen, Li, & Wang, 2009; Chen, Rubin, Li, & Li, 1999). Moreover, as China evolves toward a market-oriented society with the introduction of more individualistic values, children's shyness is increasingly being associated with peer rejection and self-reported loneliness (Chen, Cen, Li, & He, 2005). By the early part of the 21st century, as the country became more deeply immersed in a market economy, shy children—unlike their predecessors during the early 1990s—were increasingly being perceived as incompetent and being rejected by peers. In the new competitive environment, shy-inhibited behavior that may impede self-expression and active exploration is no longer regarded as adaptive and competent (Chang et al., 2005; Hart et al., 2000). Consequently, shyness becomes an undesirable characteristic in social adjustment, and shy children are at a disadvantage in obtaining social approval. An interesting finding of Chen, Cen, et al.'s study (2005) was that shyness was positively associated with both peer acceptance and rejection in 1998. The results indicate ambivalent attitudes of peers toward shy children, which, to some extent, may reflect the cultural conflict between the new values of assertiveness and traditional Chinese values of self-control during the transitional period of the social change. Finally, it has been found that in rural regions of China where traditional Chinese values are still emphasized—similar to the results during the early 1990s in urban China—shyness was favorably associated with indexes of social and psychological adjustment such as leadership and peer acceptance (Chen & Wang, in press). Thus, shy rural children are still not regarded as problematic, and, like their urban counterparts in the early 1990s, continue to obtain social approval and support from peers.

The Regulatory Function of Peer Interaction

Through the evaluation and reaction processes, social interaction may serve to regulate children's behaviors according to the norms adopted in the peer world. The regulatory function is concerned with the maintenance or modification of children's behaviors based on their understanding of the message from peer evaluations and reactions. In a study of group entry behavior, for example, Borja-Alvarez, Zarbatany, and Peper (1991) found that the attitude of the group (e.g., positive initiation, overt rejection) affected the behavioral styles and strategies of the entering child, which in turn led to different group entry outcomes. The regulatory function of peer interaction may also be indicated, in a broad sense, by the effects of different types of peer groups on individual behaviors. Researchers have found that whereas prosocial–constructive peer groups facilitate the development of cooperative and responsible behaviors, antisocial peer group activities of children may reinforce their antagonistic attitudes, inspire them to express disruptive and defiant behaviors, and enhance their development in a socially destructive direction (e.g., Chen, Chang, Liu, & He, 2008; Chung & Chen, 2009; Dishion, Piehler, & Myers, 2008; Dodge et al., 2008).

According to the self-awareness theory (e.g., Abrams, 1994; Duval & Wicklund, 1972), social situations are likely to direct one's attention toward external demands, which provide an important basis for the regulation of social behaviors. Duval and Wicklund (1972), for example, argue that people can be in a state of objective self-awareness (OSA) in which they consider themselves in much the same way that they consider other objects. In a state of OSA, people are likely to be highly conscious of social standards and their own weaknesses relative to the standards (Duval & Silvia, 2002; Heine, Takemoto, Moskalenko, Lasaleta, & Henrich, 2008). To avoid negative feelings resulting from the actual–ideal discrepancy, people may take action to ensure that they behave in line with those standards (Bersoff, 1999; Fejfar & Hoyle, 2000; Heine et al., 2008; Moskalenko & Heine, 2003). Social evaluations in peer interactions likely elicit and enhance the awareness of social expectations and standards and guide individuals in regulating their behavior.

From the contextual–developmental perspective, the regulation of peer interaction is an important mediating process of cultural influence on individual development. The process may occur gradually as children attempt to maintain or modify their behaviors during daily peer activities according to culturally directed social evaluations. In North America, for example, the negative peer feedback that shy children receive in Canada may create heightened pressure on them to alter or control their behaviors in social situations. Shy children with adequate social-cognitive abilities are likely to regulate their behaviors to improve their social status in the group (e.g., Rubin, Coplan, Fox, & Calkins, 1995). Children who fail to adjust their anxious and wary behaviors according to social expectations may experience frustration, distress, and other negative emotions and develop adjustment difficulties (e.g., Coplan et al., 2004; Fejfar & Hoyle, 2000; Gest, 1997; Rubin et al., 2009), which in turn reinforce the negative social evaluation of shy behaviors. Unlike the experience of shy children in North America, the social approval and support that shy children have traditionally received in China inform them that peers regard their wary and restrained behaviors as acceptable and appropriate (e.g., Chen et al., 1995; Chen et al., 2006). This favorable social experience is conducive to the development of self-confidence, which helps shy children maintain their prosocial behaviors in interactions. This experience may also inspire shy children to display their competencies in other areas, such as school performance (Chen, Chen, et al., 2009). As assertiveness and self-direction have become more valued during the recent social change in urban China, children may be adjusting their behaviors according to the new expectations and attempting to control their shy and wary reactions in social situations (Chen, Cen, et al., 2005)

A main source of motivational force that directs children to participate in peer interactions, attend to social evaluations, and eventually maintain or modify their behaviors to meet peer standards is the need for intimate affect and mutual support within friendship, belongingness to the group, and overall peer acceptance in the larger setting. Close relationships with peers and overall peer acceptance have been found to be associated with socioemotional well-being in children and adolescents (Rubin et al., 2006). Children who lack intimate friendships or experience peer rejection or isolation are likely to report social dissatisfaction and other symptoms of psychological problems (e.g., Asher, Parkhurst, Hymel, & Williams, 1990; Berndt, 2002; Boivin, Hymel, & Bukowski, 1995; Burks, Dodge, & Price, 1995; Ladd & Troop-Gordon, 2003; Parker & Asher, 1993). To acquire social affiliation and acceptance, it is crucial for children to engage in social activities, to understand others' expectations, and to adjust their behaviors according to the expectations.

The regulatory function of peer interaction may be affected by various personal and social factors such as children's abilities to understand social expectations and to exercise behavioral control. Among the factors that developmental and cross-cultural researchers have investigated is children's sensitivity to social evaluations. Social–evaluative sensitivity includes both cognitive and affective processes such as attention to evaluations of peers, understanding of social cues, and concern about social relationships. Research evidence has suggested that sensitivity to social evaluation may (1) promote behaviors that are encouraged by peers, (2) inhibit behaviors that may jeopardize interactions and relationships, and (3) motivate children to be attuned to social environments and actively resolve problems in interactions (Blatt, Zohar, Quinlan, Luthan, & Hart, 1996; Henirch, Blatt, Kupermine, Zohar, & Leadbeater, 2001; Rudolph & Conley, 2005).

At the individual level, according to the social information processing model (Dodge, Coie, & Lynam, 2006), children may differ in how they attend to social situations and process social cues, owing to past social experiences and personal social-cognitive abilities. Social cognitive deficits or biases in reading social cues and interpreting the intentions of others may make children inclined to choose inappropriate solutions. Research findings have shown that, despite their marked behavioral problems and difficulties in peer relationships, aggressive children, particularly in North America, tend to be less sensitive to social evaluations, have inaccurate perceptions of social information, and overestimate their social competence (Asher et al., 1990; Boivin, Thomassin, & Alain, 1989). The literature (Cross & Madson, 1997; Maccoby, 1998; Rudolph & Conley, 2005) also suggests that gender differences exist in sensitivity to social evaluations, with girls demonstrating more concern than boys about social evaluation—perhaps owing to their greater tendency to value harmonious relationships and communality (Maccoby, 1998).

Consistent with the argument that the history of social experiences determines, in part, the development of individual inclination in processing social information (Dodge et al., 2006), cultural values of self versus group orientation may affect children's social–evaluative sensitivity. In cultures where how others view the individual is regarded as more important than how the individual views himself or herself, children may be more inclined to attend to others' perceptions of themselves. Thus, children may develop greater social sensitivity and responsiveness to peer expectations in group-oriented societies that emphasize interdependence and group harmony than in self-oriented societies that emphasize personal autonomy and individuality. Cultural influence on social–evaluative sensitivity may be reflected in specific social activities. In Chinese schools, for example, children are required to engage in frequent activities in which students' performance in social, behavioral, and academic areas is jointly evaluated by peers and oneself. The activities are believed to help children acquire accurate perceptions of how they are viewed by others and to promote awareness of weaknesses, feelings of shame, and efforts at self-improvement (e.g., Heine et al., 2008; Luo, 1996). Consistent with this argument, cross-cultural researchers have found that children and adolescents in East Asian societies such as Japan display higher levels of perspective taking and social–evaluative concern (e.g., concern about "losing face") than their counterparts in North America (e.g., Cohen & Hoshino-Browne, 2005; Dong, Yang, & Ollendick, 1994; Hwang, 1985). Given their relatively higher social–evaluative sensitivity, it may not be surprising that East Asian children are more susceptible to the influence of social interaction than their Western counterparts. It is an interesting question to what extent this tendency may explain the findings that East Asian children tend to conform to social and cultural expectations and display rule-abiding behaviors (Ho, 1986; Orlick, Zhou, & Partington, 1990; Stevenson, 1991).

Children as Active Participants in Peer Interaction and Development

Although it has been argued that children may actively participate in socialization and interaction with adults, children are viewed, in general, as the recipients of socialization influence in most cross-cultural and developmental theories (e.g., Edwards et al., 2006; Rogoff, 2003). By focusing on peer interaction processes, the contextual–developmental perspective inevitably emphasizes the active role of children themselves in development. A major indication of the active role of children is their participation in adopting the existing cultures and constructing new cultures for social evaluations and other peer activities (Corsaro & Nelson, 2003). Brown (1990), for example, found that children and adolescents in the United States formed a variety of natural peer groups such as "jocks," "brains," "populars," "partyers," "nerds," and "burnouts" with distinct norms as indications of the group identity. Similarly, Chen, Chang, and He (2003) found that Chinese children often spontaneously formed groups based on their academic norms and prosocial versus antisocial orientations. The peer culture may interact with other socialization influences such as parenting in shaping children's behaviors (Chen, Chang, He, & Liu, 2005; Lansford, Criss, Pettit, Dodge, & Bates, 2003). Chen, Chang, et al. (2005) demonstrated how peer group norms moderated the effects of parents' socialization efforts; whereas prosocial-constructive groups served to facilitate parents' socialization efforts to help their children develop social and school competencies, antisocial-destructive groups undermined the contributions of parenting to child development.

The peer activities of children with different cultural backgrounds may be particularly conducive to the construction of new cultures (e.g., Azmitia & Cooper, 2004; Chen & Tse, 2008; Way, 2006). International and domestic migrations have made exposure to a variety of social and cultural beliefs and practices as well as lifestyles a part of the common experience of migrant and nonmigrant children and adolescents today. Moreover, macrolevel cultural communication and exchange during globalization have created a constantly changing environment featuring diverse values for youths in most societies in the world. While the experience of having to deal with divergent cultural expectations may engender confusion and frustration (Berry, Phinney, Sam, & Vedder, 2006), children's diverse backgrounds are actually a valuable resource for them in developing new cultures that incorporate various—and perhaps complementary—values and behavioral norms, such as responsibility, achievement, and independence (Conzen, Gerber, Morawska, Pozzetta, & Vecoli, 1992; Fuligni, 1998; Garcia Coll et al., 1996). The integrated cultural values may help children learn to maintain a balance between pursuing their own ends and establishing group harmony (e.g., Maccoby, 1998). The emergence of integrated cultures may also provide opportunities for children and adolescents to develop sophisticated social and behavioral qualities and skills that better enable them to function flexibly and effectively in different circumstances.

The active role of children in the social interaction processes needs to be understood from a developmental perspective. Research has indicated that children and adolescents' social interaction becomes more extensive and complicated as they become more interested in, and capable of, exploring diverse lifestyles in the peer world with increasing age. There are also different internal and external demands such as the display of autonomous actions in social interactions in different developmental stages. At the same time that children develop their social–cognitive abilities, they also become more competent in understanding social evaluations, actively engaging in social activities, and regulating their behaviors according to social expectations.

Culture and Social Interaction in Different Settings

In addition to providing guidance for social evaluations and responses, culture may affect the processes of interaction indirectly by specifying the nature, function, and structure of social relationships in which interaction occurs. Sharabany and Wiseman (1993) have reported that children in Kibbutz communities focus on group involvement and have only limited dyadic friendships. According to Sharabany (2006), dyadic friendships featuring high levels of affective involvement are not encouraged in at least some collectivist societies because of the availability of other sources of emotional support, the reduced privacy characteristic of collectivist lifestyles, and the potential threat that exclusive dyadic friendships pose to the cohesiveness of the larger group. Particular values of various types of peer relationships such as the close friendship versus the peer group may have an impact on peer interaction and its significance for individual development. More generally, cultural constraints on the characteristics of peer relationships, such as the functions of friendship, the norms for peer group organization, and typical experiences in peer activities in larger settings, may affect the social processes in children's interaction (Chen & French, 2008; Gaskins, 2000).

Friendship Functions: Enhancement of Self-Worth versus Instrumental Aid

Major functions of friendship such as security-protection, companionship, intimate disclosure, instrumental assistance, and enhancement of self-worth have been found in children and adolescents in many cultures (French, Lee,

& Pidada, 2006). Nevertheless, specific social and cultural conditions determine, to a large extent, which functions of friendship are emphasized in the society (Chen & French, 2008). In Korea and some other Asian nations, for example, the Confucian values of trust among friends may promote the salience of loyalty and obligation in friendships (French et al., 2006). In Latino societies, emotional expressivity is typically encouraged to convey warmth and affection in friendships (Argyle, Henderson, Bond, Iizuka, & Contarello, 1986). Consequently, cross-cultural differences exist in friendship functions that are identified and appreciated by children.

In Western cultures, support of friends is considered a major mechanism for children to develop positive self-perceptions and self-feelings (Sullivan, 1953). This function is less salient in non-Western cultures where the development of the self is not regarded as an important developmental task. It has been found that whereas one of the major reasons for friendship among North American children is that friends make them feel good about themselves, Chinese (e.g., Chen, Kaspar, Zhang, Wang, & Zheng, 2004; Cho, Sandel, Miller, & Wang, 2005) and Indonesian (French et al., 2005) children and children with an Arab and Caribbean background (Dayan, Doyle, & Markiewicz, 2001) often do not report the enhancement of self-worth as an important function of friendship.

Relative to self-validation, instrumental aid appears to be more important for friendships of children in many collectivist or group-oriented cultures (Smart, 1999; Tietjen, 1989). Way (2006), for example, found that sharing of money and protecting friends from harm were salient aspects of the friendships of low-income black and Hispanic adolescents in the United States. Instrumental assistance has also been found to be a highly salient feature of friendships in Asian and Latino societies such as China (Chen, Kaspar, et al., 2004), Cuba (Gonzalez, Moreno, & Schneider, 2004), Costa Rica (DeRosier & Kupersmidt, 1991), Indonesia (French et al., 2005), South Korea (French et al., 2006), and the Philippines (Hollnsteiner, 1979). In these societies, instrumental assistance may occur in diverse forms. For example, a theme that has often emerged from interviews with Chinese adolescents is the strong appreciation of friends' mutual assistance in school achievement (e.g., Way, 2006).

Cultural values of self-validation or instrumental aid may help children organize their activities with friends that facilitate related behaviors. Specifically, whereas friends in Western cultures may support one another to display self-confidence and develop positive self-regard, friends in some Asian cultures are likely to concentrate on helping one another attain success on social and academic tasks (Chen, Kaspar, et al., 2004). Moreover, by emphasizing particular functions of friendship, cultural values enhance the relevance of the related behaviors or characteristics in social evaluations and reinforce children's sensitivity to evaluations with regard to these behaviors or characteristics in interactions among friends.

Individual Autonomy versus Responsibility in the Peer Group

Peer group affiliation is a common phenomenon among school-age children (e.g., D'Hondt & Vandewiele, 1980; Kiesner, Poulin, & Nicotra, 2003; Salmivalli, Huttunen, & Lagerspetz, 1997). Research conducted with Western children indicates that involvement in peer groups increases from childhood to early adolescence, which is believed to be derived from the desire of youths to obtain support for personal autonomy from the family (Rubin et al., 2006). Once children enter the peer group, they are expected to learn independence while maintaining positive relationships with others. Children are encouraged to pursue personal interest and gradually develop self-identity and individuality through group activities (Brown, 1990). Intensive interaction within the small clique is the major form of peer activity in childhood but tends to decline from middle childhood to adolescence, when children start to be affiliated with multiple groups and larger crowds (e.g., Brown, 1990). During adolescence, a variety of peer groups such as those labeled as populars, nerds, and partyers (e.g., Brown & Klute, 2003) indicate that peer groups are formed mainly based on adolescents' particular interests. As adolescents increasingly seek independence, they start to feel the tension with the constraint of group norms and attempt to avoid the restriction of the group. As a result, there is a general loosening of group ties, and adolescents' sense of belongingness declines steadily with age (see Rubin et al., 2006). At the same time, the influence of group interaction on individual attitudes and behaviors may weaken in middle and late adolescence.

The tension between the pursuit of independence and personal interest and the commitment to the group undertaking may be less evident in group-oriented than self-oriented cultures. In group-oriented cultures that value commitment to social relationships, children and adolescents are encouraged to maintain strong social affiliation, identify with the group, and assume responsibility for the group (Sharabany, 2006). There is great pressure on group members to conform to group norms, which are often in accord with the general socialization goals in the society. D'Hondt and Vandewiele (1980) have noticed that peer groups in Senegalese youth are organized on social and moral principles such as solidarity, unity, and struggle against social injustices. Similarly, children and adolescents in China often describe group activities in terms of how they fit with adults' requirements and standards such as maintaining and enhancing interpersonal cooperation and school achievement (Chen et al., 2008; Sun, 1995). Particular attention is paid to whether group activities are guided by the "right" social goals and whether these activities are beneficial to children's performance on socially valued tasks. The encouragement of commitment and social orientation in group organization may promote individual awareness of responsibility in mutual evaluations during group interaction.

Play and Peer Activities in Larger Settings

Developmental researchers have investigated children's peer interactions across cultures by observing children's play activities in structured as well as naturalistic settings such as classrooms, school backgrounds, and villages. Little, Brendgen, Wanner, and Krappmann (1999) found that, compared with children in West Berlin, children in the former East Berlin experienced less fun and enjoyment with their peers, largely because of adults' greater control of children's peer interaction. However, with the changes in the educational system following German unification, peer interaction among children in East Berlin has been increasingly based more on personal choices and less controlled by adults. As a result, children in the former East Berlin are now expected to engage in more playful and intimate activities with friends, express more personal likings, and experience greater enjoyment in their peer interactions.

Cross-cultural differences have also been observed in sociodramatic activity in children's play. According to Farver et al. (1995) and Edwards (2000), sociodramatic behavior and pretense require children to control their anxiety and to express their inner interests and personal styles. Western children tend to engage in more sociodramatic activities than children in many other societies, particularly those with subsistence economies. It has been found that children in Maya societies (Gaskins, 2000), Bedouin Arab countries (Ariel & Sever, 1980), Kenya, Mexico, and India (Edwards, 2000) engage in little sociodramatic activity. Farver et al. (1995) also found that Korean American preschool children displayed less social and pretend play than Anglo-American children. Moreover, when Korean children engaged in pretend play, it contained more everyday and family role activities and less fantastic themes (e.g., actions related to legend or fairy-tale characters that do not exist) (Farver & Shin, 1997). Gosso, Lima, Morais, and Otta (2007) found in Brazil that urban children in Sao Paulo, especially from high-socioeconomic-status families, engaged in significantly more pretend or sociodramatic activities than children in an Indian village (Paranowa-ona) and a small coastal town (Seashore in São Paulo state). Apparently, the extent to which children engage in sociodramatic activities and their content are both influenced by social and cultural conditions.

Taken together, in Western and non-Western urban societies, an important socialization goal is to help children develop self-confidence, assertive behaviors, and personal styles (e.g., Smetana, 2002; Triandis, 1995). Accordingly, the social and ecological environment (e.g., the structuring of activities, physical settings) is set up for children to learn and practice self-directive and expressive skills. Social interactions in playful and sociodramatic activities may facilitate the development of these skills. Similarly, social interactions in activities such as collaboration on particular tasks in traditional societies with subsistence economies (Gaskins, 2006; de Guzman, Edwards, & Carlo, 2005) may help children develop cooperative behavior and self-control that are useful for adaptation in these societies.

Conclusions, General Issues, and Implications

Children in different societies differ considerably on socioemotional functioning such as self-expression, cooperation and responsibility, aggression, and shyness (see Chen, Chung, & French, in press, for a comprehensive review). To explain the cross-cultural differences, researchers often examine cultural backgrounds such as the broad collectivist versus individualist and independent versus interdependent orientations (e.g., Oyserman, Coon, & Kemmelmeier, 2002). As a result, our understanding of the role of culture is largely limited to its macro-level aspects that may be associated with children's social and cognitive functions in a static and mechanistic manner. Relatively little is known about the processes through which cultural beliefs and values are involved in human development. Social psychologists (e.g., Abrams, 2004; Tafjel, 1981) have suggested that the role of group norms, which are likely culturally based, is affecting individual attitudes and behaviors. However, the group norm influence is discussed mainly in terms of the self system, such as perceived membership of social groups, group identification, self-categorization, and in-group favoritism, with little attention directed at the social interaction context.

The contextual–developmental perspective emphasizes peer interaction as a context for the formation of the links between cultural values and individual socioemotional development (Chen, Chung, et al., 2009). According to this perspective, cultural norms and values provide a basis for social evaluative processes in peer interaction, which in turn serve to regulate individual behavior. Children play an active role in development by constructing new cultures to guide social evaluations and other peer activities. Culture may also guide the social interaction processes by specifying the functional and structural features of the various peer contexts such as friendships and groups in which interaction occurs. In the contextual–

developmental framework, peer interaction meditates the links of culture and development mainly through the group-level processes, including the establishment of group norms, acceptance-based peer evaluations, and peer regulation of children's behaviors. Individual-level processes such as sensitivity to social expectations may occur in the group context.

Social evaluation and regulation are common activities in peer interaction from middle childhood to adolescence. However, the social interaction processes may vary across developmental stages, owing to different internal and external demands for peer affiliation and the display of autonomous actions. For example, social interaction becomes more complicated with age, as children are more interested in, and capable of, exploring different lifestyles with peers (Brown, 1990). At the same time, children may be more competent in understanding social evaluations, integrating various values for peer activities, and regulating their behaviors. A high level of peer interaction is likely to promote the relevance of sophisticated and diverse cultures to socioemotional functioning.

Finally, the contextual–developmental perspective has implications for research and applied work. While developmental researchers should explore the cultural norms and values that guide children's social interaction in order to understand its nature and significance, it is important for cross-cultural researchers to investigate cultural influences on human development in the social interaction context. It is also interesting to examine how the regulatory function of social interaction is affected by personal, group, and situational conditions. In addition, as indicated by the contextual–developmental perspective, the social interaction processes play a crucial role in cultural influences on individual behavior. Thus, parents, educators, and professionals should take into account the social interaction context in developing culturally compatible and appropriate remediation programs for children who display behavioral and socioemotional problems.

References

Abrams, D. (2004). Social self-regulation. *Personality and Social Psychology Bulletin, 20,* 473–483.

Argyle, M., Henderson, M., Bond, M., Iizuka, Y., & Contarello, A. (1986). Cross-cultural variations in relationship rules. *International Journal of Psychology, 21,* 287–315.

Ariel, S., & Sever, I. (1980). Play in the desert and play in the town: On play activities of Bedouin Arab children. In H. B. Schwartzman (Ed.), *Play and culture* (pp. 164–175). West Point, NY: Leisure Press.

Asher, S., Parkhurst, J. T., Hymel, S., & Williams, G. A. (1990). Peer rejection and loneliness in childhood. In S. R. Asher & J. D. Coie (Eds.), *Peer rejection in childhood* (pp. 253–273). New York: Cambridge University Press.

Azmitia, M., & Cooper, C. R. (2004). Good or bad? Peer influences on Latino and European American adolescents' pathways through school. *Journal of Education for Students Placed at Risk, 6*, 45–71.

Berry, J. W., Phinney, J. S., Sam, D. L., & Vedder, P. (2006). *Immigrant youth in cultural transition: Acculturation, identity, and adaptation across national contexts.* Mahwah, NJ: Erlbaum.

Berndt, T. J. (2002). Friendship quality and social development. *Current Directions in Psychological Science, 11*, 7–10.

Bersoff, D. M. (1999). Why good people sometimes do bad things: Motivated reasoning and unethical behavior. *Personality and Social Psychology Bulletin, 25*, 28–39.

Blatt, S. J., Zohar, A., Quinlan, D. M., Luthan, S., & Hart, B. (1996). Levels of relatedness within the Dependency factor of the Depressive Experiences Questionnaire for Adolescents. *Journal of Personality Assessment, 67*, 52–71.

Boivin, M., Hymel, S., & Bukowski, W. M. (1995). The roles of social withdrawal, peer rejection, and victimization by peers in predicting loneliness and depressed mood in childhood. *Development and Psychopathology, 7*, 765–785.

Boivin, M., Thomassin, L., & Alain, M. (1989). Peer rejection and self-perception among early elementary school children: Aggressive-rejectees vs. withdrawn-rejectees. In B. Schneider, G. Attili, J. Nadel, & P. P. Weissberg (Eds.), *Social competence in developmental perspective.* Dordrecht: Kluwer.

Borja-Alvarez, T., Zarbatany, L., & Peper, S. (1991). Contributions of male and female guests and hosts to peer group entry. *Child Development, 62*, 1079–1090.

Bowlby, J. (1969). *Attachment and loss. Vol. 1. Attachment.* New York: Basic Books.

Brown, B. B. (1990). Peer groups and peer cultures. In S. S. Feldman & G. R. Elliott (Eds.), *At the threshold: The developing adolescent* (pp. 171–196). Cambridge, MA: Harvard University Press.

Brown, B. B., & Klute, C. (2003). Friendships, cliques, and crowds. In G. R. Adams & M. D. Berzonsky (Eds), *Blackwell handbook of adolescence* (pp. 330–348). Malden, MA: Blackwell.

Burks, V. S., Dodge, K. A., & Price, J. M. (1995). Models of internalizing outcomes of early rejection. *Development and Psychopathology, 7*, 683–696.

Casiglia, A. C., Lo Coco, A., & Zappulla, C. (1998). Aspects of social reputation and peer relationships in Italian children: A cross-cultural perspective. *Developmental Psychology, 34*, 723–730.

Chagnon, N. A. (1983). *Yanomamo: The fierce people.* New York: Holt, Reinhart & Winston.

Chang, L., Lei, L., Li, K. K., Liu, H., Guo, B., & Wang, Y., et al. (2005). Peer acceptance and self-perceptions of verbal and behavioural aggression and withdrawal. *International Journal of Behavioral Development, 29*, 49–57.

Chen, X. (2010). Socioemotional development in Chinese children. In M. H. Bond (Ed.), *Handbook of Chinese psychology* (pp. 37–52). Oxford, UK: Oxford University Press.

Chen, X., Cen, G., Li, D., & He, Y. (2005). Social functioning and adjustment in Chinese children: The imprint of historical time. *Child Development, 76,* 182–195.

Chen, X., Chang, L., & He, Y. (2003). The peer group as a context: Mediating and moderating effects on the relations between academic achievement and social functioning in Chinese children. *Child Development, 74,* 710–727.

Chen, X., Chang, L., He, Y., & Liu, H. (2005). The peer group as a context: Moderating effects on relations between maternal parenting and social and school adjustment in Chinese children. *Child Development, 76,* 417–434.

Chen, X., Chang, L., Liu, H., & He, Y. (2008). Effects of the peer group on the development of social functioning and academic achievement: A longitudinal study in Chinese children. *Child Development, 79,* 235–251.

Chen, X., Chen, H., Li, D., & Wang, L. (2009). Early childhood behavioral inhibition and social and school adjustment in Chinese children: A five-year longitudinal study. *Child Development, 80,* 1692–1704.

Chen, X., Chung, J., & French, D. (in press). Culture and social development. In C. Hart & P. Smith (Eds.), *Wiley Blackwell handbook of childhood social development,* 2nd ed. Malden, MA: Blackwell.

Chen, X., Chung, J., & Hsiao, C. (2009). Peer interactions and relationships from a cross-cultural perspective. In K. H. Rubin, W. M. Bukowski, & B. Laursen (Eds.), *Handbook of peer interactions, relationships, and groups* (pp. 432–451). New York: Guilford Press.

Chen, X., DeSouza, A., Chen, H., & Wang, L. (2006). Reticent behavior and experiences in peer interactions in Canadian and Chinese children. *Developmental Psychology, 42,* 656–665.

Chen, X., & French, D. (2008). Children's social competence in cultural context. *Annual Review of Psychology, 59,* 591–616.

Chen, X., Kaspar, V., Zhang, Y., Wang. L., & Zheng, S. (2004). Peer relationships among Chinese and North American boys: A cross-cultural perspective. In N. Way & J. Chu (Eds.), *Adolescent boys in context* (pp. 197–218). New York: New York University Press.

Chen, X., Li, D., Li, Z., Li, B., & Liu, M. (2000). Sociable and prosocial dimensions of social competence in Chinese children: Common and unique contributions to social, academic and psychological adjustment. *Developmental Psychology, 36,* 302–314.

Chen, X., Rubin, K. H., Li, B., & Li, Z. (1999). Adolescent outcomes of social functioning in Chinese children. *International Journal of Behavioural Development, 23,* 199–223.

Chen, X., Rubin, K. H., & Li, Z. (1995). Social functioning and adjustment in Chinese children: A longitudinal study. *Developmental Psychology, 31,* 531–539.

Chen, X., & Tse, H. C. (2008). Social functioning and adjustment in Canadian-born children with Chinese and European backgrounds. *Developmental Psychology, 44,* 1184–1189.

Chen, X., & Wang, L. (in press). Shyness-sensitivity and unsociability in rural Chinese children: Relations with social, school, and psychological adjustment. *Child Development.*

Cho, G. E., Sandel, T. L., Miller, P. J., & Wang, S. (2005). What do grandmothers think about self-esteem?: American and Taiwanese folk theories revisited. *Social Development, 14,* 701–721.

Chung, J., & Chen, X. (2009). Aggressive and prosocial peer group functioning: Effects on children's social, school, and psychological adjustment. *Social Development, 19,* 659–680.

Cohen, D., & Hoshino-Browne, E. (2005). Insider and outsider perspectives on the self and social world. In R. M. Sorrentino, D. Cohen, J. M. Olson, & M. P. Zanna (Eds.), *Culture and social behavior: The tenth Ontario symposium* (pp. 49–76). Hillsdale, NJ: Erlbaum.

Coie, J. D., Terry, R., Lenox, K., Lochman, J., & Hyman, C. (1995). Childhood peer rejection and aggression as predictors of stable patterns of adolescent disorder. *Development and Psychopathology, 7,* 697–714.

Cole, M. (1996). *Cultural psychology.* Cambridge, MA: Harvard University Press.

Cole, P. M., Bruschi, C., & Tamang, B. L. (2002). Cultural differences in children's emotional reactions to difficult situations. *Child Development, 73,* 983–996.

Cole, P. M., Tamang, B. L., & Shrestha, S. (2006). Cultural variations in the socialization of young children's anger and shame. *Child Development, 77,* 1237–1251.

Conzen, K. N., Gerber, D. A., Morawska, E., Pozzetta, G. E., & Vecoli, R. J. (1992). The invention of ethnicity: A perspective from the U.S.A. *Journal of American Ethnic History, 11,* 3–41.

Coplan, R. J. & Armer, M. (2007). A "multitude" of solitude: A closer look at social withdrawal and nonsocial play in early childhood. *Child Development Perspectives, 1,* 26–32.

Coplan, R. J., Prakash, K., O'Neil, K., & Armer, M. (2004). Do you "want" to play?: Distinguishing between conflicted-shyness and social disinterest in early childhood. *Developmental Psychology, 40,* 244–258.

Corsaro, W. A., & Nelson, E. (2003). Children's collective activities and peer culture in early literacy in American and Italian preschools. *Sociology of Education, 76,* 209–227.

Cross, S. E., & Madson, L. (1997). Models of the self: Self-construals and gender. *Psychological Bulletin, 122,* 5–37.

Dayan, J., Doyle, A. B., & Markiewicz, D. (2001). Social support networks and self-esteem of idiocentric and allocentric children and adolescents. *Journal of Social and Personal Relations, 18,* 767–784.

de Guzman, M. R. T., Edwards, C. P., & Carlo, G. (2005). Prosocial behaviors in context: A study of the Gikuyu children of Ngecha, Kenya. *Applied Developmental Psychology, 26,* 542–558.

DeRosier, M. E., & Kupersmidt, J. B. (1991). Costa Rican children's perceptions of their social networks. *Developmental Psychology, 27,* 656–662.

DeRosier, M., Kupersmidt, J., & Patterson, C. (1994). Children's academic and behavioral adjustment as a function of the chronicity and proximity of peer rejection. *Child Development, 65,* 1799–1813.

D'Hondt, W., & Vandewiele, M. (1980). Adolescents' groups in Senegal. *Psychological Reports, 47,* 795–802.

Dishion, T. J., Piehler, T. F., & Myers, M. W. (2008). Dynamics and ecology of adolescent peer influence. In M. J. Prinstein & K. A. Dodge (Eds.), *Understanding peer influence in children and adolescents* (pp. 72–93). New York: Guilford Press.

Dodge, K. A., Coie, J. D., & Lynam, D. (2006). Aggression and antisocial behavior in youth. In N. Eisenberg (Ed.), *Handbook of child psychology: Vol. 3. Social, emotional, and personality development* (pp. 719–788). New York: Wiley.

Dodge, K. A., Greenberg, M. T., Malone, P. S., & Conduct Problems Prevention Research Group. (2008). Testing an idealized dynamic cascade model of the development of serious violence in adolescence. *Child Development, 79,* 1907–1927.

Dodge, K. A., Petit, G. S., McClaskey, C. L., & Brown, M. (1986). Social competence in children. *Monographs of the Society for Research in Child Development, 51* (2, Serial No. 213).

Dong, Q., Yang, B., & Ollendick, T. H. (1994). Fears in Chinese children and adolescents and their relations to anxiety and depression. *Journal of Child Psychology and Psychiatry, 35,* 351–363.

Duval, T. S., & Silvia, P. J. (2002). Self-awareness, probability of improvement, and the self-serving bias. *Journal of Personality and Social Psychology, 82,* 49–6).

Duval, T. S., & Wicklund, R. (1972). *A theory of objective self-awareness.* New York: Academic Press.

Edwards, C. P. (2000). Children's play in cross-cultural perspective: A new look at the Six Culture Study. *Cross-Cultural Research, 34,* 318–338.

Edwards, C. P., Guzman, M. R. T., Brown, J., & Kumru, A. (2006). Children's social behaviors and peer interactions in diverse cultures. In X. Chen, D. French, & B. Schneider (Eds.), *Peer relationships in cultural context* (pp. 23–51). New York: Cambridge University Press.

Eisenberg, N., Fabes, R. A., & Spinrad, T. L. (2006). Prosocial development. In N. Eisenberg (Ed.), *Handbook of child psychology: Vol. 3. Social, emotional, and personality development* (pp. 646–718). New York: Wiley.

Eisenberg, N., Pidada, S., & Liew, J. (2001). The relations of regulation and negative emotionality to Indonesian children's social functioning. *Child Development, 72,* 1747–1763.

Farver, J. M., Kim, Y. K., & Lee, Y. (1995). Cultural differences in Korean- and Anglo-American preschoolers' social interaction and play behaviors. *Child Development, 66,* 1088–1099.

Farver, J. M., & Shin, Y. L. (1997). Social pretend play in Korean- and Anglo-American preschoolers. *Child Development, 68,* 544–556.

Fejfar, M. C., & Hoyle, R. H. (2000). Effect of private self-awareness on negative affect and self-referent attribution: A quantitative review. *Personality and Social Psychology Review, 4,* 132–142.

French, D. C., Lee, O., & Pidada, S. (2006). Friendships of Indonesian, South Korean and United States youth: Exclusivity, intimacy, enhancement of worth, and conflict. In X. Chen, D. French, & B. Schneider (Eds.), *Peer relationships in cultural context* (pp. 379–402). New York: Cambridge University Press.

French, D. C., Pidada, S., & Victor, A. (2005). Friendships of Indonesian and United States youth. *International Journal of Behavioral Development, 29,* 304–313.

Fuligni, A. J. (1998). The adjustment of children from immigrant families. *Current Directions in Psychological Science, 7,* 99–103.

Garcia Coll C., Crnic, K., Lamberty, G., Wasik, B. H., Jenkins, R., Garcia, H. V., et al. (1996). An integrative model for the study of development competencies in minority children. *Child Development, 67,* 1891–1914.

Gaskins, S. (2000). Children's daily activities in a Mayan village: A culturally grounded description. *Cross-Cultural Research, 34,* 375–389.

Gaskins, S. (2006). The cultural organization of Yucatec Mayan children's social interaction. In X. Chen, D. French, & B. Schneider (Eds.), *Peer relationships in cultural context* (pp. 283–309). New York: Cambridge University Press.

Gest, S. D. (1997). Behavioral inhibition: Stability and association with adaptation from childhood to early adulthood. *Journal of Personality and Social Psychology, 72,* 467–475.

Gonzalez, Y., Moreno, D. S., & Schneider, B. H. (2004). Friendship expectations of early adolescents in Cuba and Canada. *Journal of Cross-Cultural Psychology, 35,* 436–445.

Goodnow, J. J. (1997). Parenting and the transmission and internalization of values: From social-cultural perspectives to within-family analyses. In J. E. Grusec & L. Kuczynski (Eds.), *Handbook of parnting and the transmission of values* (pp. 333–361). New York: Wiley.

Gosso, Y., Lima, M. D., Morais, S. E., & Otta, E. (2007). Pretend play of Brazilian children: A window into different cutlural worlds. *Journal of Cross-Cultural Psychology, 38,* 539–558.

Greenfield, P. M., Suzuki, L. K., & Rothstein-Fisch, C. (2006). Cultural pathways through human development. In K. A. Renninger & I. E. Sigel (Eds.), *Handbook of child psychology: Vol. 4. Child psychology in practice* (pp. 655–699). New York: Wiley.

Hart, C. H., Yang, C., Nelson, L. J., Robinson, C. C., Olson, J. A., Nelson, D. A., et al. (2000). Peer acceptance in early childhood and subtypes of socially withdrawn behaviour in China, Russia and the United States. *International Journal of Behavioral Development, 24,* 73–81.

Hartup, W. W. (1992). Social relationships and their developmental significance. *American Psychologist, 44,* 120–126.

Heine, S. J., Takemoto, T., Moskalenko, S., Lasaleta, J., & Henrich, J. (2008). Mirrors in the head: Cultural variation in objective self-awareness. *Personality and Social Psychology Bulletin, 34,* 879–887.

Henrich, C. C., Blatt, S. J., Kuperminc, G. P., Zohar, A., & Leadbeater, B. J. (2001). Levels of interpersonal concerns and social functioning in early adolescent boys and girls. *Journal of Personality Assessment, 76,* 48–67.

Hinde, R. A. (1987). *Individuals, relationships and culture.* Cambridge, UK: Cambridge University Press.

Ho, D. Y. F. (1986). Chinese pattern of socialization: A critical review. In M. H. Bond (Ed.), *The psychology of the Chinese people* (pp. 1–37). New York: Oxford University Press.

Hollnsteiner, M. R. (1979). Reciprocity as a Filipino in value. In M. R. Hollnsteiner (Ed.), *Culture and the Filipino* (pp. 38–43). Quezon City, Phillippines: Atteneo de Manila University.

Hwang, K. K. (1985). Face and favour: The Chinese power game. *American Journal of Sociology, 92*, 944–974.

Kerr, M., Lambert, W. W., & Bem, D. J. (1996). Life course sequelae of childhood shyness in Sweden: Comparison with the United States. *Developmental Psychology, 32*, 1100–1105.

Kiesner, J., Poulin, F., & Nicotra, E. (2003). Peer relations across contexts: Individual-network homophily and network inclusion in and after school. *Child Development, 74*, 1328–1343.

Ladd, G. W., & Troop-Gordon, W. (2003). The role of chronic peer difficulties in the development of children's psychological adjustment problems. *Child Development, 74*, 1344–1367.

Lansford, J. E., Criss, M. M., Pettit, G. S., Dodge, K. A., & Bates, J. E. (2003). Friendship quality, peer group affiliation, and peer antisocial behavior as moderators of the link between negative parenting and adolescent externalizing behavior. *Journal of Research on Adolescence, 13*, 161–184.

Leontiev, A. N. (1981). The problem of activity in psychology. In J. V. Wertsch (Ed.). *The concept of activity in Soviet psychology*. Armonk, NY: Sharpe.

LeVine, R. A., Dixon, S., LeVine, S., Richman, A., Leiderman, P. H., Keefer, C. H., et al. (1994). *Child care and culture: Lessons from Africa*. New York: Cambridge University Press.

Little, T. D., Brendgen, M., Wanner, B., & Krappmann, L. (1999). Children's reciprocal perceptions of friendship quality in the sociocultural contexts of East and West Berlin. *International Journal of Behavioral Development, 23*, 63–89.

Luo, G. (1996). *Chinese traditional social and moral ideas and rules*. Beijing, China: The University of Chinese People Press.

Maccoby, E. E. (1998). *The two sexes: Growing up apart, coming together*. Cambridge, MA: Harvard University Press.

Miller, J. G. (1994). Cultural diversity in the morality of caring: Individually oriented versus duty-based interpersonal moral codes. *Cross-Cultural Research, 28*, 3–39.

Miller, J. G., Bersoff, D. M., & Harwood, R. L. (1990). Perceptions of social responsibilities in India and in the United States: Moral imperatives or personal decisions? *Journal of Personality and Social Psychology, 58*, 33–47.

Moskalenko, S., & Heine, S. J. (2003). Watching your troubles away: Television viewing as a stimulus for subjective self-awareness. *Personality and Social Psychology Bulletin, 29*, 76–85.

Orlick, T., Zhou, Q. Y., & Partington, J. (1990). Co-operation and conflict within Chinese and Canadian kindergarten settings. *Canadian Journal of Behavioral Science, 22*, 20–25.

Oyserman, D., Coon, H. M., & Kemmelmeier, M. (2002). Rethinking individualism and collectivism: Evaluation of theoretical assumptions and meta-analyses. *Psychological Bulletin, 128*, 3–72.

Parke, R. D., & Buriel, R. (2006). Socialization in the family: Ethnic and ecological perspectives. In N. Eisenberg (Ed.), *Handbook of child psychology: Vol 3*.

Social, emotional, and personality development (pp. 429–504). New York: Wiley.

Parker, J. G., & Asher, S. R. (1993). Friendship and friendship quality in middle childhood: Links with peer group acceptance and feelings of loneliness and social dissatisfaction. *Developmental Psychology, 29*, 611–621.

Piaget, J. (1932). *The moral judgment of the child*. Glencoe, IL: Free Press.

Rodkin, P. C., Farmer, T. W., Pearl, R., & van Acker, R. (2000). Heterogeneity of popular boys: Antisocial and prosocial configurations. *Developmental Psychology, 36*, 14–24.

Rogoff, B. (2003). *The cultural nature of human development*. New York: Oxford University Press.

Rothbaum, F., & Trommsdorff, G. (2006). Do roots and wings complement or oppose one another?: The socialization of relatedness and autonomy in cultural context. In J. E. Grusec & P. D. Hastings (Eds.), *Handbook of socialization: Theory and research* (pp. 461–489). New York: Guilford Press.

Rothbaum, F., Weisz, J., Pott, M., Miyake, K., & Morelli, G. (2000). Attachment and culture. *American Psychologist, 55*, 1093–1104.

Rubin, K. H., Bukowski, W., & Parker, J. G. (2006). Peer interactions, relationships, and groups. In N. Eisenberg (Ed.), *Handbook of child psychology: Vol 3. Social, emotional, and personality development* (pp. 571–645). New York: Wiley.

Rubin, K. H., Coplan, R., & Bowker, J. (2009). Social withdrawal in childhood. *Annual Review of Psychology, 60*, 141–171.

Rubin, K. H., Coplan, R. J., Fox, N. A., & Calkins, S. (1995). Emotionality, emotion regulation, and preschoolers' social adaptation. *Development and Psychopathology, 7*, 49–62.

Rudolph, K. D., & Conley, C. S. (2005). The socioemotional costs and benefits of social-evaluative concerns: Do girls care too much? *Journal of Personality, 73*, 115–137.

Salmivalli, C., Huttunen, A., & Lagerspetz, K. (1997). Peer networks and bullying in schools. *Scandinavian Journal of Psychology, 38*, 305–312.

Schneider, B., H., & Fonzi, A. (1996). La stabilita dell'amicizia: Unostudio cross-culturale Italia–Canada [Friendship stability: A cross-cultural study in Italy–Canada]. *Eta Evolutiva, 3*, 73–79.

Schneider, B. H., Fonzi, A., Tomada, G., & Tani, F. (2000). A cross-national comparison of children's behavior with their friends in situations of potential conflict. *Journal of Cross-Cultural Psychology, 31*, 259–266.

Schneider, B. H., Smith, A., Poisson, S. E., & Kwan, A. B. (1997). Cultural dimensions of children's peer relations. In S. Duck (Ed.), *Handbook of personal relationships: Theory, research and interventions* (2nd ed., pp. 121–146). Hoboken, NJ: Wiley.

Sharabany, R. (2006). The cultural context of children and adolescents: Peer relationships and intimate friendships among Arab and Jewish children in Israel. In X. Chen, D. French, & B. Schneider (Eds.), *Peer relationships in cultural context* (pp. 452–478). New York: Cambridge University Press.

Sharabany, R., & Wiseman, H. (1993). Close relationships in adolescence: The case of the kibbutz. *Journal of Youth and Adolescence, 22*, 671–695.

Smart, A. (1999). Expressions of interest: Friendship and *guanxi* in Chinese societies. In S. Bell & S. Coleman (Eds.), *The anthropology of friendship* (pp. 119–136). Oxford, UK: Berg.

Smetana, J. (2002). Culture, autonomy, and personal jurisdiction. In R. Kail & H. Reese (Eds.), *Advances in child development and behavior* (Vol. 29, pp. 52–87). New York: Academic Press.

Stevenson, H. W. (1991). The development of prosocial behavior in large-scale collective societies: China and Japan. In R. A. Hinde & J. Groebel (Eds.), *Cooperation and prosocial behaviour* (pp. 89–105). Cambridge, UK: Cambridge University Press.

Sullivan, H. S. (1953). *The interpersonal theory of psychiatry*. New York: Norton.

Sun, S. L. (1995). *The development of social networks among Chinese children in Taiwan*. Unpublished doctoral dissertation, University of North Carolina at Chapel Hill.

Super, C. M., & Harkness, S. (1986). The developmental niche: A conceptualization at the interface of child and culture. *International Journal of Behavioral Development, 9*, 545–569.

Tafjel, H. (1981). *Human groups and social categories*. Cambridge: Cambridge University Press.

Tietjen, A. (1989). The ecology of children's social support networks. In D. Belle (Ed.), *Children's social networks and social support* (pp. 37–69). New York: Wiley.

Triandis, H. C. (1995). *Individualism and collectivism*. Boulder, CO: Westview Press.

Vygotsky, L. S. (1978). M. Cole, V. John-Steiner, S. Scribner, & E. Souberman (Eds.), *Mind in society: The development of higher psychological processes*. Cambridge, MA: Harvard University Press.

Way, N. (2006). The cultural practice of close friendships among urban adolescents in the United States. In X. Chen, D. French, & B. Schneider (Eds.), *Peer relationships in cultural context* (pp. 403–425). New York: Cambridge University Press.

CHAPTER 3

Culture, Public Policy,
and Child Development

HIROKAZU YOSHIKAWA *and* MADELEINE CURRIE

Large-scale social change with consequences for children is a matter of urgency in the industrialized and majority worlds. Despite the many sources of social change that can influence children's well-being, mental health, and socioemotional development—such as industrialization, demographic or other changes resulting from globalization, technological change, natural disasters, environmental change, and armed conflict—few developmental scientists examine how large-scale social change impacts child development. Increasingly, international nongovernmental organizations (NGOs) highlight the importance of addressing the psychosocial health of children in these situations (Belfer, 2006, 2008; Betancourt & Khan, 2008; Elbert et al., 2009; Hill, 2006; Timimi, 2005; UNICEF, 2009; Wessells, 2009; Wickrama & Kaspar, 2007; World Health Organization, 2006).

Work on two macrosystem influences on children—culture and public policy—can speak to the mechanisms of effects of social change on development (Bronfenbrenner & Morris, 1998). These two systems are rarely considered together, however, despite the public policy challenges of increased diversity, owing to voluntary or forced migration and other factors, in many countries of the world. Cultural developmentalists study variations across nations, ethnic groups, or cultures in the proximal contexts of child socialization, most often the family. Primarily developmental psychologists, this group of researchers rarely integrates assessment of other macrosystems like public policy into their work. Conversely, public policy analysts consider the impacts of public policies in different nations and cultural contexts. This group, primarily informed by economics, sociology, political science, and evaluation science, generally does not integrate explicit measures of cultural beliefs, attitudes, or goals into their work. Thus, the integration of culture and public policy in developmental science falls outside the primary disciplines of the field and has been overlooked.

Recent evidence suggests, however, that the intersection of culture and public policy is important to investigate. For example, public policy that is responsive to the increasing diversity of many societies is a crucial need in an era of globalization and increased migration (M. M. Suarez-Orozco, 2007; Suarez-Orozco, Todorova, Qin, Villarruel, & Luster, 2006). Policies and programs for children in postconflict situations, similarly, must be sensitive to cultural norms regarding family structure and socialization (Gruskin & Tarantola, 2005; Ngalazu Phiri &Tolfree, 2005; United Nations, 1989; Wessells, 2009). Local meanings of "mental health" and socioemotional development vary greatly across cultures, and therefore basic research is required regarding the cultural appropriateness of specific constructs prior to the development of prevention or treatment programs (Betancourt & Khan, 2008; Kleinman, 1988; Lee, Kleinman, & Kleinman, 2007; LeVine, 1994; Stark, Boothby, & Ager, 2009). All of these examples indicate that the intersection of culture and public policy, far from being an esoteric corner of developmental research, should be central to the concerns of developmental scientists interested in informing program and policy development in the industrialized and majority worlds.

In this chapter we delineate several mechanisms by which culture and public policy together may shape children's socioemotional as well as cognitive development. First, changes in public policy can over time affect cultural beliefs, attitudes, and goals, which in turn can influence children through a variety of channels. Second, cultural beliefs, attitudes, and goals can moderate the effects of public policy on children. Third, cultural beliefs, attitudes, and goals can shape policy preferences at the societal or family levels.

In this chapter we focus on parental beliefs, attitudes, and goals as representative of cultural influences on child development. Parents' beliefs, attitudes, and goals are central in studies of culture and human development because they are instances of intentional passing on of socialization values across generations (Harwood & Schoelmerich, 1996; Harwood, Yalcinkaya, Citlak, & Leyendecker, 2006; Keller, 2003; Rogoff, 2003). In order to limit the scope of this chapter, we do not consider other proximal contexts in which cultural attitudes may be reflected, such as school, employment, or other organizational contexts. Public policy is represented by government investments in programs and policies that can affect children's socioemotional or cognitive development. Although NGOs and other private sector programs are extremely important as influences on children's development, we do not include these in our discussion.

Our conception of both culture and public policy is informed by dynamic systems theory, which provides a useful framework for considering change at multiple ecological levels that can intervene between the macro level and the individual level of the developing child (Ford & Lerner, 1992; Thelen & Smith, 1994; Yoshikawa & Hsueh, 2001). For example, relative to the influence of public policy on child development, dynamic systems theories remind us of the interdependence across systems, across ecological levels within systems, as well as across particular system functions. Culture and public policy could have a reciprocal causal relationship such that cultural change drives public policy change as well as vice versa. Families most often encounter public policy through interactions with formal service providers, or gatekeepers. These dyadic interactions are nested within policy implementation organizations, with administrative and supervisory structures that determine access at the family level to resources, incentives, and information. These organizations, in turn, are nested within larger institutions at the community or policy jurisdiction level. Interactions among levels are complex and change over time with alterations in the training of staff, regulations governing policy implementation, and ultimately legislation itself. The time scale of change in legislation does not often track very well with changes in implementation that families experience in communities. Similarly, cultural change can occur at a variety of ecological levels, including the community, a subpopulation within a particular cultural group, or across an entire society. A variety of social communication channels can transmit cultural change. Cultural change may "bubble up" from aggregate individual or social network-level change, or it may be influenced by macro-level sources such as political, economic, demographic, technological, or policy changes.

Reflecting these principles, in this chapter we discuss reciprocal influences among policies and cultural values. We also consider how changes in culture and public policy can influence multiple nested systems at lower ecological levels, including centrally focused families and socialization processes but also neighborhood processes and factors relating to parents' or youths' employment. We review a mix of nonexperimental and experimental evidence, utilizing a variety of disciplinary perspectives, including anthropology, sociology, developmental psychology, and public policy analysis.

Public Policies Bring About Change
in Cultural Beliefs, Values, and Goals

Public policy change can directly affect cultural beliefs, attitudes, and goals about children. We discuss here four examples spanning the policy areas of fertility policy, large-scale political change, immigration policy, and industrialization.

One of the most dramatic examples of public policy change altering cultural values and goals may be the institution of China's one-child policy during the years from 1979 to 1986. This policy was not driven by mass public opinion and is therefore an interesting case of a relatively exogenous or unidirectional influence on cultural values and attitudes. The one-child policy appeared to substantially alter not only childbearing patterns but also attitudes during the years following its passage. The policy, first instituted in 1979 but with widespread implementation occurring over the course of the next 7 years, restricted most urban couples to having one child. In rural areas, couples were allowed to have more than one child, as were couples who were both singletons themselves. Although there is some disagreement regarding the magnitude of the impact of the one-child policy on fertility rates, given the lack of appropriate comparison, the consensus among demographers is that the policy played a significant role in the continued rapid decline of the fertility rate following the policy's implementation (the rate was nearly halved during the first 16 years of the policy, from 2.9 to 1.7% annually; Hesketh, Lu, & Xing, 2005). The policy led to selective forced abortions, particularly in rural areas, although the exact extent of the phenomenon is unknown. Critics have also decried the first generation of only children as "little emperors," self-centered and unable to relate to others. The reality is certainly more complex; however, it is undeniable that for many families with single children the pattern of investing all the resources of the nuclear family in a single child has altered family life (Fong, 2004).

A relatively unknown aspect of the law is how powerful it was in changing public opinion and preferences regarding the ideal number of children in one's family. The one-child policy initially met with resistance, particularly from those living in rural areas, where modernization was less apparent and where more children were deemed necessary for the material support of the family. However, patterns of enforcement of the policy, along with ongoing government portrayals of the reasons for the policy—to facilitate modernization and its attendant socioeconomic benefits at both the national and personal levels—resulted in changes in parents' fertility ideals and preferences. Fong's (2004) study of over 2,000 Chinese singletons in early adolescence and their parents details the changing fertility preferences of urban parents who had entered childbearing age during the early years of the one-child policy. Many parents initially resisted the strictures of the policy after it was officially implemented and enforced beginning in 1978, relating that early in their marriages they had wanted at least two or three children. However, resistance to the policy had largely subsided by the time Fong began her fieldwork in 1997. Acceptance of the policy is corroborated historically by the fact that enforcement became less strict during the 1990s, since it was no longer necessary to guarantee conformity to the policy. The respondents in Dalian that Fong interviewed tended to express personal views supporting of the policy, generally assenting to the notion that the policy was strategically correct for China's social and economic future. Some parents cited their own large childhood families as the cause of limited resources during their own childhood. As levels of consumption increased during the 1990s, some parents said they were happy to have only one child, despite some parents' previous desire for a larger family. These urban parents had internalized a cultural model of modernization that accompanied corresponding declines in fertility rates.

Another example of public policy change influencing cultural norms comes from the reunification of Germany during the early 1990s. Rainer Silbereisen and colleagues have tracked changes in occupational preferences as residents of East Germany, without relocating themselves, have had to adapt to a new market-driven economy. Among a cohort of middle adolescents, the earlier onset of clear occupational preferences occurred in East Germany but not in West Germany shortly following reunification in 1991 (Silbereisen, 2005). In a younger adolescent cohort, such differences were not apparent, in that the respondents were too young in either pre- or postreunification contexts to express distinct occupational preferences. The difference in onset of occupational preferences for older adolescents in the former East Germany versus West Germany had declined in magnitude by 1996, as expected, as norms spread quite quickly in the new economy.

A third example of public policy changes influencing cultural norms comes from the area of immigration policy. The 1965 Hart–Celler Act in the United States abolished racially specific exclusion policies that had been in effect from the 19th century and further advanced through the 1924 Johnson–Reed Immigration Act (Ngai, 2004; Yoshikawa, 2011; Yoshikawa & Kalil, 2009). The central provision of the Hart–Celler Act was the institution of hemisphere-wide rather than country-specific quotas for legal migration to the United States. The provisions for legal migration in the act and the principal amendment to the act, passed in 1976, had a profound influence on patterns of migration to the United States. The country-specific quotas in place between 1924 and 1965 had reflected ethnic, racial, and political preferences (e.g., in the 1920s legislation, preferences for northern European immigrants rather than Asians and southern or eastern Europeans). The hemispheric approach, in which quotas were established for entire hemispheres with additional restrictions per country within the hemisphere, replaced this system. The result was a surge in immigration from Latin America, the Caribbean, and Asia rather than Europe. In recent years, immigration from Africa has also increased dramatically, influenced in part by the 1986 Immigration and Control Act (IRCA) and the Immigration Act of 1990. The IRCA granted amnesty to undocumented immigrants in the United States, and the Immigration Act of 1990 included a diversity program that provided visas to people from countries underrepresented in previous influxes of immigrants to the United States. This legislation, in general, has been instrumental in the increase of black immigrants to the United States (Shaw-Taylor, 2007).

African and Afro-Caribbean immigration to the United States presents interesting examples of how policy changes can influence cultural norms relating to race and ethnicity. Black Americans with recent histories in Africa and the Caribbean now constitute over 20% of the black population in some urban areas of the United States, and across the United States these groups accounted for close to 25% of the increase in black Americans between the 1990 and 2000 U.S. censuses (Logan, 2007). During that period, the Afro-Caribbean population increased by over 618,000 (close to 67%), and the African population grew by over 383,000 (close to 167%), nearly tripling the number of Africans in the United States (Logan, 2007, p. 52). As a result, demographic patterns of black Americans in the United States have changed considerably during the past two decades, which has implications for the demographic constitution of U.S. cities, where new immigrants are most highly concentrated, thereby affecting school populations and children's socialization experiences. Socioeconomic patterns and characteristics among black Americans have also changed as the result of shifting concentrations of subpopulations within the black American community. Among black Americans, Africans and Afro-Caribbeans have higher educational attainment and incomes and lower rates of unemployment and poverty. While Logan's (2007) analysis indicates a high degree of segregation between black and white Americans in the United States, there are also significant differences between blacks born in the United States and those that have immigrated from Africa and the Caribbean, such that they are expected to remain distinct groups rather than assimilate into preexisting groups in the United States (Kasinitz, 1992).

Through these demographic changes, notions of race, ethnicity, and transnationalism have changed in the United States (Shaw-Taylor, 2007). For example, adolescents' racial identity patterns as black youths in the United States have changed in many school contexts. On the one hand, immigrants adjusting to a society with very different interracial relations can develop a variety of identities as West Indian, Caribbean, and/or African American. These different pathways of identity development can be influenced by peer group composition, developing awareness of and attributions of discrimination experiences, and parental socialization. Caribbean youths and parents may distinguish themselves from African Americans with longer histories in the United States in part to ward off discrimination (Waters, 1999). Identity development among African American youths with deeper roots in the United States, on the other hand, may also be influenced by this influx of new immigrants from the Caribbean or Africa. Different kinds of incorporation of African and Caribbean youths into American schools can alter the range of "black identities" in family, school, and neighborhood contexts (Suarez-Orozco, 2004; Waters, 1999).

A final set of examples comes not from public policy change per se but from the study of industrialization, that is, shifts from agricultural to industrial economies or rural to urban populations. These shifts, largely complete in the most industrialized societies, have been occurring across the majority world during recent decades. Studies have found that industrialization can result in several shifts that show some consistency across societies transitioning from low-income to middle-income status. Kăgitcibaşi and Ataca (2005) have shown that the value of children shifted from primarily economic to primarily psychological (emotional) during the years between 1975 and 2003 in Turkey. In 1975, Kăgitcibaşi and Ataca surveyed a nationally representative sample of 2,305 married participants on the values they attribute to children, their reasons for having children, and corresponding fertility rates. They conducted another survey of 1,025 respondents in 2003. The authors defined the value of children (VOC) as "the sum total of psychological, social, and economic costs and benefits that parents derive from having children" (p. 318). Increased urbanization in Turkey during the years between the two surveys caused dramatic changes in the society, including increased levels of education and other alterations in family life, such as adolescents' increased financial dependence on their parents in light of increased educational demands. Between 1975 and 2003 the authors found that the psychological value of children (the potential of children to bring psychological benefits to their parents) had increased and that their economic value (including the children's ability to contribute to the family income during their childhood and their ability to provide for elderly parents) had decreased. These changes corresponded to changes in family relationship patterns between the samples. Models of *family interdependence*, common in less developed areas and involving both psychological and economic interdependence, decreased. Models of *psychological or emotional relatedness* increased. The researchers found that over the period of the study there were also changes in the reasons parents gave for wanting a child, the qualities parents wished for in their children, the economic expectations that older mothers had of their children, and parents' notions of the ideal family size.

In another example of the effect of industrialization and economic growth on perceptions of children, Xinyin Chen and colleagues have shown that teacher and peer perceptions of behaviorally inhibited children shifted from largely positive to neutral to largely negative across three cohorts of adolescents from whom data were collected across 15 years of dramatic economic growth in Shanghai, China (Chen, Cen, Li, & He, 2005). In a more recent study, Chen and colleagues found similar differences among children of urban versus rural migrant origins in China, such that behavioral inhibition was associated with positive teacher and peer perceptions among urban children but negative perceptions among rural migrant children (Chen, Wang, & Wang, 2009). Patricia Greenfield (2009), in her recent review of this literature, concludes that the process of industrialization as well as transitions from rural to urban economies "shifts cultural values in an individualistic direction and developmental pathways toward more independent social behavior and more abstract cognition" (p. 401). During such a transition, significant changes in family economies (how people earn a living) and social relationships often occur.

Cultural Beliefs, Values, and Goals Can Moderate the Impact of Public Policies on Children

A second mechanism through which culture and public policy can affect children's development relates to synergistic interactions. That is, cultural values and the goals of populations may interact with public policies to affect children's development. Most research on the impact of public policies on children does not investigate this hypothesis. Typically, public policy evaluations containing data on children explore whether the effects differ depending on such sociodemographic characteristics of the population as indicators of socioeconomic status, the parents' or children's ages (or developmental period), race or ethnicity, or other markers of developmental risk. Relatively few data show whether these differences result from these demographic characteristics per se or, rather, from differences in culturally based values, goals, and preferences.

Person–environment fit theory suggests that characteristics of the individual—for example, one's developmental stage or values—may in part determine how that individual selects or responds to various environmental demands (Eccles et al., 1993; Moos, 1984, 1987). Congruence between environmental demands and personal goals, values, and attitudes, for example, would be expected to produce higher levels of adjustment and well-being. Such theories have never been systematically applied to policy environments. However, they may be useful in helping to explain ethnic differences in the effects of welfare policies on childhood development.

Values and goals relevant to work and education are highly salient developmental concerns for parents in young adulthood. Such values and goals might interact with welfare program approaches to influence parents' responses to policy-driven mandates and their children's development (Yoshikawa, Morris, et al., 2006). Imagine, for example, a single parent on welfare who is without her general equivalency diploma (GED) but who nonetheless has high levels of motivation to pursue her own education. She might fare better in a welfare policy environment that encourages education and job training rather than immediately seeking out a job. In a policy environment that encourages immediate work, a parent who prefers working over staying at home with her children might fare better than one who believes that work may interfere with good parenting. Parents' responses to such mandates as involvement in adult education activities or employment may well influence their children through such intervening family processes as higher expectations for one's own and children's future education, cognitive stimulation, parental well-being, or monitoring.

Values and goals relating to work and education, moreover, may differ across various cultural groups. Evidence shows, for example, that the value of work among African American mothers has been historically strong, as experiences of oppression experienced by this group has generally led to a strong emphasis in their childhood socialization on social mobility and work. Similarly, the value of pursuing one's own education may be particularly strong among immigrant groups, such as low-income Latinos/Latinas, that have experienced interruption of their own education in their countries of origin to come to the United States and support their families back home through work (Yoshikawa, 2011).

In a recent set of studies, hypotheses about whether parental goals for work and education interact with work-first or education-first policy environments was tested experimentally. The data come from the National Evaluation of Welfare to Work Strategies, which utilized three-way random assignment of parents on welfare to test two approaches to welfare-to-work policy against a control condition. The two conditions consisted of a work-first condition, in which welfare recipients were mandated to find a job immediately by participating in job search activities—or risk losing their welfare benefits—and an education-first condition, in which recipients were mandated to participate in job training and adult basic education activities, or risk losing their benefits. The control condition was simply the opportunity to continue receiving welfare under the then active welfare regulations of the federal government. All children were ages 3–5 at random assignment.

In this experiment, measures of parents' goals were collected at baseline prior to random assignment. The measures consisted of multi-item scales of the preference for working (as compared to staying at home with family) and preference for pursuing one's own education. Assessments of children's behavioral development, as rated by parents and teachers, were collected at a 5-year follow-up (ages 8–10). Thus, the "match" between parental goals (for work vs. education) and policy environment (work-first or education-first demands) could be cleanly tested in a causal framework.

The patterns were strikingly consistent (Gassman-Pines, Godfrey, & Yoshikawa, 2009). When parents endorsed educational goals at high levels and experienced an education-first rather than work-first program, children were rated by teachers as displaying lower levels of externalizing behaviors and more assertion, cooperation, self-control, and school engagement. Because these results pertained to teacher reports, with teachers unaware of the programs to which parents had been assigned 5 years before, we can have confidence that the pattern of results indeed confirmed person–environment fit theory.

In an additional set of analyses, we found that these interactions between policy environment and parental goals to pursue their own education explained racial/ethnic differences in these programs' effects on children's school achievement (Yoshikawa, Morris, et al., 2006). In the experiment, impacts of the education-first program were more positive for Latino children than for white children. It turned out that this was attributable to the Latino parents' stronger preferences for pursuing their own education. In the geographic area of this experiment (Riverside County, California), the vast majority of Latino parents in the sample were of Mexican background. Mexican low-income parents in this sample, it turned out, had high rates of valuing their own education. Other ethnographic research shows that this group is in fact likely to have experienced an interrupted education in coming to the United States. Although in the Riverside sample immigration information was not collected, we may surmise that a proportion of the Mexican parents likely experienced such an interruption in the course of their migration to the United States.

Thus, values regarding important life goals such as education may differ across various cultural groups, and such differences may matter for how these groups respond to diverse policy environments. In these studies, person–environment fit theory was confirmed in the context of public policy, and the data showed how culture, parental goals and values, and the public policy approach can interact to affect children's socioemotional development.

Cultural Beliefs, Values, and Goals Can Alter Public Policy Preferences

Finally, a third mechanism through which culture and public policy can act together to alter human development concerns the direct impact of cultural beliefs, values, and goals on public policy preferences. The topic of cultural norms and public policy arises more often in the fields of political science or sociology than developmental science. For example, Ellwood (1988), an economist and public policy analyst, in his classic volume on poverty in the American family, described several conflicting cultural norms with deep-seated roots in the history of the United States that influence antipoverty policies for children and families. As many other theorists of cultural values have observed, cultural beliefs in any particular society often conflict. Ellwood, for example, uses the term "conundrums" to describe the values underlying American poverty policies. That is, values in U.S. society regarding the primacy of the family, the virtue of work, the autonomy of the individual, and the desire for community can conflict. This conflict in values can lead to inconsistent support in U.S. history for policies that primarily emphasize family-level responsibility for children's welfare, education, and well-being (such as the welfare reform legislation of 1996) or policies that primarily emphasize the responsibility of communities for supporting these outcomes (such as WIC (women, infants, children), the chief nutritional support program for women, infants, and children in the United States).

Policies that achieve widespread political support satisfy these conflicting values in a delicate balancing act. The Earned Income Tax Credit (EITC) represents an excellent example of a successful policy with bipartisan support in the United States that balances multiple potentially conflicting values (Ellwood was influential in championing the expansion of this policy during the 1980s and 1990s). Often known among working-poor communities as the "tax refund" or "rebate check," the EITC provides up to $4,000 per year in income for low-wage working families (with lower levels of benefits for single adults) in the form of a tax credit. The tax credit is refundable, which means that families receive it even if their level of earnings is low enough that they do not owe taxes. This policy has been shown to be the single most powerful U.S. federal policy in effectively reducing rates of child poverty. Data from 2002 demonstrate that without the EITC the poverty rate for children in the United States would have been one-third higher (Greenstein, 2005). By providing income contingent on earnings, the program supports the virtue of work that has roots in the Protestant work ethic. By directly reducing poverty for families through federal policy, the program also supports the value of the desire for community. By providing more income for families than for single adults, the program supports the primacy of the family. And finally, by basing benefits on the amount of individual earnings, the policy also supports the value of individual autonomy. The EITC can be compared in its successful balance of these values to cash welfare, a much less highly regarded program. Cash welfare was an entitlement program prior to 1996, and therefore for many it failed to support the virtue of work and the autonomy of the individual–despite the fact that a large majority of welfare recipients were also simultaneously working for pay (Edin & Lein, 1997; Yoshikawa, 1999).

A recent study provides some experimental support for the relationship between cultural values and public policy preferences. The goal of the study was to examine how various frames or cognitive schemas regarding children might differentially predict preferences for government policies to fight poverty and support low-wage employment.

The frames chosen for children in poverty included the following: the Vulnerable Child (a view of children in poverty as at risk and therefore deserving of government support); the Future Citizen (a view of children as future adult citizens in society and therefore deserving of government investment); and the Responsible Management frame (which postulated that responsible government policymakers should take into account research on child development in developing policies to support children and families).

Frames were inserted into statements that were read to participants in a national poll of 3,400 U.S. adults representative of the national electorate. The statements were randomly assigned. For example, the Vulnerable Child frame read as follows: "Lately there has been a lot of talk about the role of society in supporting children. In particular, people have offered various explanations of why it is important to devote societal resources to children at the very earliest stages of life. For example, some people believe that society needs to invest in programs that help the most vulnerable children, whose families struggle to make ends meet. According to this view, one way to level the playing field for children who suffer from poverty and discrimination is to financially support their access to the same high-quality early childhood programs that wealthier families can afford."

The Future Citizen framing statement read: "Lately there has been a lot of talk about the role of society in supporting children. In particular, people have offered various explanations of why it is important to devote societal resources to children at the very earliest stages of life. For example, some people believe that early childhood development is important for community development and economic development. According to this view, skills and capacities that begin developing in early childhood become the basis of a prosperous and sustainable society—from positive school achievement, to work force skills, to cooperative and lawful behavior. Have you heard of this explanation of why we should allocate societal assets to young children, because they predict our society's prosperity?"

Following the statement, support for a variety of public policies was gauged, including a set of items representing policies to directly reduce poverty or support the ability of low-wage workers to increase their earnings over time. The policies were selected based on developmental evidence that income poverty harms young children's development (Duncan & Brooks-Gunn, 1997) and that wage growth, coupled with stable, full-time employment, benefits children's development (Yoshikawa, Weisner, & Lowe, 2006). Policies included tax credits like the EITC, other approaches to income supplementation, parental paid leave, child care subsidies, and policies to support adult education. Items tapping support for each of these policies were highly correlated, and so these were combined into a single measure.

The most effective frame for increasing support for antipoverty policies was the Future Citizen frame. This frame increased support overall for these policies, but was especially effective among Republicans (an effect size of +0.23). This effect was also larger for whites than for blacks or Latinos, and larger for men than for women. The frame also increased support for a statement attributing responsibility for supporting child development to government rather than individuals, implying some mediation of the impact on policy preferences through support for government intervention.

This study showed that cultural values may shape public policy preferences and that, in particular, actively framing children as future economic contributors to society can increase support for public investment in children. This hypothesis is supported by the recent success of James Heckman's economic theory linking later educational and economic success to foundational skills in early childhood ("skills beget skills") in increasing support for government investment in preschool education (Heckman, 2006). In interesting contrast to the work of Kăgitcibaşi and Ataca (2006), it appears that an economic, rather than psychological, framing of the role of children predicts preferences for public support of families in an industrialized society.

Conclusion

This chapter shows that culture and public policy, as two powerful macrosystems that can influence socialization and child development, can have reciprocal influence on each other and can synergistically influence child development. We discussed how cultural values related to children and to contexts such as socialization, work, and education may be influenced by, and influence, policy. Child and family policy can be powerfully shaped by cultural attitudes. In addition, large-scale policy change can influence cultural attitudes over time as populations gradually adjust to new norms governing the family sphere. And parents can respond very differently to the incentives and regulations of public policy contexts, depending on their values and preferences.

Mechanisms of the influence of culture and policy on children can occur at multiple ecological levels. At the basic level of childbearing, for example, government-mandated fertility policies in China came to influence popular preferences regarding the ideal number of children in a family. Although few of the studies reviewed here explored parenting and family processes as conveyors of the dual influence of culture and public policy on child development, the studies of parental values suggest that parenting practices may be important mechanisms. Both parents' and youths' work behavior, as direct targets of public policy in the economic realm, are important mediators of the influence of cultural and policy changes. Few studies on work and family, however, have examined preferences regarding work along with work behaviors (e.g., occupational choice and career trajectories) in the study of macro-level influences on child development. Finally, perceptions of the value of children and desired behaviors in children appear to change as a consequence of economic growth and industrialization.

In future research, it would be productive to examine what types of policies drive which culturally based experiences and perceptions of child development. In the domain of culture, settings other than the home (such as child care programs, school, or workplace) could be examined in terms of how behavioral and programmatic norms vary by cultural context and the cultural composition of parents and children. In the economic realm, policies governing taxes, inheritance, foreign investment, and employment may have different kinds of influence on such perceptions. Policies outside the economic sphere that also shape family life, such as those in the areas of technology, housing, or communications, might also drive some of the changes. As globalization and access to worldwide media continue to speed the pace of social change in industrialized and majority-world societies, we should expect to see faster and more profound changes in values, attitudes, and behaviors in families and children.

References

Belfer, M. L. (2006). Caring for children and adolescents in the aftermath of natural disasters. *International Review of Psychiatry, 18*(6), 523–528.

Belfer, M. L. (2008). Child and adolescent mental disorders: The magnitude of the problem across the globe. *Journal of Child Psychology and Psychiatry, 49*(3), 226–236.

Betancourt, T. S., & Khan, K. T. (2008). The mental health of children affected by armed conflict: Protective processes and pathways to resilience. *International Review of Psychiatry, 20*(3), 317–328.

Bronfenbrenner, U., & Morris, P. A. (1998). The ecology of developmental processes. In R. Damon & R. Lerner (Eds.), *Handbook of child psychology: Vol. 1. Theoretical models of human development* (pp. 993–1028). New York: Wiley.

Chen, X., Cen, G., Li, D., & He, Y. (2005). Social functioning and adjustment in Chinese children: The imprint of historical time. *Child Development, 76,* 182–195.

Chen, X., Wang, L., & Wang, Z. (2009). Shyness-sensitivity and school, social and psychological adjustment in rural migrant and urban children in China. *Child Development, 80,* 1499–1513.

Duncan, G. J., & Brooks-Gunn, J. (Eds.). (1997). *Consequences of growing up poor.* New York: Russell Sage Foundation.

Eccles, J. S., Midgely, C., Wigfield, A. , Buchanan, C.M., Reuman, D., Flanagan, C., et al. (1993). Development during adolescence: The impact of stage–environment fit on young adolescents' experiences in schools and families. *American Psychologist, 48,* 90–101.

Edin, K., & Lein, L. (1997). *Making ends meet: How single mothers survive welfare and low-wage work.* New York: Russell Sage Foundation.

Elbert, T., Schauer, M., Schauer, E., Huschka, B., Hirth, M., & Neuner, F. (2009). Trauma-related impairment in children": A survey in Sri Lankan provinces affected by armed conflict. *Child Abuse and Neglect, 33*(4), 238–246.

Ellwood, D. T. (1988). Poor support: Poverty and the American family. New York: Basic Books.

Fong, V. L. (2004). *Only hope: Coming of age under China's one-child policy.* Palo Alto, CA: Stanford University Press.

Ford, D. H., & Lerner, R. M. (1992). *Developmental systems theory: An integrative approach.* Thousand Oaks, CA: Sage.

Gassman-Pines, A., Godfrey, E. B., & Yoshikawa, H. (2009). *Maternal preferences moderate the effects of mandatory employment and education programs on children.* Manuscript under review.

Greenfield, P. M. (2009). Linking social change and developmental change: Shifting pathways of human development. *Developmental Psychology, 45*(2), 401–418.

Greenstein, R. (2005). *The Earned Income Tax Credit: Boosting employment, aiding the working poor.* Washington, DC: Center for Budget and Policy Priorities.

Gruskin, S., & Tarantola, D. J. M. (2005). Human rights and children affected by HIV/AIDS. In G. Foster, C. LeVine, and J. Williamson (Eds.), *A Generation at Risk.* New York: Cambridge University Press.

Harwood, R. L., & Schoelmerich, A. (1996). Culture and class influences on Anglo and Puerto Rican mothers' beliefs regarding long-term socialization goals and child behavior. *Child Development, 67*(5), 2446–2461.

Harwood, R. L., Yalcinkaya, A., Citlak, B., & Leyendecker, B. (2006). Exploring the concept of respect among Turkish and Puerto Rican migrant mothers. *New Directions for Child and Adolescent Development, 2006*(114), 9–24.

Heckman, J. J. (2006). Skill formation and the economics of investing in disadvantaged children. *Science, 302,* 1900–1902.

Hesketh, T., Lu, L., & Xing, Z. W. (2005). The effect of China's one child policy after 25 years. *New England Journal of Medicine, 353,* 1171–1176.

Hill, N. E. (2006). Disentangling ethnicity, socioeconomic status and parenting: Interactions, influences and meaning. *Vulnerable Children and Youth Studies, 1*(1), 114–124.

Kğitcibaşi, C., & Ataca, B. (2005). Value of children and family change: A three-decade portrait from Turkey. *Applied Psychology: An International Review, 54*(3), 317–337.

Kasinitz, P. (1992). *Caribbean New York: Black immigrants and the politics of race*. Ithaca, New York: Cornell University Press.

Keller, H. (2003). Moving towards consensus on how to characterize culture. *Human Development, 46*(5), 328–330.

Kleinman, A. (1988). *Rethinking psychiatry: From cultural category to personal experience*. New York: Free Press.

Lee, D. T. S., Kleinman, J., & Kleinman, A. (2007). Rethinking depression: An ethnographic study of the experiences of depression among Chinese. *Harvard Review of Psychiatry, 15*(1), 1–8.

LeVine, R. A. (1994). *Child care and culture: Lessons from Africa*. New York: Cambridge University Press.

Logan, J. R. (2007). Who are the other African Americans?: Contemporary African and Caribbean immigrants in the United States. In Y. Shaw-Taylor & S. A. Tuch (Eds.), *The other African Americans: Contemporary African and Caribbean immigrants in the United States* (pp. 49–68). Lanham, MD: Rowman & Littlefield Publishers.

Moos, R. H. (1984). Context and coping: Toward a unifying conceptual framework. *American Journal of Community Psychology, 12*, 5–25.

Moos, R. H. (1987). Person–environment congruence in work, school, and health care settings. *Journal of Vocational Behavior, 31*, 231–247.

Ngai, M. (2004). *Impossible subjects: Illegal aliens and the making of modern America*. Princeton, NJ: Princeton University Press.

Ngalazu Phiri, S., & Tolfree, D. (2005). Family- and-community-based care for children affected by HIV/AIDS: Strengthening the front-line response. G. Foster (Ed.), C. LeVine (Ed.), & J. Williamson, *A Generation at Risk*: In *The Global Impact of HIV/AIDs on orphans and Vulnerable Children* (pp. TK). New York: Cambridge University Press.

Rogoff, B. (2003). *The cultural nature of human development*. Oxford, UK: Oxford University Press.

Shaw-Taylor, Y. (2007). The intersection of assimilation, race, presentation of self, and transnationalism in America. In Y. Shaw-Taylor & S. A. Tuch (Eds.), *The other African Americans: Contemporary African and Caribbean immigrants in the United States* (pp. 1–48). Lanham, MD: Rowman & Littlefield.

Silbereisen, R. K. (2005). Social change and human development: Experiences from German reunification. *International Journal of Behavioral Development, 29*, 2–13.

Stark, L., Boothby, N., & Ager, A. (2009). Children and fighting forces: 10 years on from Cape Town. *Disasters, 33*(4), 522–547.

Suarez-Orozco, C. (2004). Formulating identity in a globalized world. In M. Suarez-Orozco & D. Qin-Hilliard (Eds.), *Globalization: Culture and identity in a new millennium*. Berkeley: University of California Press.

Suarez-Orozco, C., Todorova, I., Qin, D. B., Villarruel, F. A., & Luster, T. (2006). The well-being of immigrant adolescents: A longitudinal perspective on risk and protective factors. In *The crisis in youth mental health: Critical issues and effective programs: Vol. 2. Disorders in adolescence* (pp. 53–83). Westport, CT: Praeger.

Suarez-Orozco, M. M. (Ed.). (2007). *Learning in the global era: International per-*

spectives on globalization and education. Berkeley: University of California Press.

Thelen, E., & Smith, L. (1994). *A dynamic systems approach to the development of cognition and action.* Cambridge, MA: MIT Press.

Timimi, S. (2005). Effect of globalization on children's mental health. *BMJ: British Medical Journal, 331*(7507), 37–39.

UNICEF. (2009). *Machel Study 10-Year Strategic Review: Children and conflict in a changing world.* Retrieved September 15, 2009, from *www.unhcr.org/refworld/docid/4a389ca92.html.*

United Nations. (1989). *Convention on the Rights of the Child.* United Nations Treaty Series, Vol. 1577, p. 3. Retrieved September 15, 2009, from *www.unhcr.org/refworld/docid/3ae6b38f0.html.*

Waters, M. C. (1999). Black identities: West Indian immigrant dreams and American realities. New York: Russell Sage Foundation and Cambridge: Harvard University Press.

Wessells, M. (2009). Supporting the mental health and psychosocial well-being of former child soldiers. *Journal of the American Academy of Child and Adolescent Psychiatry, 48*(6), 587–590.

Wickrama, K. A. S., & Kaspar, V. (2007). Family context of mental health risk in tsunami-exposed adolescents: Findings from a pilot study in Sri Lanka. *Social Science and Medicine, 64*(3), 713–723.

World Health Organization (WHO). (2006). *Mental health and psychosocial well-being among children in severe food shortage situations.* Retrieved on September 15, 2009, from *http://www.who.int/child_adolescent_health/documents/msd_mer_06_1/en/.*

Yoshikawa, H. (1999). Welfare and work dynamics, support services, mothers' earnings, and child cognitive development. *Child Development, 70,* 779–801.

Yoshikawa, H. (2011). *Immigrants raising citizens: Undocumented parents and their children.* New York: Russell Sage Foundation.

Yoshikawa, H., & Hsueh, J. (2001). Child development and public policy: Toward a dynamic systems perspective. *Child Development, 72,* 1887–1903.

Yoshikawa, H., & Kalil, A. (2009). *The effects of immigrant parents' documentation status on young children: A developmental research agenda.* Manuscript under review.

Yoshikawa, H., Morris, P. A., Gennetian, L. A., Roy, A. L., Gassman-Pines, A., & Godfrey, E. B. (2006). Effects of anti-poverty and employment policies on middle-childhood school performance: Do they vary by race/ethnicity, and if so, why? In A. C. Huston & M. Ripke (Eds.), *Middle childhood: Contexts of development.* New York: Cambridge University Press.

Yoshikawa, H., Weisner, T. S., & Lowe, E. (Eds.). (2006). *Making it work: Low-wage employment, family life, and child development.* New York: Russell Sage Foundation.

PART II

SOCIALIZATION
OF SOCIOEMOTIONAL
FUNCTIONING

CHAPTER 4

Parental Ethnotheories about Children's Socioemotional Development

SARA HARKNESS, CHARLES M. SUPER,
and CAROLINE JOHNSTON MAVRIDIS

"Wake up, Joey, wake up!" Diane shakes her 7-year-old son's shoulder gently. "It's time to get up for school!"

It's only 10 past seven in the morning, but the MacDonald family is already running behind schedule. Foolishly—as Diane thinks to herself now—she has accepted a request through her son's school to allow an anthropology student from a local university to come videotape a "typical morning" in their household. The student and his camera peek around the corner of Joey's bedroom just as his older sister Rachel, already fully dressed, marches into the room and shakes his whole body vigorously. *"Wake up, wake up!"*

In response, Joey retreats entirely under his covers. Rachel gives a sigh of exasperation and leaves the room as quickly as she entered. *She* is up and ready for the day!

Downstairs, the kitchen is Grand Central Station, with family members surging through as they get school backpacks and briefcases ready and toss plans for the afternoon back and forth. Rachel has soccer practice. Ron, her dad, will pick her up after school and take her there (his workplace is only a couple of blocks away), and Diane will pick her up at the end of practice, on her way home from the office. Ron will also ferry baby Melanie to her daycare center this morning, to be picked up at the last pickup time by Diane. Joey will stay for the after-school program until his mother comes to take him home.

"What do you want for breakfast?" Diane asks Rachel and Joey (who is now up and dressed, though still looking confused). Rachel wants cereal, Joey wants French toast. Diane sprints around the kitchen to accommodate both requests (luckily, the French toast is prepackaged frozen and only needs to be warmed up). Ron, meanwhile, is making coffee and quickly downing a bagel as he stands in the middle of the kitchen. Thank heavens, little Melanie sits contentedly in her highchair eating Cheerios, one by one, from the tray in front of her.

Time to go! Diane lunges for her cup of coffee on the kitchen table, takes a couple of swigs on her way to the door, and remarks to the anthropology student, "That's *my* breakfast this morning."

The anthropology student, with his video camera, follows Diane and Joey to the family minivan, and they head for Joey's school. Diane quizzes Joey—sitting in the backseat—on his weekly spelling words.

"How do you spell 'feather'?"

Joey begins, "F- E- . . . " Diane finishes with him, "A-T-H-E-R." As they approach the school, a thought suddenly occurs to her.

"Did you remember your lunch box?" she asks Joey.

"No . . . I forgot," he responds.

"But I *gave* it to you right at the door!" Diane exclaims. The car pulls up to the drop-off spot. "Never mind, it's too late now. Off you go!"

As Joey slips out of his child seat onto the floor of the car and from there to the waiting curb, Diane calls after him, "Have a good day! I love you!"

Diane drives her car around the corner and pulls over to the curb again. The anthropology student has also gotten out at Joey's school; he will walk back to campus, just a few blocks away. Diane pulls out her BlackBerry and makes an entry in Facebook to share with her friends: "Another hectic morning, just when I thought I had our schedule under control! Joey forgot his lunch—again! After going without lunch twice already, which I thought would teach him a lesson about remembering. What is this about 'consequences'? Anybody have any ideas?" She thinks of the family schedule they have posted on the refrigerator, with differently colored movable blocks for each member of the family. It's a kind of modern star chart—the kids will get a treat at the end of the week if they manage to do everything (or almost everything) on their individual lists. She'll add a new block for Joey to help him remember his lunch box. She also adds a mental "note to self: remind Joey not to forget his lunch box." At last, Diane is free and on her way to her office. When she gets there, she'll open up her BlackBerry again and read the responses from her friends. One message has already arrived: "Consider yourself lucky. Alicia is home with a fever, and it's my turn to take a personal day."

Imagine, for a moment, that the anthropology student's video recording of the MacDonald family's morning is viewed not only by his classmates but also by parents in several other cultures. Their comments on the film would be fairly predictable. A Dutch mother, for example, may seize on Joey's trouble waking up as evidence that he did not get enough sleep. The fact that he forgot his lunch box only adds further evidence for the validity of this interpretation. In her view, getting enough sleep—on a regular schedule—is the core of a healthy upbringing, one that produces alert, happy, and well-regulated children. An Italian mother, on the other hand, will focus on the moment that Joey leaves the car for school without any lunch. How can his mother even claim to love her child when she has failed to provide the most basic expression of emotional closeness and care—food? A Swedish mother may feel a quiet sense of satisfaction that social policies in her country support part-time work for parents with elementary school-age children, thus making it possible for mothers like herself to be engaged in both the world of work and the family. A Spanish mother might wonder why the MacDonalds seem to have so little help in taking care of their children. Can't Diane's mother or sister take care of the baby during the day? Why do the children have to be sent outside the family? A Korean father notices that Diane is doing a good job of coaching her son in spelling—a basic responsibility of mothers. But shouldn't Joey be getting more instruction outside of school than this? Does he go to an afterschool academy, or does this educational responsibility fall entirely on the mother's shoulders? Finally, Diane's own mother, who raised her family during a different era in America's rapidly changing work environment, feels that she is viewing a strange and different style of family life, where most of the things she took for granted—from family breakfast to sending the children off to school on the school bus—seem to have disappeared.

Just as the culturally informed perspectives of viewers from other cultures can be anticipated with some confidence, the unfolding scenario of the MacDonalds' morning is predictable—in at least two ways. First, although this morning seems hectic to both participants and observers, it is not atypical of a weekday morning in the MacDonald family. The scene we observe looks too tiring to be sustained over a long period of time—in Weisner's (2002) felicitous phrase, it does not seem to be a "sustainable daily routine." Unlikely as it may seem, however, something like this scenario is in fact repeated over the course of weeks, months, and even years. It is part of the culture of the MacDonald family. Second—and of greater interest for present purposes—the MacDonalds' morning routine is not unique to them as a family; rather, it has much in common with the morning routines of many of their contemporaries. As such, this scenario is the instantiation of a cultural script. The apparent chaos and struggle are in fact organized by cultural ideas and exigencies about being a good parent that are widely shared among American middle-class families, in which—normatively—both parents work outside the home while being fully dedicated to raising happy, healthy, and successful children. Without understanding how parents think about their children's development (as well as their own personal careers), we cannot parse the elements of their morning routine into a meaningful system. Relatedly, without a clear concept of what ideas drive parents' choices in childrearing, we cannot expect to provide any effective help. Ironically, however, this aspect of parenting has received relatively little attention in the research literature until recently. Parents' theories are in essence the "black box" of child development.

As Goodnow and Collins (1990) note, research perspectives on parental beliefs have changed over the last century, from early optimism about the importance of parents' expectations and attitudes, to a narrowed focus on behavior in the 1960s, and then to renewed interest in beliefs as essential for understanding parents' behavior. The "cognitive revolution" of the 1970s also contributed to greater interest in studying not only the way parents act but also the way they think as a window into the broader culture (Harkness & Super, 1996). More recently, globalization and the increasing cultural diversity of populations in many countries have forced researchers to consider the reality—and the implications—of often incompatible ideas living side by side in family, community, and organizational contexts.

In this chapter, we consider research across several academic disciplines that has addressed the topic of parents' beliefs about children's social and emotional development in cultural context. Beginning with classical ethnographic studies in which parental beliefs were reported in a holistic "emic" framework (Berry, 1989), we then proceed to more recent cross-cultural approaches within the anthropological tradition. From there, we continue to a consideration of the vast new cross-cultural literature on parental beliefs that has been mainly produced by psychologists. Most of this recent research is "etic" in that it uses one or more of the transcultural models that have been created to make sense of the rich variety of parental beliefs and practices around the world (Berry, 1989). Our approach, however, reflects our interest in understanding the actual content of parental ethnotheories in their own culturally "emic" terms.

A Theoretical Framework
for the Study of Parental Ethnotheories

Parents' ideas exist on many levels, from the most general and abstract to the specific and concrete. They also vary in how available they are for identification and explanation by the parents who hold them, with the most general often existing as implicit assumptions about the nature of children and the role of parents. Furthermore, cultural beliefs about the self, the family, and one's children often have strong motivational properties (D'Andrade & Strauss, 1992)—they are not just representations of the way that things *are* but also of the way things *should be*. Parental ethnotheories play a crucial role in the child's culturally structured developmental niche (Super & Harkness, 1986), a theoretical framework for understanding the child's development in cultural context. In this framework, the culturally constructed environment of the child is seen as consisting of three mutually interacting subsystems that directly interface with the growing individual: the physical and social settings of everyday life, the customary practices of child care, and the psychology of the caretakers, including shared beliefs, or parental ethnotheories. Each of these subsystems is influenced by, and often closely integrated with, aspects of the wider culture. Nevertheless, parents' cultural beliefs are powerful influences on the two other subsystems of the developmental niche. That is, within the constraints given by the wider environment, parents make choices, often implicit, about the best ways to take care of their children, and these choices tend to follow culturally recognizable patterns.

Parental beliefs and practices can be further represented by a heuristic model (Harkness & Super, 2005). At the top of the model are the most general, implicit ideas about the nature of the child, parenting, and the family. Below this triad are ideas about specific domains, such as infant sleep or social development. These ideas are closely tied to ideas about appropriate practices, and further to imagined child or family outcomes. Ideas are translated into behavior as mediated by factors such as child characteristics, parent characteristics, situational variables, and competing cultural models and their related practices. The final results can be seen in actual parental practices or behaviors and actual child and family outcomes.

Implicit Beliefs: Cultural Images of Children and the Family in Ethnographic Studies

Parental beliefs about their children's social and emotional development in classical ethnographic studies are often presented as holistic cultural models (corresponding to the top level in our heuristic model), which are either illustrated by particular behavioral vignettes or, in some cases, extrapolated from them. Margaret Mead (1928), who created the prototype for this kind of approach to the study of parenting and children in other cultures, described the cultural image of children in her Samoan field site as "little adults although lacking in experience and sometimes sadly devoid of common sense" (p. 23). Images such as these require a contrast for clarity, and ethnographers have traditionally made use of general comparisons with their own culture of origin. Interestingly, however, the classic anthropologists—who were meticulously attentive in collecting detailed observations of other cultures upon which to base their cultural insights—showed no such need to do the same at home: their generalizations about "our culture" were based on assumed common knowledge. At the same time, paradoxically, the question of how generalized the observed patterns were *beyond* the community studied was generally not addressed; rather, the cultural community was presented in its own emic terms. For example, Phoebe Ottenberg (1965, p. 21) described childrearing among the Afikpo Ibo of eastern Nigeria with this opening statement:

> Socialization and child training in Afikpo are informal and noncoercive. This seems to be associated with the belief that although an infant already has a soul at the time of birth—the reincarnation of one or more persons who have died—the spirit may change its mind about living and decide to "go back," causing the body to die.

Essentially the same belief about the tentative commitment to life on earth of the infant's soul has been more recently described in extensive detail in Alma Gottlieb's developmentally oriented ethnographic study of another West African people, the Beng of the Ivory Coast (Gottlieb, 2004). Thus, it would appear that this belief may be characteristic of a number of West African cultures and that it has remained robust over historical time.

Emic Meets Etic: The Search for General Principles of Cultural Variability

In addition to regionally specific patterns in parental ethnotheories, ethnographic studies across a wide variety of cultures have repeatedly encountered similar themes. One basic cross-cultural dimension of contrast is whether development is imagined as a process that unfolds on its own, driven by inner forces, or as one that requires supervision or overt teaching in order to turn out right. Based on her ethnographic studies of the Utku people of northern Canada, Jean Briggs (1972, p. 189) states "The Utku believe that a child's mind, his mental faculties, and understanding grow only gradually, so there is no point in trying to discipline a small child; he is incapable of learning or remembering." In a strikingly similar vein, Gaskins (2000) writes of the Mayan people of southern Mexico:

> The Maya believe that the source of development is internal and preprogrammed—it just "comes out by itself." Development and socialization are both thought to be ongoing, gradual, and continuous processes. Parents are not particularly concerned with monitoring children's develop-

mental progress nor with structuring experiences to improve or hasten it (p. 282).

Levy's (1996) ethnographic study of a small fishing village in Tahiti again echoes the same theme:

> Children [in Piri], it is believed, learn to perform tasks, for the most part, by themselves, in accordance with the gradual maturational unfolding of their abilities. Differences in achievements among children are due to differences in their inner natures. No one teaches them very much. They learn by watching and by playful trial and error that the adults often find amusing but sometimes annoying." (p. 128)

Levy contrasts this cultural model with views expressed by residents in the temple city of Bhaktapur, Nepal: "In Bhaktapur, everything seems to have to be taught and learned, and the rules and techniques for teaching are quite overt and widely shared" (p. 130). Levy suggests that these contrasting socialization beliefs are widely relevant to "such 'psychological' forms as thinking, fantasy, self, and morality in the two places" (p. 135).

Why should such similar parental beliefs turn up in such different parts of the world? Based on his own ethnographic fieldwork in Tahiti and Nepal, Levy (1996) suggested that there is a general explanation relating to differences in "cultural complexity"—that is, "simpler" societies lacking organizational hierarchies and differentiated economic and social roles beyond the family tend to favor a nativist view of development, in contrast to more culturally "complex" societies that emphasize the importance of teaching young children a variety of social and technical skills.

In order to test the validity of this interpretation, of course, one would need to look at a larger sample of societies. The Human Relations Area Files (HRAF), created from careful cataloging of ethnographic information on over 100 cultural communities around the world, were designed to answer such questions by examining patterns of co-occurrence of various cultural characteristics (Ember, 2007). Although this resource continues to be used to explore possible explanations for patterns of cultural difference and similarity, it may be that its greatest contribution has been to establish a worldwide comparative perspective that can be applied to the study of any given culture. How is a cultural community similar to others, and how is it unique? On what basis can we expect certain kinds of beliefs and behavior in a particular cultural place? At what level do generalizations about a culture hold up under comparative scrutiny?

These questions have guided a great deal of comparative ethnographic research, most notably the work of John and Beatrice Whiting and their associates. Interestingly in the present context, however, the "Whiting model" (J. W. M. Whiting, 1977) did not include parents' belief systems as part of a proposed chain of antecedents and consequences; rather, the model proposed a direct link from a society's "maintenance systems" (its socioeconomic structure), to mothers' workload, and from there to the assignment of developmental "settings" characterized in terms of different places, companions, and activities where children would learn how to be competent members of their culture. Nevertheless, the Whitings did recognize that parents had ideas; as B. B. Whiting observed about the "training mothers" of sub-Saharan Africa:

> The Ngeca mothers [in a community outside Nairobi] we interviewed are typical: they believe that they should train a child to be a competent farmer, herdsman, and child nurse and that a child from age 2 on should be assigned chores that increase in complexity and arduousness with age. They punish their children for failure to perform these tasks responsibly or for stubbornly refusing to do what their elders request of them. They allow much of their children's learning to occur through observation and imitation; only occasionally do they instruct them explicitly. Moreover, mothers seldom praise their children lest they become proud, a trait that is unacceptable. They allow the major rewards for task performance to be intrinsic. (B. B. Whiting & Edwards, 1988, p. 95)

In contrast to the African cultural model of good parenting, the Whitings proposed that the implicit ideas guiding middle-class American parents, as they observed them in the mid-20th century, would foster both competitiveness and self-doubt. This cultural contrast fit into a larger cross-cultural framework that emerged from the Whitings' "Six Culture" Study in which two dimensions of cultural variability—cultural complexity and household structure—were found to relate to children's social behavior, an indirect indication of differences in parents' ideas and socialization practices (B. B. Whiting & Whiting, 1975).

Specific Beliefs: Psychology Meets Culture

Forces of globalization and increased ethnic diversity within societies have made it impossible to ignore the cultural dimensions of ideas and practices that underlie all behavior—including that which is usually taken for granted as normal within the cultural communities to which many researchers belong. Lacking training, time, and perhaps interest in exploring the ethnotheories of diverse cultural groups, however, many psychologists interested in cross-cultural research have instead adopted existing theoretical frameworks that seem to offer an attractively simple way to explain cultural variability. The individualism–collectivism dichotomy (or relatedly, independence–interdependence), in particular, is heavily represented in cross-cultural research on parents' ideas about their children's development even though researchers frequently report that the framework does not comfortably fit their data. In response, modifications of the theory have been proposed, such as the idea that individualism and collectivism can coexist in both cultures and individuals (Tamis-LeMonda et al., 2007). Kăgitcibaşi's (2007) model, in which "independence" is separated into two separate dimensions representing relatedness versus separateness, and agency (autonomy) versus lack of control (heteronomy), has also been found to be a useful alternative for capturing cross-cultural variability.

In a somewhat similar approach, Keller (2007) suggests that there are two basic prototypes of communities and their respective psychologies: the "rural agrarian context" (found in developing contries), and the "urban, educated context" (in Western postindustrial societies). The first type of community (exemplified by the Nso village in Cameroon that she and her colleagues have studied extensively) fosters the development of the "interdependent self," who "defines himself or herself" as part of a social system (mainly the family), seeks harmonious relationships, accepts hierarchy (mainly age and gender based), values cooperation and conformity, and is identified with his or her role in the social environment" (p. 32). In contrast, the individual who grows up in the second kind of cultural context (typified by middle-class communities in Germany) develops an "independent self," one that is "self-contained, competitive, separate, unique, and self-reliant; has an inner sense of owning opinions; and is assertive" (p. 32), as well as having "personal qualities supporting self-enhancement, self-expression, and self-maximization" (p. 33). Similarly, Greenfield's (2009) theory of social change focuses on the global socioeconomic transition from small, rural subsistence-based communities to large, complex cities where wealth is accumulated, with resulting changes in children's learning environments. As both Keller and Greenfield acknowledge, their theories reflect the heritage of the Whitings' work.

Yet a third approach evident in the cross-cultural literature on parents' beliefs is to apply Baumrind's categories of parenting styles (Authoritative, Authoritarian, and Permissive), which were developed to study individual differences among middle-class European American parents (Baumrind & Black, 1967). Here, too, researchers have grappled with the poorness of fit between the model and differences observed at the cultural level in parents' beliefs about their children's social and emotional development (for example, see Chao, 1994). A fuller discussion of these frameworks is beyond the scope of the present chapter. In the present context, however, we are primarily concerned with the actual findings on parental beliefs in diverse cultures, regardless of the theoretical approach used. For the remainder of this chapter, thus, we invite the reader to accompany us on a virtual "world tour" through some major cultural regions that are distinguished by their own constellations of parental beliefs.

Around the World with Parental Ethnotheories

Our tour will consist of visits to four major cultural/geographic regions where researchers have produced a rich array of information and insights about parents' ideas regarding children's social and emotional development. Our first stop will be Asia; from there we head to sub-Saharan Africa, then across the Atlantic to the Hispanic cultures of the Americas. The large cultural region often referred to as "the West" is our next destination: We first visit western Europe before finally heading "home" to the United States, hopefully the wiser for our travels.

Asia

Parents across the Asian continent are consistently described by researchers (both Asian and non-Asian) in terms of a few themes that are important for children's social and emotional development. Primary among them is emotional interdependence, especially between a mother and her children, and relatedly, harmony within the social group. According to Lebra (1994), Japanese parents believe that these qualities can be encouraged by treating the young child with indulgence and by modeling the sensitivity they expect the child to display later in broader social contexts (Osterweil & Nagano-Nakamura, 1992). Once this basic empathy is established in the child, mothers can begin to discipline, and compliance is achieved by getting the child to empathize with her wishes (Lebra, 1994). In the meantime, aggressive behavior is regarded as offering "teachable moments" for guiding the child to work on needed social skills. Teachers as well as parents stress the importance of fostering empathic, harmonious relationships. Hayashi, Karasawa, and Tobin (2009) found that preschool teachers in Kyoto seek to foster a feeling of *omoiyari* in children, meaning the urge to respond to others' displays of emotional need or *amae*. In one instance, these authors observed a teacher urging children in her class to eat their carrots so that the carrots would not be "sad" over not having been eaten like all the other vegetables!

The role of the social reference group (teachers, neighbors, and others in the community) is seen as important for learning valued qualities. White and LeVine (1986, p. 57) state that in Japan "no conflict exists between goals of self-fulfillment and goals of social integration." Relatedly, in Taiwan, Fung (1999) found that one aspect of socioemotional competence is learning to feel the appropriate sense of shame over one's behavioral transgressions. Based on her study of families in Taipei, Fung reports that, by the time the child is about 2.5 years old, parents elicit the child's confession and repentance for various kinds of wrongdoing by way of "opportunity education"—learning from concrete events rather than from talk. Thus, mothers point out the child's misdeed to others such as nonrelatives and even bring up events from the past. Although to Western eyes this practice may seem harsh, Fung points out that the feeling of shame is not seen as a developmental end in itself but rather as a vehicle for the child's social and moral education; it serves the purpose of helping the child to be socially integrated, not set apart. Other research suggests that Asian parents' beliefs are not entirely focused on fostering obedience and group harmony, however. Parents in a Taiwanese city studied by Tamis-LeMonda and her colleagues (Tamis-LeMonda, Wang, Koutsouvanou, & Albright, 2002) stressed the importance of following social rules, being polite, honest, respectful, and responsible, and getting along with others. Yet these parents also discussed concepts of independence—even more so than U.S. parents. As the authors note, these findings challenge a simple categorization of Taiwanese parenting ideas as "collectivistic" (Tamis-LeMonda et al., 2002).

Parents' ideas about children's socioemotional development in mainland China bear a good deal of similarity to those of parents in Japan and Taiwan. Mothers in urban areas emphasize the importance of preschoolers' social skills—specifically, sharing, controlling negative emotions around peers, and helping others—nearly always in terms of conforming with social conventions (Cheah & Rubin, 2003). Relatedly, Chinese parents' ideas about shyness have been the focus of research by Chen and his colleagues (see Chen, Chapter 2, this volume). It may be that the trait of shyness in young children, previously appreciated as fulfilling social norms of politeness and respect, has more recently become a source of concern for Chinese parents who worry about whether their child will be able to compete in globalized today's environment (Chen & Bond, 2010).

Like Japanese and Taiwanese parents, Chinese parents studied by Cheah and Rubin (2003) favored the use of direct instruction, or "training," versus modeling (or suggestions) for teaching valued social skills. As with the shaming instances described in Taiwan by Fung (1999), however, "training" is done in the broader context of care and concern, not for the purpose of dominating the child or inflicting negative feelings. The concept of "training" as explained by Chao (1994) is a key aspect of Chinese parental ethnotheories, as it resolves an apparent paradox of "authoritarian" childrearing beliefs among Asian parents. Recognition of this Chinese cultural construct also reveals the culture-bound nature of Baumrind's original formulation, in which strictness (as an aspect of authoritarian parenting) is intertwined with hostility.

Although ideas about learning might seem less related to children's social or emotional development than to cognitive development, Li (2001) found that ideas about learning, as explained by adults from various parts of China, were often related to aspects of emotional engagement and social membership. In addition to hard work and achievement, a central focus was the concept of "heart and mind for wanting to learn," that is, a passion for learning. Thus, the concept of "concentration" has an emotional aspect as it includes the notion of full engagement of mind *and heart* in one's studies. These adults also spoke of the social contribution of learning. Gaining knowledge and skills is not only for personal betterment, they said, but "is part of and a step toward the well-being of the larger society" (Li, 2001, p. 128). In the same vein, good efforts at learning lead to strong moral character, which includes many social qualities, such as a sense of honor, shame, and filial piety. These ideas, as Li points out, are heavily influenced by Confucian and other classic writings.

Training for both emotional interdependence and academic learning can start very early, as demonstrated by Harkness and her colleagues (2007), who documented Korean mothers' ideas and practices related to their 2-month-old babies. One mother described the process of putting her baby down to sleep:

> My baby has to be worked on . . . for about thirty minutes. I can put her to sleep in thirty minutes but it takes longer to leave her. My baby prefers to be held vertically rather than horizontally. She likes to put her arms around my shoulder. I hold her with one arm and with the other I pat her. At the same time I sing to her, then she yawns. Then she will rub her face on my shoulder and go to sleep. I hold her for a while and slowly sit down. I pat her sitting down on a sofa. I keep singing to her to make her sleep better. When she is sound asleep I put her down in the bed. If she wakes up again, I have to do this routine from the beginning all over again. (in Harkness et al., 2007, p. 29)

Many of these mothers reported that either they or the babysitter would actually sleep alongside the baby, maintaining physical contact so that the baby would feel secure. These same mothers, however, also devoted themselves to showing their babies pictures in order to "stimulate their brain development," and one reported playing audiotapes for her baby in Korean and English, commenting that "the earlier she starts, the better." The themes of closeness and education are related—literally so, as the mother has to hold the baby upright in order to look at the many educational pictures mounted on the walls.

The literature on infancy in Asian settings demonstrates an additional point that is not so evident in the literature on older children—with its focus on such abstract concepts as "politeness" and "harmony with the group"—namely, that "seeing" these values in child behavior is an attributional process, one governed largely by parents' cultural belief systems. Shwalb, Shwalb, and Shoji (1994) discovered both similarities and differences between the United States and Japan in the fundamental dimensions of socioemotional behavior as indicated by mothers' ratings of specific infant behaviors. Both groups identified behaviors reflecting "Intensity of expression," for example, "Joyful when bathed" and "Cries when things are not his/her own way." The Japanese mothers, however, also formulated a unique cluster labeled "stability/gentleness." Similarly, Nakagawa and Sukigara (2005) were unable to replicate the U.S. factor structure of a widely used temperament questionnaire (Gartstein & Rothbart, 2003), and when they asked Japanese mothers to sort the questionnaire's behavioral items into their usual 14 categories, the results were dramatically different. Nearly half of the infant behaviors belonging to the dimension of Activity Level, for example, were considered by Japanese mothers to represent instead Distress to Limitations. Infant distress inevitably engages maternal concern, and that returns us to the overarching cultural model of socioemotional interdependence. Unlike the core Western idea that development means separation and individuation, the traditional Japanese image has the infant born as separate, and the goal of successful mothering is to engage and ensure interdependence (Rothbaum, Weisz, Pott, Miyake, & Morelli, 2000; Shwalb & Shwalb, 1996). In this light, Japanese mothers are less focused on security as a platform for independent exploration, and they interpret negative reactions to the stresses of separation not as aggressive or retaliatory, but as attempts to reestablish the security of interdependence (Rothbaum, Kakinuma, Nagaoka, & Azuma, 2007). Thus, the U.S. mother may find herself in a confrontation with her infants, whereas the Japanese mother is positioned to foster soothing accommodation.

Sub-Saharan Africa

The research literature on parents' ideas in sub-Saharan Africa includes a rich heritage of anthropological studies carried out over more than a century. African children were the first outside Europe and the United States to be studied, and for decades reports from Africa dominated the cross-cultural developmental literature (Super, Harkness, Barry, & Zeitlin, 2011). LeVine and colleagues (2008) point out that Western researchers' perceptions of African customs of infant and child care (and the beliefs they instantiate) have mirrored historical changes in the researchers' own societies. During the years preceding World War II, they note, Western observers often perceived African customs of care involving close mother–infant physical contact and an extended period of breast-feeding (up to 3 years of age) as overly indulgent. Later, however,

> The same practices, insofar as they were not accompanied by visual and verbal expressions of the mother's love that were familiar to Western observers, were occasionally interpreted as neglectful of the infant's

emotional needs. . . . Do African mothers "indulge" their infants too much—or too little? Both the question and its answers reflect the biases of observers rather than the indigenous contexts that shape infant experience. (p. 56)

In the context of this critique, it seems fitting that the two main bodies of research related to African parents' ideas about their children's social and emotional development both involve Afrocentric responses to the inaccuracies created by "imposed etic" research brought to the continent from overseas. The first, on mother–child attachment, was originally stimulated by Bowlby's proposition that there is a "strong bias for attachment behavior to become directed mainly towards one particular person" (Bowlby, 1969, p. 308). Many scholars were convinced that caretaking by multiple persons would threaten the essential attachment process, and Ainsworth's (1967) observations of mothers and infants in Uganda were presented in support of this position. In contrast, the Leidermans (1974), who carried out their research in neighboring Kenya, found that older siblings who were active caretakers of infants also functioned as a "secure base." Multiple caretaking arrangements involving persons other than siblings have also been widely documented in African societies. Tronick, Morelli, and Winn (1987), for example, describe a pattern of infant care that includes breast-feeding by other mothers as part of a general pattern of shared child care. Child fostering is a practice common in many African societies (Verhoef & Morelli, 2007). Although this practice is not always seen as a positive alternative to keeping the child with its mother, there appears to be less concern about maintaining the mother's relationship with the child. As one mother in the Kipsigis community of Kokwet (Kenya), commented to the first author, "I would not worry about leaving my child with my sister if I go abroad because I know she would take care of him the same way I would."

A second recent focus of research in Africa has been local conceptualizations of intelligence and their differences from Western ideas. "Socially responsible intelligence" is said to be a key organizing cultural model for parents across much of sub-Saharan Africa. It is called *n'glouélé* by Baoulé of the Ivory Coast (Dasen et al., 1985), *nzelu* by the Chewa of Zambia (Serpell, 1993), and *ng'om* by the Kipsigis of western Kenya (Harkness & Super, 1992). As the English term implies, the concept has a cognitive component, but the African terms add a social dimension that includes both awareness of the social surroundings and a readiness to act. "Social cognition translates into responsible intelligence, not in abstraction," according to Nsamenang (2006, p. 296), "but primarily as it enhances the attainment of social ends." The word has a distinct utility for parents who make daily decisions whether a child is sufficiently mature, or "socially intelligent," to carry a message across the village, to care for a 1-year-old for part of the day, or to negotiate prices in the market. As Weisner (1989, p. 86) comments, among the Abaluhyia of rural Kenya, "Mothers use evidence that a child has the ability to give and receive social support, and assist others, as markers of a child's more general developmental level, in the same way as an American parent might use literacy skills . . . or verbal facility" to indicate maturity. Among Kipsigis mothers in Kenya, a child's ability to carry out an errand unsupervised was closely matched with their perception of whether the child's personality had emerged (Harkness et al., 2009). Similar reports come from the Kpelle of Liberia (Lancy, 1996) and the Yoruba of Nigeria (Zeitlin, 1996). More broadly, this conceptualization of social intelligence is part of an orientation characterized by Nsamenang (2006) as "sociogenic," an understanding that emotional, social, and cognitive development are as much the result of becoming part of the social group as they are of internal growth.

Latin America

In contrast to the historical depth of research on children in Africa, the literature on Latin America (at least in English) is relatively recent, and much of it focuses on immigrant families in the United States. Despite its smaller scope, however, closely related themes relating to training for obedience, responsibility, and good manners have frequently been noted. Harwood and her colleagues, who have carried out several studies of Puerto Rican mothers and infants both on the island and in the United States (Harwood, Miller, & Irizarry, 1995; Harwood, Schölmerich, Ventura-Cook, & Schulze, 1996), refer to this complex as a concern with inculcating "proper demeanor" (including being cooperative, showing respect toward others, and fulfilling role obligations), in contrast to a focus on "self-maximization" (e.g., being self-confident, developing one's personal potential, and becoming psychologically independent)—found more typically among European-American mothers. These culturally structured goals are expressed through a variety of parenting practices related to feeding, sleeping, and toilet training, such that the Puerto Rican mothers in Harwood's studies favored more mother-directed strategies (Schulze, Harwood, Schölmerich, & Leyendecker, 2002). The cultural differences, however, are moderated by social class and mothers' education: more educated Puerto Rican mothers expressed greater concern with the development of their child's own capacities and emotional independence (although still less than their European American counterparts) (Harwood, Super, & van Tijen, 2000; Miller & Harwood, 2002).

Research with Mexican families in both Mexico and the United States has found a similar emphasis on good moral values, obedience and responsibility, and respect for elders (Arcia & Johnson, 1998), as captured in the term *bien educado* (literally, "well-educated"—but meaning something more like "well-brought-up"). This concept is further elaborated in Cooper and colleagues' study of Mexican immigrant parents (Cooper, Brown, Azmitia, & Chavira, 2005). Their explanation of what constitutes *el buen camino de la vida* (the good path of life), included "showing proper demeanor, living a moral and responsible life, being a respectful person, and developing oneself spiritually" (p. 367) while also avoiding bad influences and doing well in school and work. Delgado-Gaitan (1994) found in a study of Mexican immigrants residing in California that, regardless of whether they were first- or second-generation (that is, recent immigrants or the children of immigrants), parents expressed high expectations for respect from their children. Second-generation immigrants, however, allowed their children more autonomy in relation to routine contexts like watching TV and they encouraged more critical thinking, whereas the concept of respect became construed more narrowly. As research by LeVine, Miller, Richman, and LeVine (1996) shows, changes in parenting ideas and practices are not limited to immigrants: Mexican mothers living in the city of Cuernavaca who had more years of school (from 1 to 9 years) reported earlier ages at which they thought the baby could recognize their voice—which in turn was associated with talking more with the baby.

"The West": Europe and the United States

The idea of a distinctive "Western mind" has been widely accepted by researchers on both sides of the northern Atlantic Ocean. Such a mind, as the anthropologist Clifford Geertz (1984) famously wrote, is housed in a "self" that is sharply differentiated from the environment:

> The Western conception of the person as a bounded, unique, more or less integrated motivational and cognitive universe, a dynamic center of awareness, emotion, judgment, and action organized into a distinctive whole and set contrastively both against other such wholes and against its social and natural background is, however incorrigible it may seem to us, a rather peculiar idea within the context of the world's cultures (p. 126).

This cultural conception of the person as described by Geertz maps closely onto the individualism side of the I/C divide, and much research on parents' ideas in both European and North American societies has applied this framework in comparative studies with "non-Western" parents. Nevertheless, a closer look at parents' ideas within Europe and North America reveals many (although sometimes subtle) differences—such that it may be more accurate to conceptualize parental ethnotheories in terms of "themes and variations" (Harkness & Super, 2005) that are evident as one traverses the European continent from north to south, from east to west, and especially as one hops across "the pond" to the United States and Canada.

Variability in parental ethnotheories within the Western world is evident in the culturally distinctive ways that parents describe their children, as documented by Harkness and Super and their international collaborative group (Harkness & Super, 2005). Parents of infants and young children in six Western cultural groups (in Australia, Italy, the Netherlands, Spain, Sweden, and the United States) all frequently described their children as sociable, loving, active, and strong-willed. Beyond these common themes, however, each cultural sample had its own profile of characteristic child descriptions. The U.S. parents focused on cognitive qualities (such as being intelligent or cognitively advanced), and they also described their children as independent and even rebellious. Parents in the European samples, in contrast, talked about their children's cognitive competence much less and spoke more about their children's positive social and emotional qualities, such as being happy, well balanced, and even-tempered. Other specific cultural patterns were also evident, with the Dutch parents more commonly describing their children as "regular" in habits (or needing a "regular" environment), while the Spanish parents emphasized qualities of good character, and the Italian parents focused on qualities of being both self-directed and "simpatico." The Swedish parents presented an image of the child as, above all, happy and secure while also being easy to manage, while the Australian parents' descriptions focused about equally on cognitive and socioemotional qualities (Harkness & Super, 2005; Harkness et al., 2010). The cultural differences between the Dutch and the U.S. parents' descriptions of their children are supported in a study categorizing descriptors into the "Big Five" factors of personality, in which Dutch parents more frequently described their children in relation to emotional stability, whereas the American parents talked more about intellectual qualities and openness to experience (Kohnstamm, Halverson, Havill, & Mervielde, 1996).

Another study of mothers' ideas about infant care and development (Harkness et al., 2007), carried out with different samples of mothers of 2-month-old infants, produced similar results for samples of mothers in Italy, the Netherlands, Spain, and the United States. The U.S. mothers were most concerned about promoting their baby's cognitive development by providing adequate "stimulation," whereas the Dutch mothers were most attentive to helping their baby to establish a regular and restful routine. The Italian mothers saw their babies as needing emotional closeness and social stimulation in interaction with other people; the Spanish mothers also stressed the importance of social contacts and, in addition, were closely attuned to the baby's physical needs.

A study of parental ethnotheories of children's temperament (Super et al., 2008) adds further to this picture of culturally distinctive patterns in seven Western cultural communities (those already cited, plus Poland). Parents from all sites generally rated their children young similarly in relation to six of the nine Thomas and Chess (1977) dimensions (Activity, Approach, Adaptability, Intensity, Mood, and Persistence; there were small differences with regard to Regularity, Distractibility, and Threshold). There were cultural differences in which dimensions of temperament were associated with higher difficulty ratings and in how the dimensions intercorrelated with each other. Most distinctively, although children in most of the samples who were perceived as less adaptable and more negative in mood tended to be rated as more difficult, the Italian mothers did not seem to find negative mood problematic; rather, they found shyness in social situations (such as a large family gathering), as represented by the Approach dimension, to be a difficult quality to deal with. Also, low persistence was related to difficulty in only the Dutch and Swedish samples. In the U.S. sample, children rated as highly active and intense (in addition to being less adaptable and more frequently negative in mood) were often seen as difficult. Interestingly, the correlation between Activity and difficulty appears also in the Australian sample, even though the social ecologies of children in these two middle-class samples probably were more spacious, with more room (inside and out) for children to play actively.

Other research is generally consistent with the work we have described here, but it adds further dimensions. For example, a comparison of Dutch and American parents found that the Dutch cultural concept of "the three Rs" (standing for rest, regularity, and cleanliness) was applied to ideas about sleep management; in contrast, the American parents struggled with a conflict between a desire to be responsive to their baby's individual needs and their own need to get a good night's sleep (Super et al., 1996). Another study of the same samples found that American parents worried about both independent and dependent behavior in their young children, whereas Dutch parents accepted both as natural for that age (Harkness et al., 2000).

In Sweden, parents are reported to take a similarly accepting attitude toward the developmental needs of their young children for physical and emotional closeness, specifically with regard to co-sleeping, which is also seen (uniquely) as a "right" of the child (Welles-Nyström, 2005). One parent asked rhetorically, "She is a part of us—why wouldn't we like to have her next to us?" A similar cultural emphasis on easing developmental transitions toward independence was found among Norwegian parents (Aukrust, Edwards, Kumru, Knoche, & Kim, 2003), who favored long-term stability in relationships with preschool teachers and peers and a home-like school setting—in contrast to U.S. parents, who were not concerned about such continuity and viewed preschool more in terms of its academic mission.

Several studies in Italy suggested that parents' common practice of sharing their bed or bedroom with their baby appears to be part of a general strategy of supporting the baby's perceived needs for physical and emotional closeness (New, 1988; Wolf, Lozoff, Latz, & Paludetto, 1996). New and Richman (1996) reported that mothers in central Italy stressed the infant's early social participation in the life of the family. They instantiated this belief by keeping the baby up with the family until he fell asleep on his own and by making sure that the baby could participate in family meals even if it meant waking him or her up from a nap. Edwards, Gandini, and Giovaninni's (1996) study of parents' and teachers' developmental expectations showed that U.S. middle-class parents generally had expectations for the earlier mastery of many skills, including compliance and politeness in addition to emotional maturity, independence, school-related skills, and particularly social skills with peers as well as verbal assertiveness.

Studies of parenting in France reveal yet another variation on Western themes of childrearing. For example, Suizzo's (2002) research on mothers of infants and toddlers in Paris identified "awakening and exposing the child to diverse stimuli"—including introducing the child to a variety of different foods, giving them massages, and reading to them—as a major socialization goal. Other goals for the child's development included "proper presentation" (cleanliness, good manners, and emotional self-regulation); at the same time, the mothers also wanted to avoid becoming a "slave" to the baby. The author observed that ideals related to social competence and bettering oneself as an individual seemed to coexist comfortably for these mothers: "Although Parisian mothers stress the importance of developing individual pleasures and qualities, and of being self-assured and autonomous, these goals are justified through the ultimate goal of being able to join groups" (p. 315). Suizzo (2004) suggests that "stimulation" may mean different things in different cultures, with European-American middle class mothers focusing more narrowly on cognitive rather than social or physical stimulation (Suizzo, 2004).

European-American parents are generally portrayed in the research literature as concerned primarily with their children's cognitive development, less so with the establishment and maintenance of social relationships outside the family. Yet, other themes also emerge as distinctively American. In particular, as Miller and her colleagues (Miller, Wang, Sandel, & Cho, 2002) have demonstrated, American mothers are highly concerned about their young children's "self-esteem," which the authors describe as "extremely important because it promotes the development of a whole array of psychological strengths, including resilience, respect for others, and realization of one's own potential" (p. 210). The American "folk theory" of self-esteem, as the authors term it, is dependent on the ways that important others demonstrate love and appreciation for the child, thus revealing a sense of the child's vulnerability to environmental threats. The authors contrast this belief with childrearing ideas held by Taiwanese mothers, who seek opportunities for moral education of their children by talking about the child's misdeeds. In another study of American parents' beliefs and practices, DeCaro and Worthman (2007) identify two conflicting cultural models of childrearing—one favoring stimulation and enrichment, the other emphasizing protection and simplification. Likewise, Weisner has discussed B. Whiting's conceptualization of the "American dependency conflict," which involves socializing children for two incompatible goals, autonomy and attention seeking (Weisner, 2001). The varying components of American parents' ethnotheories are also discussed by Tamis-LeMonda and colleagues (2002), who found that self-esteem was a key childrearing goal in a group of American parents of preschoolers (by comparison with their Greek and Taiwanese counterparts); further, although the American mothers valued qualities such as assertiveness and creativity, they also emphasized the importance of good manners and compassion for others. As the authors put it, these parents stressed the individual—"but not at the expense of others' feelings" (p. 200). Clearly, American parents are concerned about much more than just promoting individualism and cognitive development in their children.

Summary and Conclusions

As illustrated by the theoretical framework introduced at the beginning of this chapter, parental ethnotheories play an essential directive role in the ways that parents understand their own children and how they shape children's social and emotional development. The importance of such belief systems and their relationship to practices has long been recognized by ethnographic researchers who sought coherence and meaning in the minutiae of the exotic cultures they studied. More recently, some scholars have turned an ethnographic eye to their own societies, sometimes finding the exotic in the familiar. The rapidly increasing documentation of beliefs and practices in diverse cultural places has brought to light regularities in parental beliefs, both within cultural regions and related to different types of cultures. Building on this observation, a recent development in cross-cultural studies of parental ethnotheories has been the construction of dimensions or prototypes of societies that, in theory, should explain cultural differences in parental ethnotheories and practices. As the application of these frameworks in research repeatedly shows, however, cultures are inevitably more complicated than the framework that is supposed to explain them—

even in cases where the framework is applied back to the cultural context in which it was originally developed. Finding the right level of generalization, both within and across cultures, is one of the most interesting challenges that faces researchers concerned with the connections between culture and human development. We know that we meet this challenge successfully when we can understand others as they see themselves and when we can understand ourselves as others see us.

References

Ainsworth, M. D. S. (1967). *Infancy in Uganda: Infant care and the growth of love*. Baltimore: Johns Hopkins University Press.

Arcia, E., & Johnson, A. (1998). When respect means to obey: Immigrant Mexican mothers' values for their children. *Journal of Child and Family Studies, 7*, 79–95.

Aukrust, V. G., Edwards, C. P., Kumru, A., Knoche, L., & Kim, M. (2003). Young children's close relationships outside the family: Parental ethnotheories in four communities in Norway, United States, Turkey, and Korea. *International Journal of Behavioral Development, 27*(6), 481–494.

Baumrind, D., & Black, A. E. (1967). Socialization practices associated with dimensions of competence in preschool boys and girls. *Child Development, 38*(2), 291–327.

Berry, J. W. (1989). Imposed etics - emics - derived etics: The operationalization of a compelling idea. *International Journal of Psychology, 24*, 721–735.

Bowlby, J. (1969). *Attachment and loss. (Vol. 1). Attachment.* New York: Basic Books.

Briggs, J. L. (1972). The issues of autonomy and aggression in the three-year-old: The Utku Eskimo case. *Seminars in Psychiatry, 4*(4), 317–329. (Reprinted in LeVine, R. A., & New, R. (Eds.), (2008). *Anthropology and child development: A cross-cultural reader* (pp. 2187–2197). Malden, MA: Blackwell.)

Chao, R. K. (1994). Beyond parental control and authoritarian parenting style: Understanding Chinese parenting through the cultural notion of training. *Child Development, 65*(4), 1111–1119.

Cheah, C. S. L., & Rubin, K. H. (2003). European American and mainland Chinese mothers' socialization beliefs regarding preschoolers' social skills. *Parenting: Science and Practice, 3*, 1–21.

Chen, X., & Bond, M. H. (2010). Socio-emotional development in Chinese children. In *The Oxford handbook of Chinese psychology* (pp. 37–52). New York: Oxford University Press.

Cooper, C. R., Brown, J., Azmitia, M., & Chavira, G. (2005). Including Latino immigrant families, schools, and community programs as research partners on the good path of life (*el buen camino de la vida*). In T. S. Weisner (Ed.), *Discovering successful pathways in children's development: Mixed methods in the study of childhood and family life.* (pp. 359–385). Chicago: University of Chicago Press.

D'Andrade, R., & Strauss, C. (1992). *Human motives and cultural models*. New York: Cambridge University Press.

Dasen, P. R., Barthelemy, D., Kan, E., Kouame, K., Daouda, K., Adjei, K. K., et al. (1985). N'glouélé, l'intelligence chez les Baoulé [N'glouélé, intelligence among the Baoulé]. *Archives de psychologie, 53*, 295–324.

DeCaro, J. A., & Worthman, C. M. (2007). Cultural models, parenting behavior, and young children's experience in working American families. *Parenting: Science and Practice, 7*, 177–203.

Delgado-Gaitan, C. (1994). Socializing young children in Mexican-American families: An intergenerational perspective. In P. M. Greenfield & R. R. Cocking (Eds.), *Cross-cultural roots of minority child development* (pp. 55–86). Hillsdale, NJ: Erlbaum.

Edwards, C. P., Gandini, L., & Giovaninni, D. (1996). The contrasting developmental timetables of parents and preschool teachers in two cultural communities. In S. Harkness & C. M. Super (Eds.), *Parents' cultural belief systems: Their origins, expressions, and consequences* (pp. 270–288). New York: Guilford Press.

Ember, C. R. (2007). Using the HRAF collection of ethnography in conjunction with the standard cross-cultural sample and the ethnographic atlas. *Cross-Cultural Research: The Journal of Comparative Social Science, 41*(4), 396–427.

Fung, H. (1999). Becoming a moral child: The socialization of shame among young Chinese children. *Ethos, 27*(2), 180–209.

Gartstein, M. A., & Rothbart, M. K. (2003). Studying infant temperament via the Infant Behavior Questionnaire. *Child Development, 26*(1), 64–86.

Gaskins, S. (2000). Children's daily activities in a Mayan village: A culturally grounded description. *Cross-Cultural Research, 34*, 375–389. Reprinted in LeVine, R. A., & New, R. (Eds.). (2008). *Anthropology and child development: A cross-cultural reader* (pp. 2281–2288). Malden, MA: Blackwell.

Geertz, C. (1984). "From the native's point of view": On the nature of anthropological understanding. In R. A. Shweder & R. A. LeVine (Eds.), *Culture theory: Essays on mind, self, and emotion* (pp. 123–136). New York, Cambridge University Press.

Goodnow, J. J., & Collins, W. A. (1990). *Development according to parents: The nature, sources, and consequences of parents' ideas*. Hillsdale, NJ: Erlbaum.

Gottlieb, A. (2004). *The afterlife is where we come from*. Chicago: University of Chicago Press.

Greenfield, P. M. (2009). Linking social change and developmental change: Shifting pathways of human development. *Developmental Psychology, 45*(2), 401–418.

Harkness, S., & Super, C. M. (1992). Parental ethnotheories in action. In I. Sigel, A. V. McGillicuddy-DeLisi, & J. Goodnow (Eds.), *Parental belief systems: The psychological consequences for children* (2nd ed., pp. 373–392). Hillsdale, NJ: Erlbaum.

Harkness, S., & Super, C. M. (1996). Introduction. In S. Harkness & C. M. Super (Eds.), *Parents' cultural belief systems: Their origins, expressions, and consequences* (pp. 1–23). New York: Guilford Press.

Harkness, S., & Super, C. M. (2005). Themes and variations: Parental ethnotheories in Western cultures. In K. H. Rubin & O.-B. Chung (Eds.), *Parental beliefs, parenting, and child development in cross-cultural perspective* (pp. 61–79). New York: Psychology Press.

Harkness, S., Super, C. M., Barry, O., Zeitlin, M., Long, J., & Sow, S. (2009). Assessing the environment of children's learning: The developmental niche in Africa. In E. Grigorenko (Ed.), *Multicultural psychoeducational assessment* (pp. 133–155). New York: Springer.

Harkness, S., Super, C. M., Moscardino, U., Rha, J.-H., Blom, M. J. M., Huitrón, B., et al. (2007). Cultural models and developmental agendas: Implications for arousal and self-regulation in early infancy. *Journal of Developmental Processes, 1*(2), 5–39.

Harkness, S., Super, C. M., Rios Bermudez, M., Moscardino, U., Blom, M. J. M., Rha, J.-H., et al. (2010). Parental ethnotheories of children's learning. In D. F. Lancy & S. Gaskins (Eds.), *The anthropology of learning in childhood* (pp. 65–81). Lanham, MD: Alta-Mira Press.

Harkness, S., Super, C. M., & van Tijen, N. (2000). Individualism and the "Western mind" reconsidered: American and Dutch parents' ethnotheories of children and family. In S. Harkness, C. Raeff, & C. M. Super (Eds.), *Variability in the social construction of the child* (New Directions for Child and Adolescent Development series, no. 87, pp. 23–39). San Francisco: Jossey-Bass.

Harwood, R. L., Miller, J. G., & Irizarry, N. L. (1995). *Culture and attachment: Perceptions of the child in context.* New York: Guilford Press.

Harwood, R. L., Schölmerich, A., & Schulze, P. A.. (2000). Homogeneity and heterogeneity in cultural belief systems. In S. Harkness, C. Raeff, & C. M. Super (Eds.), *Variability in the social construction of the child* (New Directions for Child and Adolescent Development series, no. 87, pp. 41–57). San Francisco: Jossey-Bass.

Harwood, R. L., Schölmerich, A., Ventura-Cook, E., & Schulze, P. A. (1996). Culture and class influences on Anglo and Puerto Rican mothers' beliefs regarding long-term socialization goals and child behavior. *Child Development, 67*(5), 2446–2461.

Hayashi, A., Karasawa, M., & Tobin, J. (2009). The Japanese preschool's pedagogy of feeling: Cultural strategies for supporting young children's emotional development. *Ethos, 37*(32–49).

Kăgitcibaşi, Ç. (2007). *Family, self, and human development across cultures: Theory and applications* (2nd ed.). Mahwah, NJ: Erlbaum.

Keller, H. (2007). *Cultures of infancy.* Mahwah: Erlbaum.

Kohnstamm, G. A., Halverson, C. F., Havill, V. L., & Mervielde, I. (1996). Parents' free descriptions of child characteristics: A cross-cultural search for the developmental antecedents of the Big Five In S. Harkness & C. M. Super (Eds.), *Parents' cultural belief systems: Their origins, expressions, and consequences* (pp. 27–55). New York: Guilford Press.

Lancy, D. F. (1996). *Playing on the mother ground: Cultural routines for children's development.* New York: Guilford Press.

Lebra, T. S. (1994). Mother and child in Japanese socialization: A Japan–U.S. comparison. In P. M. Greenfield & R. R. Cocking (Eds.), *Cross-cultural roots of minority child development* (pp. 259–274). Hillsdale, NJ: Erlbaum.

Leiderman, P. H., & Leiderman, G. F. (1974). Affective and cognitive consequences of polymatric infant care in the East African Highlands. In A. D. Pick (Ed.), *Minnesota symposiumn on child psychology* (Vol. 8). Minneapolis: University of Minnesota Press.

LeVine, R. A., Dixon, S., LeVine, S. E., Richman, A., Keefer, C. H., Liederman, P. H., et al. (2008). The comparative study of parenting. In R. A. LeVine & R. S. New (Eds.), *Anthropology and child development: A cross-cultural reader* (pp. 55–65). Malden, MA: Blackwell. Excerpted from LeVine, R. A., Dixon, S., LeVine, S., Richman, A., Leiderman, P. H., Keefer, C. H., & T. B. Brazelton. (1994). *Child care and culture: Lessons from Africa* (pp. 97–21). New York: Cambridge University Press.

LeVine, R. A., Miller, P. M., Richman, A. L., & LeVine, S. (1996). Education and mother–infant interaction: A Mexican case study. In S. Harkness & C. M. Super (Eds.), *Parents' cultural belief systems: Their origins, expressions, and consequences* (pp. 254–269). New York: Guilford Press.

Levy, R. (1996). Essential contrasts: Differences in parental ideas about learners and teaching in Tahiti and Nepal . In S. Harkness & C. M. Super (Eds.), *Parents' cultural belief systems: Their origins, expressions, and consequences* (pp. 123–142). New York: Guilford Press.

Li, J. (2001). Chinese conceptualization of learning. *Ethos, 29*(2), 111–137.

Mead, M. (1928, November/December). Samoan children at work and play. *Natural History*, pp. 103–104. Reprinted in LeVine, R. A., & New, R. (Eds.), (2008). *Anthropology and child development: A cross-cultural reader* (pp. 22–24). Malden, MA: Blackwell.

Miller, A. M., & Harwood, R. L. (2002). The cultural organization of parenting: Change and stability of behavior patterns during feeding and social play across the first year of life. *Parenting: Science and Practice, 2*(3), 241–272.

Miller, P. J., Wang, S., Sandel, T., & Cho, G. E. (2002). Self-esteem as folk theory: A comparison of European American and Taiwanese mothers' beliefs. *Parenting: Science and Practice, 2*, 209–239.

Nakagawa, A., & Sukigara, M. (2005). How are cultural differences in the interpretation of infant behavior reflected in the Japanese Revised Infant Behavior Questionnaire? *Japanese Journal of Educational Psychology, 53*(4), 491–503.

New, R. S. (1988). Parental goals and Italian infant care. In R. A. LeVine, P. M. Miller, & M. M. West (Eds.), *Parental behavior in diverse societies* (New Directions in Child Development series, no. 40, pp. 51–63). San Francisco: Jossey-Bass.

New, R. S., & Richman, A. L. (1996). Maternal beliefs and infant care practices in Italy and the United States. In S. Harkness & C. M. Super (Eds.), *Parents' cultural belief systems: Their origins, expressions, and consequence.* (pp. 385–404). New York: Guilford Press.

Nsamenang, A. B. (2006). Human ontogenesis: An indigenous African view on development and intelligence. *International Journal of Psychology, 41*(4), 293–297.

Osterweil, Z., & Nagano-Nakamura, K. (1992). Maternal views on aggression: Japan and Israel. *Aggressive Behavior, 18*, 263–270.

Ottenberg, P. (1965). The Afikpo Ibo of Eastern Nigeria. In J. L. Gibbs, Jr. (Ed.), *Peoples of Africa* (pp. 3–39). New York: Holt, Rinehart & Winston.

Rothbaum, F., Kakinuma, M., Nagaoka, R., & Azuma, H. (2007). Attachment and AMAE: Parent-child closeness in the United States and Japan. *Journal of Cross-Cultural Psychology, 38*(4), 465–486.

Rothbaum, F., Weisz, J., Pott, M., Miyake, K., & Morelli, G. (2000). Attachment and culture: Security in the United States and Japan. *American Psychologist, 55*(10), 1093–1104.

Schulze, P. A., Harwood, R. L., Schölmerich, A., & Leyendecker, B. (2002). The cultural structuring of parenting and universal developmental tasks. *Parenting: Science and Practice, 2*(2), 151–178.

Serpell, R. (1993). *The significance of schooling: Life-journeys in an African society.* New York, Cambridge University Press.

Shwalb, B. J., Shwalb, D. W., & Shoji, J. (1994). Structure and dimensions of maternal perceptions of Japanese infant temperament. *Developmental Psychology, 30*(2), 131–141.

Shwalb, D. W., & Shwalb, B. J. (1996). *Japanese childrearing: Two generations of scholarship.* New York: Guilford Press.

Suizzo, M. (2002). French parents' cultural models and childrearing beliefs. *International Journal of Behavioral Development, 26,* 297–307.

Suizzo, M. (2004). Mother-child relationships in France: Balancing autonomy and affiliation in everyday interactions. *Ethos, 32*(3), 293–323.

Super, C. M., Axia, G., Harkness, S., Welles-Nyström, B., Zylicz, P. O., Rios Bermudez, M., et al. (2008). Culture, temperament, and the "difficult child" in seven Western cultures. *European Journal of Developmental Science., 2*(1–2), 136–157.

Super, C. M., & Harkness, S. (1986). The developmental niche: A conceptualization at the interface of child and culture. *International Journal of Behavioral Development, 9,* 545–569.

Super, C. M., Harkness, S., Barry, O., & Zeitlin, M. (2011). Think locally, act globally: Contributions of African research to child development. *Child Development Perspectives.*

Super, C. M., Harkness, S., van Tijen, N., van der Vlugt, E., Fintelman, M., & Dykstra, J. (1996). The three R's of Dutch childrearing and the socialization of infant arousal. In S. Harkness & C. M. Super (Eds.), *Parents' cultural belief systems: Their origins, expressions, and consequences.* (pp. 447–466). New York: Guilford Press.

Tamis-LeMonda, C. S., Wang, S., Koutsouvanou, E., & Albright, M. (2002). Childrearing values in Greece, Taiwan, and the United States. *Parenting: Science and Practice, 2,* 185–208.

Tamis-LeMonda, C. S., Way, N., Hughes, D., Yoshikawa, H., Kalman, R. K., & Niva, E. Y. (2007). Parents' goals for children: The dynamic coexistence of individualism and collectivisim in cultures and individuals. *Social Development, 17*(1), 183–209.

Thomas, A., & Chess, S. (1977). *Temperament and development.* New York: Brunner/Mazel.

Tronick, E. Z., Morelli, G., & Winn, S. (1987). Multiple caretaking of Efe (Pygmy) infants. *American Anthropologist, 89,* 96–106. Reprinted as Multiple care-giving in the Ituri forest, in LeVine, R. A., & New, R. S. (Eds.), (2008). *Anthropology and child development: A cross-cultural reader* (pp. 173–183). Malden, MA: Blackwell.

Verhoef, H., & Morelli, G. (2007). "A child is a child": Fostering experiences in northwestern Cameroon. *Ethos, 35*(1), 33–64.

Weisner, T. S. (1989). Cultural and universal aspects of social support for children: Evidence from the Abaluyia of Kenya. In D. Belle (Ed.), *Children's social networks and social supports* (pp. 70–90). New York: Wiley.

Weisner, T. S. (2001). The American dependency conflict: Continuities and discontinuities in behavior and values of countercultural parents and their children. *Ethos, 29*(3), 271–295.

Welles-Nyström, B. (2005). Co-sleeping as a window into Swedish culture: Considerations of gender and health care. *Scandinavian Journal of Caring Sciences, 19*(4), 354–360.

White, M. I., & LeVine, R. A. (1986). What is an *ii ko* (good child)? In H. W. Stevenson, H. Azuma & K. Hakuta (Eds.), *Child development and education in Japan* (pp. 55–62). New York: Freeman.

Whiting, B. B., & Edwards, C. P. (1988). *Children of different worlds: The formation of social behavior.* Cambridge, MA: Harvard University Press.

Whiting, B. B., & Whiting, J. W. M. (1975). *The children of six cultures: A psychocultural analysis.* Cambridge, MA: Harvard University Press.

Whiting, J. W. M. (1977). A model for psychocultural research. In P. H. Leiderman, S. R. Tulkin, & A. Rosenfeld (Eds.), *Culture and infancy: Variations in the human experience.* New York: Academic Press.

Wolf, A. W., Lozoff, B., Latz, S., & Paludetto, R. (1996). Parental theories in the management of young children's sleep in Japan, Italy, and the United States. In S. Harkness & C. M. Super (Eds.), *Parents' cultural belief systems: Their origins, expressions, and consequences* (pp. 364–384). New York: Guilford Press.

Zeitlin, M. (1996). My child is my crown: Yoruba parental theories and practices in early childhood. In S. Harkness & C. M. Super (Eds.), *Parents' cultural belief systems: Their origins, expressions, and consequences* (pp. 407–427). New York: Guilford Press.

CHAPTER 5

Pathways to Emotion Regulation
Cultural Differences in Internalization

FRED ROTHBAUM *and* NATALIE RUSK

Cultural research on emotion regulation sometimes yields seemingly contradictory findings. For example, emotion suppression typically leads to negative outcomes among European Americans but to positive outcomes for East Asians (Butler, Lee, & Gross, 2009; Matsumoto, Yoo, & Nakagawa, 2008). Why would the same strategies have different effects in different cultures? How do caregiving practices contribute to these differences? To address these questions, we examine the developmental pathway of people who place relatively greater priority on the interdependent self and of people who place relatively greater priority on the independent self. We build on prior efforts to link culture, caregiving practices, and emotion (Higgins, 2008; Mesquita & Albert, 2007; Miller, 2003; Tsai, 2007), but we focus on different notions of internalization, different caregiving practices, and different emotion regulation processes.

We distinguish between two pathways to children's emotion regulation. One pathway is rooted in caregiving practices that foster autonomy and related goals such as seeking independence and environmental mastery. The second pathway is rooted in caregiving practices that foster harmony and related goals, such as seeking to fulfill complementary roles and to adhere to norms that bind people to one another and their contexts.

Our major claim is that children internalize—willingly engage in—strategies for managing their emotions when there is fit, or congruence, between those strategies and their goals. Strategies for changing negative emotional situations (e.g., by expressing one's feelings) fit with the goal of autonomy. Strategies for accepting negative emotional situations (e.g., by suppressing one's feelings) fit with the goal of harmony. The greater the fit between strategies and goals, the more likely it is that people will internalize both. Trying to use a strategy that does not fit with one's goal is often counterproductive (Higgins, 2008).

The pathway of autonomy is associated with the pursuit of personal happiness. In cultures that promote autonomy and independence, caregivers tend to foster happiness, particularly high-intensity happiness, as a goal (e.g., Heine, Lehman, Markus, & Kitayama, 1999; Tsai, 2007). Happiness is a cue that one is making progress toward fulfilling one's personal and freely chosen preferences, needs, and purpose in life (e.g., Heine et al., 1999; Lutz, 1987; Mesquita & Albert, 2007). In contrast, cultures that promote harmony tend to foster emotional calm and balance. To function harmoniously, people need to attend to the emotions of others. Calmness is associated with knowledge that all is well with others and that the self has met its role obligations (Kitayama, Mesquita, & Karasawa, 2006; Lee, Aaker, & Gardner, 2000; Lu & Gilmour, 2004; Mesquita & Albert, 2007; Miller, 2003; Tsai, 2007; Uchida & Kitayama, 2009).

On Culture, Self, and Control

To understand cultural aspects of emotion regulation, we adopt a developmental sociocultural perspective that focuses on children's sense of self and their control as they participate in culturally organized practices and routines (Rogoff, 1990). Like other sociocultural theorists, we assume that individuals' ways of thinking, feeling, and acting influence and are influenced by prevailing meaning systems, practices, and settings (D'Andrade, 1990; Markus & Kitayama, 2003; Shweder et al., 2006).

The cultures we contrast are those in which the independent self and the interdependent self are prioritized. People prioritizing the independent self rely heavily on their own preferences, desires, judgments, and other internal attributes to exert influence (Kitayama, Duffy, & Uchida, 2007). Relationships with other people are essential to their well-being, but largely to foster the self's agenda (Rothbaum, Morelli, & Rusk, 2010; Rothbaum & Trommsdorff, 2007). People focused on an independent self typically pursue primary control—changing the world to fit the self (Kitayama et al., 2007; Morling & Evered, 2006; Weisz, Rathbaum, & Blackburn, 1984). The independent self is maintained by a first-person perspective (Cohen, Hoshino-Browne, & Leung, 2007).

In contrast, people prioritizing an interdependent self are more focused on the expectations, desires, and needs of others. When encountering difficulties, they are likely to adjust their actions to accommodate others and the larger context. They are more likely to pursue secondary control—changing the self to fit the world—and to view the world from a third-person perspective (see references in previous paragraph). Conceptions of self are supported by beliefs that other people hold similar conceptions of themselves (Zou et al., 2009)

Since most research on conceptions of self and control has contrasted peoples from European and American communities (especially in the United States, but also in northern and western European countries, and Canada and Australia, which are largely composed of European immigrants) with peoples from East Asian communities (especially Japan, China, and South Korea), we too focus on the contrast between these groups. Most of this research has been limited to urban middle-class samples. People in non-industrialized agricultural communities also tend to have interdependent selves, and we borrow from research on those communities as well.

Conceptions of self and control are within-culture and within-individual, as well as between-culture variables. While the independent self is dominant for most European Americans, there are many situations, such as team sports, where European Americans' interdependent self is particularly accessible. Similarly, there are situations (e.g., involving individual competition) where East Asians access an independent self. People differ in the extent to which each type of self is typically accessible, largely because of situations that are common in their community (Kitayama, Markus, Matsumoto, & Norasakkunkit, 1997).

Organization of This Chapter

The remainder of this chapter is divided into four sections. First, we describe how our notion of internalization is similar to and different from prevailing notions. Second, we review research on childrearing practices from infancy to adolescence, focusing on parenting influences. Of particular importance is the distinction between (1) practices fostering the independent self, involving distal warmth, separations and reunions, and autonomy promotion, and (2) practices fostering the interdependent self, involving continuous contact, indulgence of dependency needs, and high levels of control. The evidence suggests that these differences in childrearing practices give rise to distinctive goals and strategies.

In the third section, we show how, when there is a fit between goals and strategies, internalization of both is facilitated. We focus on fit between goals and strategies involving emotions. We show how the goals of autonomy and happiness fit with strategies for changing emotional situations (i.e., altering them in ways one prefers) and how the goals of harmony and calmness fit with strategies for accepting and adjusting to emotional situations (i.e., aligning with others' emotions and situational demands). The research we review is primarily concerned with constructive strategies because those strategies are most common and most informative about interventions to promote positive socioemotional development. We briefly consider implications in the fourth and final section.

Differences in Internalization

Internalization has been a long-standing concern of leading developmental researchers (Aronfreed, 1969; Baumrind, 1996; Grusec, 2002; Hoffman, 1975; Kochanska, 2002; Maccoby, 1992; Ryan & Deci, 2000). It refers to the process whereby socialization agents are able to "hand off" responsibility for children's adoption of culturally prescribed values and behaviors to the children themselves. These investigators view behaviors as internalized when children willingly engage in them. During the early stages of internalization, most of the heavy lifting is performed by caregivers; parents', teachers', and older siblings' incentives, monitoring, modeling, and instruction are needed to foster desired behavior. Later, children exhibit the behaviors in the absence of adults' influence because they are committed to them.

Probably the most influential theory of internalization, self-determination theory (SDT), posits three fundamental needs: autonomy, relatedness, and competence (Deci & Ryan, 2000). SDT depicts autonomy as key to internalized behavior in that children are likely to personally endorse behavior when they have *freely* chosen it. The theory further claims that children everywhere willingly engage in behavior and function well when their basic need for autonomy is met.

In support of SDT, several studies indicate that autonomy relates to well-being in interdependent as well as independent cultures (Chirkov, Ryan, Kim, & Kaplan, 2003; Chirkov, Ryan, & Willness, 2005; Vansteenkiste, Zhou, Lens, & Souenens, 2005). In those studies the concepts of autonomy and internalization are used interchangeably, because autonomy is seen as the central feature of internalized behavior. Behavior is deemed autonomous when it is freely chosen, when people are committed to it, and when it is internally motivated—that is, when it is internalized.

Other cultural theorists dispute whether autonomy is central to well-being in all cultures (Heine et al., 1999; Iyengar & Lepper, 1999; Kitayama, Karnsawa, & Mesquita, 2004; Markus & Kitayama, 1991; Mesquita & Albert, 2007; Rothbaum, Putt, Azuma, Miyake, & Weisz, 2000; Schwartz, 2006; Triandis, 1989; Weisz et al., 1984). While SDT equates autonomy with volition and free choice and distinguishes it from individualism and other manifestations of independence, these other cultural researchers link autonomy with individualism and independence as well as volition and free choice. These cultural researchers claim that people from European American communities are more likely to actively pursue the goal of autonomy and to commit themselves to behaviors that fulfill that goal than are people from most other communities, particularly people from East Asia.

SDT investigators have found that autonomy, which they conceptualize as willingness, free choice, and internalization, predicts well-being in diverse cultures. We agree that internalization leads to well-being, but we focus on cultural differences as well as universal features of internalization. Unlike SDT proponents, but consistent with most cultural theorists, we regard the goal of autonomy as closely linked to individuation and independence.

Borrowing from all of the foregoing theorists, we define internalization as the process whereby a goal or behavior is integrated with one's sense of self.[1] When such integration occurs, people feel an ownership of their behaviors and goals and willingly endorse them. We claim that, in many communities, behavior is internalized even when it is influenced by external agents and settings and when it is experienced as obligatory. When internalization is based on harmony, people willingly engage in obligations (Miller, 2003).

Table 5.1 summarizes research by cultural investigators who study links between people's conceptions of self and control, on the one hand, and their goals and strategies, on the other. The table indicates general goals (autonomy and harmony) and general strategies (for change and acceptance), as well as corresponding goals for emotion (to be happy and to be calm) and the emotion regulation strategies that fit with those goals.

TABLE 5.1. How Conceptions of Self and Types of Control Relate to Goals and Strategies

Conceptions of self:	Independent self	Interdependent self
Types of control:	Primary control	Secondary control
General goals:	Autonomy	Harmony
Emotion goals:	Happy; absence of sadness	Calm; absence of anxiety
General strategies:	Change the situation: initiate and determine outcomes; self-agency	Accept the situation: attend and adjust to larger context; group agency
Emotion regulation strategies:	Ways to become happy (e.g., express emotions; redirect attention from negative to positive emotion)	Ways to become calm (e.g., suppress emotions; redirect attention from self's to others' emotions)

Our thesis, that fit between goals and strategies increases the internalization of both, borrows from regulatory fit theory, which focuses on the fit between regulatory orientations (promotion or prevention) and regulatory means (eager or vigilant) in adults. We focus on the fit between goals (harmony, autonomy) and strategies (acceptance, change), and on childrearing practices that contribute to these goals and strategies.[2] Regulatory fit theorists provide evidence that, in cases of fit, there is an increase in people's valuation of activities in which they are engaged, in their automatic and persistent use of strategies, and in their feeling "right" (Higgins, 2006, 2008; Lee et al., 2000). We suggest that a goal–strategy fit leads to similar benefits (cf. Heine et al, 1999; Morling & Evered, 2006; Weisz et al., 1984).

One type of goal–strategy fit, common among people with independent selves, involves the goal of autonomy and strategies for changing the situation. For example, when people with the independent goal of autonomy choose their own tasks as opposed to having trusted others make those choices, they show more persistence, positive emotion, and other markers of willing engagement (Iyengar & Lepper, 1999). More generally, we suggest that the goals of autonomy and happiness fit with strategies for effecting change and increasing self-confidence.

Another type of fit, common among people with interdependent selves, involves the goal of harmony and strategies for accepting the situation. When people with the interdependent goal of harmony have trusted others make choices for them, they show more signs of internalization, including preference for, enjoyment of, and persistence in behavior (Iyengar & Lepper, 1999). More generally, we suggest that goals of harmony and calmness fit with strategies for accepting other people and circumstances and increasing self-improvement.

Childrearing Antecedents of Goals and Strategies

According to the model proposed here, socialization agents instill goals and strategies for emotion. Fit between these goals and strategies fosters the internalization of both. When caregivers instill the goal of harmony, which relates to the pursuit of calm emotions, their children are likely to internalize acceptance-based and adjustment-based emotion regulation strategies. Examples of such strategies include suppressing emotional expressions so as not to disturb others, redirecting attention to others' emotions, and selecting conventional situations that one is expected to select. By contrast, children encouraged to pursue the goals of autonomy and high-intensity happy emotions are likely to internalize change-based emotion regulation strategies. Examples include expressing the self's emotions, redirecting attention from negative to positive emotions, and choosing situations that lead to success and that lift the self's feelings.

Infancy and Preschool Years

From infancy, caregivers provide care that sets the stage for valuing harmony or autonomy. While caregivers everywhere are sensitive to children's needs and foster children's security, the nature of sensitivity and security is colored by the goals parents seek to instill.

The crowning achievement of the caregiver–infant attachment relationship is the development of the secure base—use of the caregiver as a foundation from which to explore the environment. We have suggested elsewhere that attachment theorists' conceptualization of the secure base reflects Western investigators' emphasis on the development of autonomy (Rothbaum et al., 2000b). Exploration is an early manifestation of children's efforts to individuate and gain independence and autonomy. Exploration involves manipulating objects and gaining mastery; it is the way in which very young children learn to change their situations. Behavior that is autonomous—fully owned and uniquely authored by the self—often elicits high-intensity happiness, and those feelings in turn energize renewed autonomous behavior (Mesquita & Albert, 2007).

Japanese experts are more circumspect about the early importance of autonomy. As noted by Takahashi (1990, p. 29), "Mothers' effectiveness in serving a secure base function well represents the quality of attachment only in the American culture, in which social independence or self-reliance is emphasized." Rather than fostering children's autonomy and high-intensity happiness, the primary function of the secure base in Japan has more to do with fostering children's harmony with, accommodation to, and fitting in with others and the larger context (Rothbaum, Weisz, Pott, Miyake, & Morelli, 2000; Rothbaum, Morelli, & Rusk, 2010). Emotions typically associated with harmony are calmness, relaxation, and relief from anxiety (Mesquita & Albert, 2007; Tsai, 2007).

According to attachment theorists, security entails a balance between attachment, on the one hand, and exploration and autonomy, on the other. The importance of this balance has been confirmed in many studies of European American families. Exploration and autonomy are associated with feelings of enthusiasm and excitement. For interdependent Puerto Rican families, by contrast, the more important balance is between attachment and calm, respectful attentiveness (Harwood, Miller, & Irizarry, 1995). By closely attending to and imitating the practices that their caregivers deem acceptable, children are able to fulfill the goal of harmony that is emphasized in many interdependent communities. While attachment is linked to exploration and autonomy in all communities, we suggest that the strength of this link as well as the strength of the link between attachment and both harmony and accommodation varies from culture to culture (Morelli & Rothbaum, 2007; Rothbaum et al., 2010).

Infant–caregiver relationships among European Americans are characterized by frequent separations and reunions. Separations occur when caregivers leave children with unfamiliar babysitters, and when they allow children time for solitary play throughout the day, in playpens or safe areas removed from the caregiver. Older children experience preschools, sleepovers, overnight camps, and age-segregated social events that remove them from the everyday supervision of caregivers (Rothbaum & Trommsdorff, 2007). Frequent separations from the caregiver, in safe situations where the caregiver is available if needed, are seen as important by European American caregivers because they afford young children opportunities for increased autonomy and playful exploration, especially exploration of novel impersonal objects in new settings. Such opportunities reinforce children's sense of agency, pride, and self-esteem and induce emotions of excitement and high-intensity happiness because they lead to individual-authored rather than group-authored outcomes (Mesquita & Albert, 2007).

Separations are more common and more valued by caregivers invested in the independent as contrasted with the interdependent self (Chen et al., 1998; Rothbaum & Trommsdorff, 2007; Weisner, 1984). In Japan, many parents find the idea of leaving toddlers alone in unfamiliar settings, and with unfamiliar adults, difficult to fathom. The Strange Situation paradigm, which has been employed so successfully to assess security of attachment in U.S. children, is regarded as excessively stressful by Japanese parents (Rothbaum, Kakinuma, Nagaoka, & Azuma, 2007).

Cultures that emphasize the interdependent self, labeled "back and hip cultures," provide more continuous proximity and prolonged body contact than do cultures emphasizing the independent self, labeled "crib and cradle cultures" (Whiting, 1990, p. 160; see also Rogoff, 2003; Roopnarine & Carter, 1992). Children with interdependent selves are coached to care for others and attend to others' emotions more than to identify their own preferences and emotions (Rothbaum, Pott, et al., 2000). Their ability to determine "the face color" of others (i.e., to read others' emotions) and to behave accordingly is highly valued (Wang & Leichtman, 2000).

Perhaps the most striking example of differences in closeness is that European American caregivers keep their children apart from them during naps and nighttime sleep, while co-sleeping is the norm in most of the world (Morelli, Rogoff, Oppenheim, & Goldsmith, 1992). European

American caregivers and experts believe that separation fosters children's autonomous regulation—that is, self-initiated change in emotion forms the foundation for later regulation (Ferber, 1985). They also believe that parents must facilitate the progression from dependence to autonomy and self-efficacy and that too much dependence or too much delay in shifting to independence undermines self-determined regulation (Shweder et al., 2006).

Caregivers elsewhere believe that close body contact is essential for successful emotion regulation (Keller et al., 2004) and that separate sleeping arrangements are unthinkable. Mayan caregivers are shocked when shown films of infants sleeping alone (Morelli et al., 1992; see also Shweder, Jensen, & Goldstein, 1995). Adults with interdependent selves view emotion regulation as having more to do with aligning self with others (and thus connecting with and accepting others' emotions) than with changing emotions to fit one's preferences. They are focused on the goal of regulating the self harmoniously, in cooperation with others, and relying on others for safety, protection, and feelings of calm, as contrasted with the goal of regulating the self autonomously, apart from others, and relying on self's preferences to increase self's positive emotions (Cohen et al., 2007; Kitayama et al., 2004; Morelli & Rothbaum, 2007).

For European Americans, achieving autonomy does not mean less relatedness, because wings and roots complement one another (Feeney, 2007; Rothbaum & Trommsdorff, 2007). Independent selves' "distal" forms of closeness are seen as creating an optimal blend of separation and contact that is needed to foster both autonomy and relatedness. Distal closeness is made possible by props, such as infant seats, and practices such as brief and demonstrative expressions of warmth (e.g., eye contact, hugging, kissing, and praise), as compared to proximal and prolonged contact, as seen in co-sleeping, co-bathing, and lengthy periods of breastfeeding, holding, and carrying (Rothbaum & Trommsdorff, 2007).

The nature of caregivers' sensitivity also differs. Japanese caregivers' emphasis on harmony leads them to discern others' subtle cues, to anticipate others' needs, and thereby to prevent negative emotions. By contrast, European Americans value and practice forms of sensitivity characterized by waiting for children to explicitly express their needs and by responsiveness as needed (Morelli & Rothbaum, 2007; Rothbaum, Nagaoka, & Ponte, 2006). For example, in stressful situations Japanese mothers often redirect the child's attention before the child expresses frustration, whereas German mothers wait for the child's signals of distress before responding (Trommsdorff & Friedlmeier, 2009). Responsive sensitivity is consistent with an emphasis on autonomous regulation initiated by the child. Interestingly, both Japanese and U.S. caregivers maintain that adults' anticipation is more likely to foster children's interdependence (empathy, propriety, and compliance) than independence (exploration, autonomy, and self-assertion) and that adults' responsiveness is more likely to foster independence than interdependence (Rothbaum et al., 2007).

Similar cultural differences are observable for praise. Chinese American parents give praise in anticipation of desired behavior so as to induce it or in response to compliant, accommodative behavior, while European American parents give praise in response to young children's self-initiated behavior (Wang, Wiley, & Chiu, 2008; see Dennis, Cole, Zahn-Waxler, & Mizuta, 2002, for similar findings comparing European American and Japanese parents). While roots (closeness) and wings (autonomy) complement one another in European American communities, in East Asian and many other communities gains in closeness and harmony are often accompanied by losses in autonomy—restrictions on infants' movements, promotion of passivity, and indulgence of dependency needs (Edwards, 1995; Rothbaum & Trommsdorff, 2007; Saarni, Mumme, & Campos, 1998).

Extreme closeness fosters harmony in large part because it increases empathy. Choi (1992) reports a communications pattern in which Korean mothers and young children are "attuned to one another in a fused state," in contrast to Canadian mothers who "withdraw themselves . . . so that the children's reality can remain autonomous" (p. 38). High levels of empathy have been found among the Javanese (Mulder, 1992) and Japanese (Azuma, 1986; Clancy, 1986; Fogel, Stevenson, & Messinger, 1992). The high level of empathy training in these communities is likely to be seen by European Americans as undermining autonomy.

European American caregivers, as compared to Puerto Rican caregivers, encourage children to attend more to their own wishes, thoughts, and desires (Harwood, Leyendecker, Carlson, Ascencio, & Miller, 2002). In so doing, they reinforce the child's natural "first-person" perspective— viewing the world from inside their own head. Cohen et al. (2007) found that this perspective intensifies felt emotion. They also found that people who prioritize the interdependent, as compared to the independent, self more often adopt a "third-person generalized other" perspective that shifts attention from one's own to others' emotions. The shift from an egocentric first-person perspective to a decentered third-person perspective over the years 5–12 was much more pronounced among Asian American than U.S. children (Cohen et al., 2007).

Perhaps as a consequence of greater perspective taking, Japanese preschoolers respond to hypothetical situations involving interpersonal conflict and distress with fewer references to anger and aggression than North American preschoolers (Zahn-Waxler, Friedman, Cole, Mizuta, & Hiruma, 1996). Japanese mothers have earlier expectations for children's modulation of emotions than do U.S. caregivers (Hess, Kashiwagi, Azuma, Price, & Dickson, 1980), and Chinese parents discourage expressivity (Chen et al., 1998).

Tsai (2007) reviews evidence that East Asian caregivers directly foster more low-arousal positive emotion (calm, peaceful) as compared to European American caregivers, who foster more high-arousal positive emotion (excitement and elation). Her review indicates greater soothing of infants by Asian caregivers and greater stimulating by U.S. caregivers in studies on physical contact, play, and vocalizations. As children mature, U.S. parents use more positive emotions with their children than do Asian parents. Tsai links differences in emotion socialization to European Americans' tendency to act on the environment and exert influence and East Asians' tendency to adjust the self and fit in with the environment.

Middle Childhood and Adolescence

Cultural differences in incentives for children to obtain autonomy from their caregivers and family continue into adolescence. Teens' and their caregivers' expectations regarding the timing of autonomy are earlier for European Americans than many other groups, especially with regard to separation (Dubas & Gerris, 2002; Kwak, 2003; Smetana, 2002). German as compared to Japanese and Balinese teens' autonomy is expedited by their lesser harmony and greater number of conflicts with parents (Trommsdorff, 1995).

While there are earlier expectations regarding autonomy for European American children, there are earlier expectations regarding social forms of responsibility for East Asian children. Children in East Asian and other non-Western communities more often care for their siblings, take on communal chores, and assume other household duties and obligations motivated by the goal of social harmony as opposed to the goal of personal autonomy (Rothbaum & Trommsdorff, 2007). While some studies do not report higher expectations by parents in East Asia than in the United States, East Asians' expectations are more specific and thus more difficult to fulfill (Oishi & Sullivan, 2005).

Authoritative caregiving, which includes overt affection and autonomy support, constitutes the most common, as well as the most effective, pattern of caregiving for European Americans. This pattern entails firm but negotiated control, with parents providing ample opportunities for children to communicate their own perspectives, feelings, and needs. Authoritarian caregiving, which predicts poor social functioning in European American children, entails high levels of control and low levels of nurturance and acceptance (Baumrind, 1989).

Research in other cultures, especially in East Asia, provides less evidence that the authoritative pattern, as compared to the authoritarian pattern, is common or optimal. The most effective pattern includes elements of both, combining high control and high caring. Among the Chinese, parental control and criticism of the child are often accompanied by behaviors indicating concern, caring, and involvement. This combination of caregiving qualities best predicts social harmony in Chinese families (Chao & Tseng, 2002). Parental control and warmth are positively related in many if not most communities (Kim & Rohner, 2002; Rohner & Pettengill, 1985; Trommsdorff & Freidlmeier, 1993); the inverse relationship obtained in European American samples is the exception to the worldwide pattern. In traditional Chinese society, control, or training ("guan"), is viewed as fostering family hierarchy, moral behavior, fulfillment of obligations, self-discipline, self-sacrifice, and other qualities associated with harmony (Chao, 1994). Chao & Tseng (2002) cite more than 20 studies indicating greater parental control and exercise of authority and less encouragement of autonomy in several Asian groups than in Caucasians.

In contrast to these findings, some investigators report that children in all communities benefit from authoritative parenting (Sorkhabi, 2005) and, in particular, from autonomy support (Chirkov et al., 2005; Vansteenkiste et al., 2005). When compared with authoritarian or dominating control, that observation is undoubtedly true—because those types of control are usually defined in terms of hostile, punitive, and coercive practices that undermine children's well-being in *all* communities.

The more interesting question is whether there are cultural differences in patterns of caregiving that are unrelated to these negative practices. The evidence indicates that among European American as compared to East Asian parents there is more explicit praise, fostering of self-esteem, encouragement of emotional communication, and other features of autonomy support and authoritative caregiving. East Asian caregivers are more likely to encourage self-effacement than self-esteem, and they more often foster suppression than expression of emotion (Chen et al., 1998; Lin & Fu, 1990; Rothbaum, Morelli, Pott, & Liu-Constant, 2000). Suppression—including dampening of such positive feelings as pride and happiness—promotes interpersonal harmony. East Asians value moderation of emotional experience more than experiences of high-intensity positive emotions (Kitayama et al., 2006; see also Tsai, 2007). While expressions of shame and certain socially engaging positive emotions, such as friendliness and respect, are encouraged in East Asia, emotional expression is typically reserved. The purpose of emotion regulation in East Asia is to preserve harmony.

Interviews with children point to similar conclusions. Traditional Indian children, who are more interdependent relative to middle-class Indian children (who are more independent), perceive others as unaccepting of emotional expression and report greater control of felt emotion (Raval, Martini, & Raval, 2007). They express their negative feelings indirectly if at all: "Withdrawal responses (sitting in a corner, being quiet and not wanting to talk and/or pointing) were among the most common methods of expressing anger and sadness" (p. 49). Raval et al. explain: "Expression of anger or sadness may convey a discomfort with the social world that is harmful to . . . group harmony. . . . The expression of anger or sadness indicates an acknowledgement of one's personal goals . . . the assertion of [which] could be harmful to group cohesion" (p. 95). Similarly, Nepalese children either appraise their negative emotions (especially anger) as not very significant or mask expression of them (Cole, Bruschi, & Tamang, 2002; Cole & Tamang, 1998).

Psychological control by parents is seen as especially undermining of autonomy, and thus of well-being, among European Americans (Barber, 2002). As compared to caregivers in many other cultures, European Americans rely less on both positive (e.g., empathy training) and negative (shame and anxiety induction) forms of psychological control (Fung, 1999; Trommsdorff & Kornadt, 2003). Taiwanese as compared to European American parents are more likely to tell stories in which they cast young children as transgressors, and they seek out opportunities to correct and shame young children so as to impart the moral code and foster self-improvement. By contrast, European American mothers focus on their children's successes, their positive emotional experiences, and what children are able to accomplish (Miller, Fung, & Mintz, 1996). They recall events that highlight their children's preferences, autonomy, and emotions (Wang & Ross, 2007). Psychological control is seen as harmful because it instills in children a reluctance to question authority, express themselves, or manifest other forms of autonomy (Barber, 2002).

Parents are not the only socialization influences. Older children's and adolescents' adoption of the goal of autonomy versus harmony is influenced by several factors including: (1) an educational system that emphasizes freedom of thought as contrasted with a strict moral code; (2) the freedom to select work opportunities; and (3) the freedom to select mates and to part from them (Rothbaum & Trommsdorff, 2007). More distal influences include: (1) the degree of material prosperity, which makes choice attractive (choosing which need to forego is aversive; Snibbe & Markus, 2005); (2) a political structure that ensures freedoms and rights rather than long-standing tradition; and (3) religious beliefs that center on the individual's personal relationship with a deity and high-intensity emotions rather than on a sense of unity with external forces and low-intensity emotions (Tsai, 2007). Cultures differ in the relative number of situations supporting freedom and the goal of autonomy versus external constraint and the goal of harmony (Kitayama et al., 1997).

Fit between Goals
and Emotion Regulation Strategies

The research reviewed previously shows how childrearing practices influence goals and strategies pertaining to emotion. In this section we examine the *fit* between those goals and strategies (cf. Mesquita & Albert, 2007). We focus on emotion regulation strategies and on emotional components of the goal of autonomy versus harmony, namely, the pursuit of happiness versus calmness (Kitayama et al., 2006; Mesquita & Albert, 2007). Our thesis is that when people have goals for autonomy and happiness, they more readily internalize strategies for changing the emotional situation, and that when people have goals for harmony and calmness, they more readily internalize strategies for accepting the emotional situation. As shown in Table 5.2, we focus on five points in the emotion regulation process identified by Gross (1998): selecting situations, modifying situations, deploying attention, meaning making (cognitive change), and response modulation.

TABLE 5.2. How Goals Relate to Emotion Regulation Strategies

	Goals: Autonomy and High-Intensity Happiness	Goals: Harmony and Calmness/ Balanced Emotions
Situation selection	Choose situations that self prefers and that elevate positive emotions	Select moral situations in which people fulfill obligations and proper roles
Situation modification	Change the world to fit the self	Change the self to fit the world
Attention deployment	Distract self from negative to positive thoughts; attend to what self wants; first-person perspective	Distract self from own to others' emotions; attend to situational demands; third-person perspective
Meaning making and reappraisal	View stressors as opportunities to grow and gain mastery; find "silver lining" and shift perspective so as to make self feel better	View stressors as chances to improve self, to make self a better person, to self-sacrifice, and to practice endurance or forbearance
Response modulation	Verbally express positive and negative emotions, including socially disengaged emotions; strive for genuineness and authenticity	Suppress expression of emotions or express emotions indirectly; allow socially engaging emotions (empathy, shame)

The five emotion regulation processes are from Gross (1998, 2007).

At each point in the regulatory process, we identify relatively more change-based and more acceptance-based strategies.

Situation Selection: Choosing Preferred Activities and Selecting Obligatory Activities

When stressed, children with the goal of autonomy select situations that allow them to overcome their negative emotions. The goal of autonomy inspires children to choose situations that are interesting and appealing and that lead to personal success and high-intensity happiness (Higgins, 2008; Rothbaum, Pott, et al., 2000; Tsai, 2007). Children motivated by autonomy seek to change their emotional situation—from a stress-inducing one to an exciting and happy one. For example, following failure, students with autonomy and happiness goals are more likely to seek tasks on which they previously succeeded; students with harmony and calmness goals are more likely to persevere at the tasks on which they have failed (Heine et al., 2001).

People with the interdependent goal of harmony are less experienced in choosing situations. They less often freely pursue personal desires and more often rely on others when selecting activities (Iyengar & Lepper, 1999). When stressed, their priority is to restore their own and others' sense of calm rather than to seek excitement and personal happiness. They are likely to select situations that allow them to redouble efforts to fulfill role obligations and to engage in proper behavior. Situations allowing for self-improvement and self-sacrifice (e.g., cram schools, sports leading to family honor) are likely to be pursued rather than situations involving personal advancement and individual satisfaction (e.g., interest areas, self-care).

According to Confucian philosophy, situation selection shapes character (see Slingerland, 2003). The mother of Mencius is said to have moved three times until she found a community that would model proper conduct and scholarly pursuits (Van Norden, 2008). She was moving to avoid inappropriate settings rather than to suit her personal preference. Relative to European Americans, Asian Americans benefit more emotionally from fulfilling expectations of parents and friends and benefit less from seeking personal fun and enjoyment (Oishi & Diener, 2001).

Situation Modification: Changing the World and Changing the Self

According to Gross (2002), situation modification resembles primary control—changing the world to fit the self. When people cannot select a less stressful situation, they often seek to modify the current situation. Primary control strategies involving self-assertion are more common, more preferred, and more beneficial to European Americans than to many other groups (Morling & Evered, 2006; Weisz et al., 1984). Morelli cites an example of primary control in her work with U.S. children: when Sara was frustrated by her mother's lack of attention (her mother was engaged in conversation with the researcher), she marched back and forth between her mother and the researcher, chanting "Look at me" (reported in Morelli & Rothbaum, 2007). Explicitly requesting help, insisting on "my turn," and rearranging the setting to suit the self are among many ways that children change the emotional situation and thereby elevate their mood.

Whereas primary control is connected with the independent goal of autonomy and increasing self's happiness, secondary control is connected with the interdependent goal of harmony and increasing calm—in self *and others*. To regulate negative emotions, Efe children in the same situation as Sara used more subtle accommodative behaviors such as closer proximity, gentle touch, and postural shifts that did not disrupt the flow of adult activity. Children with the goal of harmony see themselves as embedded in, as opposed to apart from, the situation, and they seek to change themselves to fit the situation. They practice forms of situation modification that foster harmony with norms, role obligations, and fate as well as with other people. Mothers model this kind of situation modification when they indulge rather than resist children's dependent behavior (e.g., whining) so as to reduce conflict (Rothbaum & Trommsdorff, 2007). Mothers' accommodative practices teach children to accommodate to other people and, in so doing, to reduce others' distress.

Attention Deployment: Positive Distraction and Wider Awareness

European Americans frequently rely on positive distractions to cope with stressors. Diverting attention from negative thoughts toward more neutral or positive thoughts leads to recovery from negative moods among both children (Eisenberg, Spinrad & Smith, 2004; Kochanska, Murray, & Harlan, 2000; Mischel & Ayduk, 2004) and adults (Nolen-Hoeksema, Wisco, & Lyubomirsky, 2008). Whereas dwelling on unwanted thoughts fuels worry and rumination, shifting to pleasant thoughts about enjoyable images, events, and activities effectively changes the emotional situation. Attentional strategies serve the independent goal of autonomy—they are self-initiated, involve the self's interests and preferences, and are executed on one's own.

Instead of relying on distractors involving positive thoughts, children with the interdependent goal of harmony are likely to engage in forms of distraction involving perspective taking (e.g., "imagine myself floating off from my pain"; Cohen et al., 2007). That is, they shift from their immediate egocentric concerns to a third-party perspective from which they gain a more distant view of self and a greater awareness of other people and the surrounding context. The emotions of people with the goal of harmony are highly influenced by others' emotions (Cohen et al., 2007; Masuda et al., 2008; Mesquita & Leu, 2007; Oishi, Diener, Scollon, & Biswas-Diener, 2004).

For people with the goal of harmony, distraction has less to do with replacing negative experience with positive experience, or with achieving happiness, and more with attaining calmness and a greater appreciation of the balance between, and relatedness of, positive and negative experiences (Mesquita & Leu, 2007; Trommsdorff & Rothbaum, 2008). Present awareness is an example of East Asians' everyday attention deployment strategies.

Meaning Making: Reappraisals Involving Self-Enhancement and Self-Improvement

People often regulate emotions by reappraising the meaning of stressful events and thereby rendering them less stressful. Cultural differences in reappraisal resemble cultural differences in attention deployment. For people with an independent goal of autonomy, reappraisal is often aimed at changing from a negative to a positive view of a situation, for example, viewing failure as an opportunity for increasing self-efficacy and feeling better about the self (Tweed, White, & Lehman, 2004). Examples of enhancement-oriented reappraisals are interpreting a failure as a challenge to achieve more, to outperform others, or to fulfill one's dreams. People with the goal of autonomy reinterpret negative events as potentially positive ones.

For people with the interdependent goal of harmony, reappraisal has more to with accepting negative events than interpreting them positively. Acceptance-based emotion regulation involves increased openness to experience (letting in negative feelings and letting them go rather than dwelling on them), creating a space for those emotions (and realizing they will subside) and increased compassion—especially compassion to others who are responsible for those events (Neff, Pisitsungkagarn, & Hsieh, 2008). The type of acceptance that fits with the goal of harmony has more to do with not judging others than not judging self (Rothbaum & Wang, 2011). Accordingly, reappraisals often involve self-improvement—findings ways to strengthen one's character. Examples include reappraising negative events as opportunities for forbearance (to maintain a "stiff upper lip"), for transcending self's egocentric concerns, for accepting the negative emotional situation, and for improving the broader emotional climate, rather than as opportunities for self-enhancement and improving self's emotions (Chu,

2007; Constantine, Okazaki, & Utsey, 2004; Li, 2002; Tweed et al., 2004; Wong, Wong, & Scott, 2006; Yue, 2001).

Response Modulation: Emotional Expression and Emotional Suppression

Gross (1998) maintains that response modulation differs from the four other types of emotion regulation in that it occurs after emotion has been experienced. Emotions are more effectively regulated early in their formation; trying to modulate their expression after they are fully formed is difficult and costly. Research with European American samples indicates that suppressing negative thoughts and emotions drains people's energy and increases their vulnerability to the reemergence of those thoughts when they are least able to cope with them (Wenzlaff & Luxton, 2003). Yet, there are striking cultural differences in the costs and benefits of suppression; East Asians find it easier and less costly to suppress (Butler, Lee, & Gross, 2009).

Several studies indicate that people who express themselves—that is, engage in coherent narrative retellings of stressful events—experience reduced stress (Pennebaker, 1997). Despite some inconsistencies, most European American studies confirm that people benefit from the expression of emotions (Kennedy-Moore & Watson, 2001). Emotional expression fits with the goal of autonomy that entails ownership and assertion of deeply felt personal preferences (LaGuardia & Ryan, 2007; Masuda et al., 2008; Morelli & Rothbaum, 2007). In adults, open expression of emotions about close relationships is a sign of "autonomous" (secure) attachment (Cassidy & Shaver, 2008).

In most groups to which European Americans are compared, self-expression is more costly. Other peoples' greater emphasis on harmony makes suppression of expression more valued and practiced. Individuals are discouraged from explicitly expressing emotions because doing so tends to disrupt harmony and calmness (Kim & Markus, 2002). East Asians more often rely on strategies involving listening attentively to others than expressing themselves clearly, and their emotions are more influenced by the emotions of others (Cohen et al., 2007; Masuda et al., 2008). Several large-scale cultural studies have documented greater suppression of emotion, and increased automaticity and lesser costs of suppression, in people who prioritize the interdependent goal of harmony rather than the independent goal of autonomy (Butler et al., 2007, 2009; Matsumoto et al., 2008). When harmony is valued, emotional maturity has more to do with openness to others' emotions and less to do with self-assertion and emotional expression.[3]

Implications

Our thesis is that childrearing practices lead children in different cultures to adopt different goals and strategies, and internalization is likely when there is fit between goals and strategies. Underlying this thesis is the assumption that cultures differ in the types of situations they provide. European American cultures offer more situations that call for independence and primary control (e.g., show-and-tell activities in school, individual competition, free elections); in those situations, the goal of autonomy and change-based strategies are adaptive. By contrast, East Asian cultures provide more situations that require interdependence and secondary control (e.g., intergroup competitions; traditional ceremonies, school activities requiring the admission of faults); in those situations, the goal of harmony and acceptance-based strategies are adaptive (Mesquita & Albert, 2007; Rothbaum, Pott, et al., 2000). Since all cultures have situations that support both autonomy and harmony, there are within-culture as well as between-culture differences in the situations children experience. We suggest that adaptation is greatest when children learn which goals are most appropriate in different situations.

Consider what happens when European American children, who are accustomed to a fairly steady diet of autonomy-fostering situations, are exposed to situations involving very clear expectations and norms for appropriate behavior, such as when playing a role in a religious ceremony. In those situations, the goal of harmony is more adaptive than the goal of autonomy because it motivates internalization of appropriate regulatory strategies, such as suppression of emotional expression. The notion that adaptation is greatest when people's goals are matched to the situations that elicit them differs from the notion more commonly emphasized by cultural researchers—namely, that East Asian children are most competent when they rely on the goal of harmony and that European American children are most competent when they rely on the goal of autonomy.

Educating parents and children about the benefits of matching their goals to the situation at hand could increase children's adoption of more situation-appropriate goals, which in turn would lead them to more readily internalize appropriate strategies (Cheng, 2003). We suspect that parents often focus on behavioral strategies rather than goals, whereas goals are more central to conceptions of self and thus to the internalization process. When children's goals are well tailored to the situations in which they find themselves, they readily adopt emotion regulation strategies deemed appropriate. Efforts to change children's strategies without changing their situation-specific goals is an endeavor worthy of Sisyphus.[4]

Summary

Our main point is that behavior is likely to feel right, to persist, and to be automatic when it fits with one's goals. Childrearing practices involving continuous closeness, prolonged contact, and high levels of control lead to the goal of harmony that fits with strategies for *accepting* emotional situations. Conversely, practices involving more distal contact, repeated separations and reunions, and the fostering of overt communication and self-esteem lead to the goal of autonomy that fits with strategies for *changing* emotional situations. Children with interdependent selves typically pursue calm emotions and use strategies in which they: select normative, appropriate situations; change themselves to accommodate situations; direct attention away from their own emotions and toward others' emotions; appraise negative situations as opportunities to improve self-control and practice forbearance; and inhibit emotional expression. Children with independent selves pursue high-intensity positive emotions and use strategies in which they: choose situations that they find personally desirable; change situations to suit their emotions; direct attention away from unwanted emotions; appraise negative situations as opportunities to gain increased self-esteem; and express their unique individual selves. While we focus on the goal–strategy fit, our larger concern is the fit among goals, strategies, *and* situations.

Notes

1. Since there are substantial cultural differences in conceptions of self (Markus & Kitayama, 1991), there are correspondingly substantial cultural differences in internalization.

2. While any goal may be pursued with a promotion or prevention orientation, the goal of autonomy is more likely to be pursued with a promotion orientation because both are concerned with seeking ideals, maximizing the self, and personal accomplishments. The goal of harmony, by contrast is more likely to be pursued with a prevention orientation because both are concerned with obligations, avoiding negative outcomes (especially outcomes that adversely affect others), and security. Eager means resemble change-based strategies in that they entail risk taking, exploration, and self-enhancement. Vigilant means resemble acceptance-based strategies in that both entail caution, accommodation, and self-improvement (Higgins, 2008; Lee & Semin, 2009).

3. In claiming that European Americans are emotionally expressive, we do not mean that they are effusive. One can be taciturn and at the same time more expressive than is deemed appropriate by East Asians. John Wayne was not effusive, but he was also not suppressing his desires and feelings. Everyone around him knew what he wanted and what he stood for because he made his desires known with a minimum of words. He was clear about his preferences and did

not hesitate to express them even when they were in conflict with others' preferences.

4. Interdependence may be linked with different goals in different cultures. While we focus on the goal of harmony, which pertains to community, duty, and hierarchy, Indian interdependence pertains more to divinity and sacred and natural order (Shweder et al., 2006), and Latino interdependence pertains more to proper demeanor (Harwood et al., 1995). Assuming that there are only two higher-order goals underlying internalization perpetuates the problem that this chapter is intended to address—a too-limited notion of how internalization occurs.

References

Aronfreed, J. (1969). The concept of internalization. In D. A. Goslin (Ed.), *Handbook of socialization theory and research* (pp. 263–322). Chicago: Rand McNally.

Azuma, H. (1986). Why study child development in Japan? In H. W. Stevenson, H. Azuma, & K. Hakuta (Eds.), *Child development and education in Japan* (pp. 3–12). New York: Freeman.

Barber, B. (Ed.). (2002). *Intrusive parenting: How psychological control affects children and adolescents*. New York: American Psychological Association.

Baumrind, D. (1989). *Child development today and tomorrow*. San Francisco: Jossey-Bass.

Baumrind, D. (1996). The discipline controversy revisited. *Family Relations, 45,* 405–505.

Butler, E. A., Lee, T. L., & Gross, J. J. (2007). Emotion regulation and culture: Are the social consequences of emotion suppression culture-specific? *Emotion, 7,* 30–48.

Butler, E. A., Lee, T. L., & Gross, J. J. (2009). Does expressing your emotions raise or lower your blood pressure? The answer depends on cultural context. *Journal of Cross-Cultural Psychology, 40,* 510–517.

Cassidy, J., & Shaver, P. R. (Eds.). (2008). *Handbook of attachment: Theory, research, and clinical applications* (2nd ed.). New York: Guilford Press.

Chao, R. K. (1994). Beyond parental control and authoritarian parenting style: Understanding Chinese parenting through the cultural notion of training. *Child Development, 65,* 1111–1119.

Chao, R., & Tseng, V. (2002). Parenting of Asians. In M. H. Bornstein (Ed.), *Handbook of parenting: Vol. 4. Social conditions and applied parenting* (2nd ed., pp. 59–93). Mahwah, NJ: Erlbaum.

Chen, X., Hastings, P. D., Rubin, K. H., Chen, H., Cen, G., & Stewart, S. L. (1998). Child-rearing attitudes and behavioral inhibition in Chinese and Canadian toddlers: A cross-cultural study. *Developmental Psychology, 34,* 677–686.

Cheng, C. (2003). Cognitive and motivational processes underlying coping flexibility: A dual-process model. *Journal of Personality and Social Psychology, 84,* 425–438.

Chirkov, V., Ryan, R. M., Kim, Y., & Kaplan, U. (2003). Differentiating autonomy from individualism and independence: A self-determination theory perspective on internalization of cultural orientations and well-being. *Journal of Personality and Social Psychology, 84,* 97–109.

Chirkov, V. I., Ryan, R. M., & Willness, C. (2005). Cultural context and psychological needs in Canada and Brazil: Testing a self-determination approach to internalization of cultural practices, identity and well-being. *Journal of Cross-Cultural Psychology, 36,* 423–443.

Choi, S. H. (1992). Communicative socialization processes: Korea and Canada. In S. Iwawaki, Y. Kashima, & K. Leung (Eds.), *Innovations in cross-cultural psychology* (pp. 103–121). Lisse, Netherlands: Swets & Zeitlinger.

Chu, P. S. (2007). *The impacts of culture on social support, communication, values, and coping strategies.* Master's thesis, Kansas State University, Manhattan, KS.

Clancy, P. M. (1986). The acquisition of communicative style in Japanese. In B. B. Schieffelin & E. Ochs (Eds.), *Language socialization across cultures* (pp. 213–250). New York: Cambridge University Press.

Cohen, D., Hoshino-Browne, E., & Leung, A. K.-Y. (2007). Culture and the structure of personal experience: Insider and outsider phenomenologies of the self and social world. In M. P. Zanna (Ed.), *Advances in experimental social psychology* (Vol. 39, pp. 1–67). San Diego, CA: Elsevier.

Cole, P. M., Bruschi, C. J., & Tamang, B. L. (2002). Cultural differences in children's emotional reactions to difficult situations. *Child Development, 73,* 983–996.

Cole, P. M., & Tamang, B. L. (1998). Nepali children's ideas about emotional displays in hypothetical challenges. *Developmental Psychology, 34,* 640–646.

Constantine, M. G., Okazaki, S., & Utsey, S. O. (2004). Self-concealment, social self-efficacy, acculturative stress, and depression in African, Asian, and Latin American international college students. *American Journal of Orthopsychiatry, 74,* 230–241.

D'Andrade, R. (1990). Some propositions about the relations between culture and human cognition. In J. W. Stigler, R. A. Shewder, & G. Herdt (Eds.), *Cultural psychology: Essays on comparative human development* (pp. 48–65). Cambridge, UK: Cambridge University Press.

Deci, E. L., & Ryan, R. M. (2000). The "what" and "why" of goal pursuits: Human needs and the self-determination of behavior. *Psychological Inquiry, 11,* 227–268.

Dennis, T. A., Cole, P. M., Zahn-Waxler, C., & Mizuta, I. (2002). Self in context: Autonomy and relatedness in Japanese and U.S. mother–preschooler dyads. *Child Development, 73,* 1803–1817.

Dubas, J. S., & Gerris, J. R. (2002). Longitudinal changes in the time parents spend in activities with their adolescent children as a function of age, pubertal status, and gender. *Journal of Family Psychology, 16,* 415–426.

Edwards, C. P. (1995). Parenting toddlers. In M. H. Bornstein (Ed.), *Handbook of parenting: Vol. 1. Children and parenting* (pp. 41–63). Mahwah, NJ: Erlbaum.

Eisenberg, N., Spinrad, T. L., & Smith, C. (2004). Emotion-related regulation:

Its conceptualization, relations to social functioning and socialization. In P. Philippot & R. S. Feldman (Eds.), *The regulation of emotion* (pp. 277–306). Mahwah, NJ: Erlbaum.

Feeney, B. C. (2007). The dependency paradox in close relationships: Accepting dependence promotes independence. *Journal of Personality and Social Psychology, 92,* 268–285.

Ferber, R. (1985). *Solve your child's sleep problems.* New York: Simon & Schuster.

Fogel, A., Stevenson, M. B., & Messinger, D. (1992). A comparison of the parent–child relationship in Japan and the United States. In J. L. Roopnarine & D. Bruce (Eds.), *Annual advances in applied developmental psychology: Vol. 5. Parent–child socialization in diverse cultures* (pp. 25–51). Norwood, NJ: Ablex.

Fung, H. (1999). Becoming a moral child: The socialization of shame among young Chinese children. *Ethos, 27,* 180–209.

Gross, J. J. (1998). The emerging field of emotion regulation: An integrative review. *Review of General Psychology, 2,* 271–299.

Gross, J. J. (2002). Emotion regulation: Affective, cognitive, and social consequenes. *Psychophysiology, 39,* 281–291.

Gross, J. J. (2007). *The handbook of emotion regulation.* New York: Guilford Press.

Grusec, J. E. (2002). Parenting socialization and children's acquisition of values. In M. H. Bornstein (Ed.), *Handbook of parenting: Vol. 5. Practical issues in parenting* (2nd ed., pp. 143–167). Mahwah, NJ: Erlbaum.

Harwood, R. L., Leyendecker, B., Carlson, V., Ascencio, M., & Miller, A. M. (2002). Parenting among Latino families in the U.S. In M. H. Bornstein (Ed.), *Handbook of parenting: Vol. 4: Social conditions and applied parenting* (2nd ed., pp. 21–46). Mahwah, NJ: Erlbaum.

Harwood, R. L., Miller, J. G., & Irizarry, N. L. (1995). *Culture and attachment: Perceptions of the child in context.* New York: Guilford Press.

Heine, S. J., Kitayama, S., Lehman, D. R., Takata, T., Ide, E., Leung, C., et al. (2001). Divergent consequences of success and failure in Japan and North America: An investigation of self-improving motivations and malleable selves. *Journal of Personality and Social Psychology, 81,* 599–615.

Heine, S. J., Lehman, D. R., Markus, H. R., & Kitayama, S. (1999). Is there a universal need for positive self-regard? *Psychological Review, 106,* 766–794.

Hess, R. D., Kashiwagi, K., Azuma, H., Price, G. G., & Dickson, W. P. (1980). Maternal expectations for mastery of developmental tasks in Japan and the United States. *International Journal of Psychology, 15,* 259–271.

Higgins, E. T. (2006). Value from hedonic experience and engagement. *Psychological Review, 113,* 439–460.

Higgins, E. T. (2008). Culture and personality: Variability across universal motives as the missing link. *Social and Personality Psychology Compass, 2,* 608–634.

Hoffman, M. L. (1975). Moral internalization, parental power, and the nature of parent–child interaction. *Developmental Psychology, 11,* 228–239.

Iyengar, S. S., & Lepper, M. R. (1999). Rethinking the value of choice: A cultural perspective on intrinsic motivation. *Journal of Personality and Social Psychology, 76*, 349–366.

Keller, H., Lohaus, A., Kuensemueller, P., Abels, M., Yovsi, R. D., Voelker, S., et al. (2004). The bio-culture of parenting: Evidence from five cultural communities. *Parenting: Science and Practice, 4*, 25–50.

Kennedy-Moore, E., & Watson, J. C. (2001). How and when does emotional expression help? *Review of General Psychology, 5*, 187–212.

Kim, H. S., & Markus, H. R. (2002). Freedom of speech and freedom of silence: An analysis of talking as a cultural practice. In R. Shweder, M. Minow, & H. R. Markus (Eds.), *Engaging cultural differences: The multicultural challenge in liberal democracies* (pp. 432–452). New York: Russell Sage Foundation.

Kim, K., & Rohner, R. P. (2002). Parental warmth, control, and involvement in schooling: Predicting academic achievement among Korean American adolescents. *Journal of Cross-Cultural Psychology, 33*, 127–140.

Kitayama, S., Duffy, S., & Uchida, Y. (2007). Self as cultural mode of being. In S. Kitayama & D. Cohen (Eds.), *Handbook of cultural psychology* (pp. 136–174). New York: Guilford Press.

Kitayama, S., Karasawa, M., & Mesquita, B. (2004). Collective and personal processes in regulating emotions: Emotion and self in Japan and the United States. In P. Philippot & R. S. Feldman (Eds.), *Regulation of emotion* (pp. 251–273). Mahwah, NJ: Erlbaum.

Kitayama, S., Markus, H. R., Matsumoto, H., & Norasakkunkit, V. (1997). Individual and colletive processes in the construction of the self: Self enhancement in the United States and self-depreciation in Japan. *Journal of Personality and Social Psychology, 91*, 890–903.

Kitayama, S., Mesquita, B., & Karasawa, M. (2006). Cultural affordances and emotional experience: Socially engaging and disengaging emotions in Japan and the United States. *Journal of Personality and Social Psychology, 91*, 890–903.

Kochanska, G. (2002). Committed compliance, moral self, and internalization: A mediational model. *Developmental Psychology, 38*, 339–351.

Kochanska, G., Murray, L. T., & Harlan, E. T. (2000). Effortful control in early childhood: Continuity and change, antecedents, and implications for social development. *Developmental Psychology, 36*, 220–232.

Kwak, K. (2003). Adolescents and their parents: A review of intergenerational family relations for immigrant and non-immigrant families. *Human Development, 46*, 15–136.

La Guardia, J. G., & Ryan, R. M. (2007). Why identities fluctuate: Variability in traits as a function of situational variations in autonomy support. *Journal of Personality, 75*, 1205–1228.

Lee, A. Y., Aaker, J. L., & Gardner, W. L. (2000). The pleasures and pains of distinct self-construals: The role of interdependence in regulatory focus. *Journal of Personality and Social Psychology, 78*, 1122–1134.

Lee, A. Y., & Semin, G. R. (2009). Culture through the lens of self-regulatory orientations. In R. S. Wyer, C. Y. Chiu, & Y. Y. Hong (Eds.), *Understanding culture: Theory, research, and application* (pp. 271–288). New York: Psychology Press.

Li, J. (2002). A cultural model of learning: Chinese "heart and mind for wanting to learn." *Journal of Cross-Cultural Psychology, 33*, 248–269.

Lin, C. C., & Fu, V. R. (1990). A comparison of child-rearing practices among Chinese, immigrant Chinese, and Caucasian-American parents. *Child Development, 61*, 429–433.

Lu, L., & Gilmour, R. (2004). Culture and conceptions of happiness: Individual oriented and social oriented SWB. *Journal of Happiness Studies, 5*, 269–291.

Lutz, C. (1987). Goals, events, and understanding in Ifaluk emotion theory. In D. Holland & N. Quinn (Eds.), *Cultural models in language and thought* (pp. 290–312). New York: Cambridge University Press.

Maccoby, E. E. (1992). The role of parents in the socialization of children: An historical overview. *Developmental Psychology, 28*, 106–117.

Markus, H. R., & Kitayama, S. (1991). Culture and the self: Implications for cognition, emotion, and motivation. *Psychological Review, 98*, 224–253.

Markus, H. R., & Kitayama, S. (2003). Culture, self, and the reality of the social. *Psychological Inquiry, 14*, 277–283.

Masuda, T., Ellsworth, P. C., Mesquita, B., Leu, J., Tanida, S., & van de Veerdonk, E. (2008). Placing the face in context: Cultural differences in the perception of facial emotion. *Journal of Personality and Social Psychology, 94*, 365–381.

Matsumoto, D., Yoo, S. H., & Nakagawa, S. (2008). Culture, emotion regulation, and adjustment. *Journal of Personality and Social Psychology, 94*, 925–937.

Mesquita, B., & Albert, D. (2007). The cultural regulation of emotions. In. J. J. Gross (Ed.), *Handbook of emotion regulation* (pp. 486–503). New York: Guilford Press.

Mesquita, B., & Leu, J. (2007). The cultural psychology of emotion. In S. Kitayama & D. Cohen (Eds.), *Handbook of cultural psychology* (pp. 734–759). New York: Guilford Press.

Miller, J. G. (2003). Culture and agency: Implications for psychological theories of motivation and social development. In V. Murphy-Berman & J. Berman (Eds.), *Nebraska Symposium on Motivation: Cross-cultural differences in perspectives on the self* (Vol. 49, pp. 59–99). Lincoln: University of Nebraska Press.

Miller, P. J., Fung, H., & Mintz, J. (1996). Self-construction through narrative practices: A Chinese and American comparison of early socialization. *Ethos, 24*, 237–280.

Mischel, W., & Ayduk, O. (2004). Willpower in a cognitive–affective processing system: The dynamics of delay of gratification. In R. F. Baumeister & K. D. Vohs (Eds.), *Handbook of self-regulation: Research, theory, and applications* (pp. 99–129). New York: Guilford Press.

Morelli, G. A., Rogoff, B., Oppenheim, D., & Goldsmith, D. (1992). Cultural variation in infants' sleeping arrangements: Questions of independence. *Developmental Psychology, 28*, 604–613.

Morelli, G. A., & Rothbaum, F. (2007). Situating the person in context: Attachment relationships and self-regulation in young children. In S. Kitayama & D. Cohen (Eds.), *Handbook of cultural psychology* (pp. 500–527). New York: Guilford Press.

Morling, B., & Evered, S. (2006). Secondary control reviewed and defined. *Psychological Bulletin, 132,* 269–296.

Mulder, N. (1992). *Individual and society in Java: A cultural analysis.* Yogyakarta, Indonesia: Gadjah Mada University Press.

Neff, K. D., Pisitsungkagarn, K., & Hsieh, Y. P. (2008). Self-compassion and self-construal in the United States, Thailand, and Taiwan. *Journal of Cross-Cultural Psychology, 39,* 267–285.

Nolen-Hoeksema, S., Wisco, B. E., & Lyubomirsky, S. (2008). Rethinking rumination. *Perspectives on Psychological Science, 3,* 400–424.

Oishi, S., & Diener, E. (2001). Goals, culture, and subjective well-being. *Personality and Social Psychology Bulletin, 27,* 1674–1682.

Oishi, S., Diener, E., Scollon, C. N., & Biswas-Diener, R. (2004). Cross-situational consistency of affective experiences across cultures. *Journal of Personality and Social Psychology, 86,* 460–472.

Oishi, S., & Sullivan, H. W. (2005). The mediating role of parental expectations in culture and well-being. *Journal of Personality, 73,* 1267–1294.

Pennebaker, J. W. (1997). Writing about emotional experiences as a therapeutic process. *Psychological Science, 8,* 162–166.

Raval, V. V., Martini, T. S., & Raval, P. H. (2007). "Would others think it is okay to express my feelings?" Regulation of anger, sadness and physical pain in Gujarati children in India. *Social Development, 16,* 79–105.

Rogoff, B. (1990). *Apprenticeship in thinking.* New York: Oxford University Press.

Rogoff, B. (2003). *The cultural nature of human development.* New York: Oxford University Press.

Rohner, R., & Pettengill, S. M. (1985). Perceived parental acceptance-rejection and parental control among Korean adolescents. *Child Development, 56,* 524–528.

Roopnarine, J. L., & Carter, D. B. (1992). *Parent–child socialization in diverse cultures.* Norwood, NJ: Ablex.

Rothbaum, F., Kakinuma, M., Nagaoka, R., & Azuma, H. (2007). Attachment and amae: Parent–child closeness in the United States and Japan. *Journal of Cross-Cultural Psychology, 38,* 465–486.

Rothbaum, F., Morelli, G., Pott, M., & Liu-Constant, Y. (2000). Immigrant-Chinese and Euro-American parents' physical closeness with young children: Themes of family relatedness. *Journal of Family Psychology, 14,* 334–348.

Rothbaum, F., Morelli, G., & Rusk, N. (2010). Attachment, learning and coping: The interplay of cultural similarities and differences. In M. Gelfand, C. Y. Chiu & Y. Y Hong (Eds.), *Advances in culture and psychology* (Vol. 1, pp. 154–215). New York: Oxford University Press.

Rothbaum, F., Nagaoka, R., & Ponte, I. C. (2006). Caregiver sensitivity in cultural context: Japanese and U.S. teachers' beliefs about anticipating and responding to children's needs. *Journal of Research in Childhood Education, 21,* 23–41.

Rothbaum, F., Pott, M., Azuma, H., Miyake, K., & Weisz, J. (2000). The development of close relationships in Japan and the United States: Path of symbiotic harmony and generative tension. *Child Development, 71,* 1121–1142.

Rothbaum, F., & Trommsdorff, G. (2007). Do roots and wings complement or oppose one another?: The socialization of relatedness and autonomy in cultural context. In J. E. Grusec & P. Hastings (Eds.), *The handbook of socialization: Theory and research.* (pp. 461–489). New York: Guilford Press.

Rothbaum, F., & Wang, Y. Z. (2011). Cultural and developmental pathways to acceptance of self and acceptance of the world. In L. A. Jensen (Ed.) *Bridging cultural and developmental approaches to psychology: New syntheses in theory, research, and policy* (pp. 187–211). Oxford: Oxford University Press.

Rothbaum, F., Weisz, J., Pott, M., Miyake, K., & Morelli, G. (2000). Attachment and culture: Security in Japan and the U.S. *American Psychologist, 55*, 1093–1104.

Ryan, R. M., & Deci, E. L. (2000). Self-determination theory and the facilitation of intrinsic motivation, social development, and well-being. *American Psychologist, 55*, 68–78.

Saarni, C., Mumme, D. L., & Campos, J. (1998). Emotional development: Action, communication, and understanding. In N. Eisenberg (Ed.) & W. Damon (Series Ed.), *Handbook of child psychology: Vol. 3. Social, emotional, and personality development* (5th ed., pp. 237–309). New York: Wiley.

Schwartz, S. H. (2006). A Theory of cultural value orientations: Explication and applications. *Comparative Sociology, 5*, 137–182.

Shweder, R. A., Goodnow, J., Hatano, G., LeVine, R. A., Markus, H., & Miller, P. (2006). The cultural psychology of development: One mind, many mentalities. In W. Damon & R. M. Lerner (Eds.), *Handbook of child psychology*, (Vol. 1, 6th ed., pp. 716–792). New York: Wiley.

Shweder, R. A., Jensen, L. A., & Goldstein, W. M. (1995). Who sleeps by whom revisited: A method for extracting the moral goods implicit in practice. *New Directions for Child and Adolescent Development, 67*, 21–39.

Slingerland, E. (2003). *Confucian analects.* Indianapolis, IN: Hackett.

Smetana, J. G. (2002). Culture, autonomy, and personal jurisdiction in adolescent–parent relationships. In H. W. Reese and R. Kail (Eds.), *Advances in child development and behavior* (Vol. 29, pp. 51–87). New York: Academic Press.

Snibbe, A. C., & Markus, H. R. (2005). You can't always get what you want: Educational attainment, agency, and choice. *Journal of Personality and Social Psychology, 88*, 703–720.

Sorkhabi, N. (2005). Applicability of Baumrind's parent typology to collective cultures: Analysis of cultural explanations of parent socialization effects. *International Journal of Behavioral Development, 29*, 552–563.

Takahashi, K. (1990). Are the key assumptions of the "Strange Situation" procedure universal?: A view from Japanese research. *Human Development, 33*, 23–30.

Triandis, H. C. (1989). The self and social behavior in differing cultural contexts. *Psychological Review, 96*, 506–520.

Trommsdorff, G. (1995). Person–context relations as developmental conditions for empathy and prosocial action: A cross-cultural analysis. In T. A. Kindermann & J. Valsiner (Eds.), *Development of person–context relations* (pp. 113–146). Hillsdale, NJ: Erlbaum.

Trommsdorff, G., & Friedlmeier, W. (1993). Control and responsiveness in Japanese and German mother–child interactions. *Early Development and Parenting, 2*, 65–78.

Trommsdorff, G., & Friedlmeier, W. (2009). Preschool girls' distress and mothers' sensitivity in Japan and Germany. *European Journal of Developmental Psychology*.

Trommsdorff, G., & Kornadt, H. J. (2003). Parent–child relations in cross-cultural perspective. In L. Kuczynski (Ed.), *Handbook of dynamics in parent–child relations* (pp. 271–306). Thousand Oaks, CA: Sage.

Trommsdorff, G., & Rothbaum, F. (2008). Development of emotion regulation in cultural context. In M. Vandekerckhove, C. von Scheve, S. Ismer, S. Jung, & S. Kronast (Eds.), *Regulating emotions: Culture, social necessity, and biological inheritance* (pp. 85–120). Malden, MA: Blackwell.

Tsai, J. L. (2007). Ideal affect: Cultural causes and behavioral consequences. *Perspectives on Psychological Science, 2*, 242–259.

Tweed, R. G., White, K., & Lehman, D. R. (2004). Culture, stress, and coping: Internally- and externally-targeted control strategies of European Canadians, East Asian Canadians, and Japanese. *Journal of Cross-Cultural Psychology, 35*, 652–668.

Uchida, Y. & Kitayama, S. (2009). Happiness and unhappiness in east and west: Themes and variations. *Emotion, 9*, 441–456.

Van Norden, B. W. (2008). Introduction. In Mencius, *Mengzi: With selections from traditional commentaries*, trans. B. W. Van Norden (pp. xiii–xliv). Indianapolis, IN. Hackett.

Vansteenkiste, M., Zhou, M., Lens, W., & Soenens, B. (2005). Experiences of autonomy and control among Chinese learners: Vitalizing or immobilizing? *Journal of Educational Psychology, 96*, 755–764.

Wang, Q., & Leichtman, M. D. (2000). Same beginnings, different stories: A comparison of American and Chinese children's narratives. *Child Development, 71*, 1329–1346.

Wang, Q., & Ross, M. (2007). Culture and memory. In H. Kitayama & D. Cohen (Eds.), *Handbook of cultural psychology* (pp. 645–667). New York: Guilford Press.

Wang, Y. Z., Wiley, A. R., & Chiu, C.-Y. (2008). Independence-supportive praise versus interdependence-promoting praise. *International Journal of Behavioral Development, 32*, 13–20.

Weisner, T. S. (1984). A cross-cultural perspective: Ecocultural niches of middle childhood. In A. Collins (Ed.). *The elementary school years: Understanding development during middle childhood*. Washington, DC: National Academy Press.

Weisz, J. R., Rothbaum, F. M., & Blackburn, T. C. (1984). Standing out and standing in: The psychology of control in America and Japan. *American Psychologist, 39*, 955–969.

Wenzlaff, R. M., & Luxton, D. D. (2003). The role of thought suppression in depressive rumination. *Cognitive Therapy and Research, 27*, 293–308.

Whiting, J. W. M. (1990). Adolescent rituals and identity conflicts. In J. W. Stigler, R. A. Shweder, & G. Herdt (Eds.), *Cultural psychology. Essays on compara-*

tive human development (pp. 357–365). New York: Cambridge University Press.

Wong, P. T. P.,Wong, L. C. J., & Scott, C. (2006). Beyond stress and coping: The positive psychology of transformation. In P. T. P. Wong & L. C. J. Wong (Eds.), *Handbook of multicultural perspectives on stress and coping* (pp. 1–26). New York: Springer.

Yue, X. (2001). Culturally constructed coping among university students in Beijing. *Journal of Psychology in Chinese Societies, 2*, 119–137.

Zahn-Waxler, C., Friedman, R. J., Cole, P. M., Mizuta, I., & Hiruma, N. (1996). Japanese and United States preschool children's responses to conflict and distress. *Child Development, 67*, 2462–2477.

Zou, X., Tam, K., Morris, M. W., Lee, S., Lau, I. Y., & Chiu, C. Y. (2009). Culture as common sense: Perceived consensus vs. personal beliefs as mechanisms of cultural influence. *Journal of Personality and Social Psychology, 97*, 579–597.

PART III

SOCIOEMOTIONAL PROCESSES

CHAPTER 6

Emotion, Self-Regulation, and Social Behavior in Cultural Contexts

GISELA TROMMSDORFF *and* PAMELA M. COLE

The question of how a cultural perspective informs the development of children's self-regulation and social development remains somewhat neglected. In this chapter, we address this topic, emphasizing cultural influences on the socialization of emotion as they bear on the development of children's self-regulation and therefore social behavior. We share the view that individual differences in emotion regulation and social behavior are best explained by a developmental psychological perspective that integrates cultural context into its account. We also emphasize early childhood as an important period during which to study this integrative perspective. To be successful in school and in life, children must learn to engage in social behavior that conforms to social standards, which requires balancing their agentic and relationship motivations. This balance is achieved through skill at self-regulation, particularly its emotional aspects, which helps children engage in prosocial behavior even when agentic and relationship goals conflict. The behavioral standards to which children must conform are often culturally specific. We emphasize the importance of early caregiving as a means of transmitting cultural values through socialization practices, and we address caregivers' naïve theories and socialization goals that may organize their practices as they strive to foster children's social competence.

Our chapter has four sections. In the first section, we discuss the role of emotion and emotion regulation in social development. Second, we deal with caregivers' socialization of children's emotions and social behavior, focusing on the role of self-regulation in social development. Third, we address the role of culture in the socialization of emotions, emotion regulation, and social development. In the fourth section, we summarize our major points and suggest a cultural model of emotion regulation and social development. Finally, we offer suggestions for topics for future research.

The Role of Emotion and Emotion Regulation in Social Development

Functional Relations between Emotional and Social Development

Emotional Development

Generally, it is assumed that emotions are composed of several components, including feelings, physiological activity, and cognitions. Our view of emotions is influenced heavily by contemporary theories that emphasize these components as associated aspects of emotions, but not their defining characteristics. These aspects are not always discernible and may not always correlate with one another. Rather, we assume that emotions represent motivations to achieve goals (Barrett & Campos, 1987). That is, emotions emerge as a person strives to maintain or regain a sense of well-being, that is, to achieve goals that are of significance for well-being. In this regard, emotions are not located in a person and may not involve feelings (awareness of emotion) or explicit thoughts. We further assume that biological factors undergird the ability to be emotional, and this requirement includes being able to perceive changes in well-being, to organize a goal-oriented response, and to act accordingly, including selecting actions (and inhibiting actions) that are consonant with sociocultural standards.

Regarding the development of emotions, two theoretical approaches are to be distinguished. The *structural* approach (e.g., Ekman, Friesen, & Ellsworth, 1972) is rooted in evolutionary thinking (Darwin, 1859) and assumes that a biologically based adaptive value is accorded to emotions. Further, an integrated pattern of physiological responses early in infancy is also assumed (Izard, Ackerman, Schoff, & Fine, 2000). The first basic emotions are observed at birth, and others emerge during the first year of life. These various emotional expressions appear to be biologically rooted, as they appear so early in life and are displayed in similar ways cross-culturally (Izard, 1994). Emotion theories taking a *functionalist perspective* assume that the emotional life of newborns and infants is characterized by global positive or negative experiences (Sroufe, 1996) and that emotions shape goal-directed action (Eisenberg & Spinrad, 2004). The display of emotions has a communicative function that serves goal attainment; in infancy, for example, emotional expressions clearly influence the caretaker's behavior, and in this way the infant's emotional communication indicates the infant's goals that conditions be maintained or modified in order to regain or sustain well-being.

Because the desire to achieve one's personal goals can come into conflict with relationship goals, and each type of goal can come into conflict with sociocultural standards, successful goal achievement requires adequate *emotion regulation*. Circumstances often require the modulation of emotional experience or expression in order for a person to act in socially appropriate ways. For example, inadequately modulating the experience and expression of anger when one's goals are frustrated may lead to aggressive or rude behavior, which may have undesirable consequences such as social rejection. The regulation of anger can help a child achieve a desired goal that has been thwarted while maintaining a positive social relationship (Cole, Martin, & Dennis, 2004; Trommsdorff, 2006).

The topic of emotion regulation has gained much interest in recent years (Cole, Dennis, Martin, & Hall, 2008; Cole et al. 2004; Holodynski & Friedlmeier, 2006; Thompson, 1994). Although it is a topic of its own, from a broader perspective, *emotion* regulation can be regarded as an aspect of *self-regulation*. Self-regulation is the motivation and ability to regulate thought and action, as well as emotion, as part of goal-directed behavior (Blair, 2002; Calkins & Williford, 2009; Kopp, 1982; Trommsdorff, 2009a). That is, self-control in such forms as delay of gratification and inhibition of aggressive or antisocial behavior involves the conjoint regulation of emotion, cognition, and action. The early childhood integration of the domains that contribute to self-regulation is critical because these contribute to a child's school readiness; as early as first grade, children in formal schooling in most places in the world are expected to show persistence in learning new information, to cooperate with their classmates even when there are conflicting goals, and to comply with classroom rules (Blair, 2002). According to Eisenberg and Spinrad (2004), emotion-related self-regulation involves the processes "of initiating, avoiding, inhibiting, maintaining, or modulating the occurrence, form, intensity, or duration" of emotion-related physiological, motivational, cognitive, and/or behavioral responses in the service of affect-related biological or social adaptation in order to achieve individual goals.

A major aspect of self-regulation is effortful control, often conceptualized as a dimension of *temperament*. Effortful control from this perspective is conceptualized as the means by which children regulate their emotionality, defined as "the efficiency of executive attention—including the ability to inhibit a dominant response and/or to activate a subdominant response, to plan, and to detect errors" (Rothbart & Bates, 2006, p. 129). Effortful control first emerges during the late toddler years as the neural underpinnings of the executive attention system mature. In addition to attentional control, effortful control includes the ability to inhibit prepotent responses and to plan actions, skills that also serve self-regulation (Posner & Rothbart, 2007; also see Garon, Bryson, & Smith, 2008). To summarize, emotion regulation is a part of *self-regulation* and entails the recruitment of effortful control, by which the component domains of action, thought, and emotion are coordinated to effect appropriate social behavior (Blair, 2002). In line with functionalist theories of emotion, we take an agentic perspective on self-regulation; that is, we view the emotional aspects of self-regulation as goal-directed and influencing action that is aimed at achieving those goals, appreciating that the goals involved in complex social behavior can be, and often are, multiple (Cole et al., 2004; Eisenberg & Spinrad, 2004; Trommsdorff, 2009a). Therefore, the importance of emotion regulation for the effective self-regulation of social behavior is evident.

Social Development

Emotional competence, including emotion regulation, is regarded as an important accomplishment of a child's development because of its importance to social competence (Brownell & Kopp, 2007; Chen & French, 2008; Denham, 1998; Rubin, Bukowski, & Parker, 1998; Saarni, 1999). Denham and colleagues (Denham et al., 2003) investigated the degree to which early emotional competence paves the pathway to later social competence. Using a longitudinal design, they showed that three components of 3- and 4-year-olds' emotional competence (competent emotional expressivity, competent emotional knowledge, and competent emotion regulation) predicted subsequent social adjustment and social competencies that emerged during the preschool and kindergarten years. Generally speaking, evidence suggests the importance of early emotional development, particularly the ability to regulate and understand emotional responses, in promoting children's prosocial behavior and reducing the likelihood of aggressive behavior.

Evolutionary theorizing assumes biological roots of *aggression* and of emotions such as anger that motivate aggression. However, much recent work on aggression was influenced by social-cognitive theories, such as Bandura's (1989) social learning theory and Dodge and Pettit's (2003) social information-processing model. These approaches, however, tended to neglect the role of emotion and emotion regulation (Lemerise & Arsenio, 2000). In contrast, motivational theories on aggression assume that biological factors (genetic dispositions), emotions (e.g., anger), and cognitive processes (e.g., attributions about the other person's intentions) influence aggressive behavior and its development while empathy and sympathy inhibit aggressive responses (Kornadt, 2002, 2007). Accordingly, the regulation of emotions in the anger family and the activation of other-oriented emotions, such as empathy, should reduce aggressive behavior and foster social competence.

Prosocial behavior has often been regarded as a desirable aspect of social development and an important domain of social competence. Again, the role of emotions is of crucial importance for the study of prosocial behavior. Studies based on evolutionary assumptions have pointed out the survival value of prosocial behavior, especially in terms of reciprocity and cooperation (Tomasello, Carpenter, Call, Behne, & Moll, 2005). These authors have underlined the importance of emotions for prosocial behaviors such as cooperation. According to Tomasello et al. (2005), emotions such as anxiety, joy, and anger have similar features in humans and primates, but the joy that arises from sharing with others is uniquely human. A basic prerequisite of prosocial behavior may be the ability to understand what another person is thinking, feeling, and doing, an ability mediated in part by mirror neuron mechanisms (Gallese, Fadiga, Fogassi, & Rizzolatti, 1996; Rizzolatti & Fabbri-Destro, 2008). These enable humans to understand others' emotions without complex cognitive elaboration. According to this biologically rooted theory, empathy—which is often assumed to motivate prosocial behavior—is a universal capacity.

As with theories about the development of aggression, theories of prosocial behavior traditionally emphasized the cognitive aspects of prosociality. The functional value of emotions emerged from observational studies of infant and early childhood development. For example, an infant's crying can evoke distress in young children who observe the crying (Zahn-Waxler & Robinson, 1995). The young child's emotional reaction to another's distress is regarded as promoting the development of prosocial behavior. In some studies, the empathic responses and prosocial behavior of 2-year-olds is conceived of and measured as the same phenomenon (Bischof-Köhler, 2000).

However, evidence has shown that the quality of emotional reactions when witnessing another person in need or distress differs among individuals. Underwood and Moore (1982) first reported that there was no empirical evidence of relations between empathy and prosocial behavior. However, the early research may have failed to distinguish sympathy from personal distress (Eisenberg & Fabes, 1990). Sympathy consists of feelings of concern or sorrow for the other person. Personal distress is a self-focused aversive emotional reaction. According to Batson (1991), sympathy is associated with the motivation to reduce the other person's distress, which thereby leads to altruistic behavior. In contrast, personal distress is associated with the motivation to reduce one's own distress, which may result in avoiding contact with the person in need. This view was supported in studies with adult participants (Batson, 1991) and with child participants, including young children. Eisenberg and Fabes (1990) used several methods (self-reports, physiological and facial markers) to measure the emotional reactions when observing another person in need. In case of other-oriented emotions, children are inclined to "help" their peer by comforting, caring, or sharing. These studies underline the functional importance of sympathy (feeling with the victim) for altruistic or prosocial behavior (see review by Eisenberg, Fabes, & Spinrad, 2006; Eisenberg, 2007). In our own studies we have observed processes of emotional reactions when witnessing another person in need; the primary emotional reaction of empathy could evolve into sympathy, or other- or self-focused distress (Trommsdorff, 1995). These emotional reactions were associated with different behavior that was differentiated in line with Barbee (1990) as approach-type helping (solve and support) versus avoidance–type helping (dismiss and escape); or problem-focused helping (solve and dismiss) versus emotion-focused helping (support and escape) (Friedlmeier, 1996). Together, these studies underline the importance of emotion development and regulation in the development of prosocial behavior.

These studies also highlight the role of emotion in goal-directed behavior, thus underscoring our agentic approach. We incorporate a theoretical framework of the development of self and agency in cultural context, borrowing from research on the development of self-construal. Agency is related to control (control of self or control of environment) and to belief in self-efficacy (Bandura, 2001). It is a potent motivating force that is influenced by the socialization of emotion and social behavior, leading to culturally appropriate emotion regulation and social skills. Agency is related to how one construes the self, which differs according to the cultural model of the self (Miller, 2003; Trommsdorff, 2007). Parents socialize their children in line with the predominant cultural values for agency (e.g., of autonomy or relatedness) and the self—for example, as independent or interdependent. As the child acquires a culturally specific self-construal, children's emotion regulation and social behavior will follow different developmental pathways.

Aspects of Social Competence

One task of emotional development is learning to establish and maintain positive social relationships, including the ability to initiate and maintain friendships and to respect and comply with the authority of adults. Emotion regulation, including the ability to express emotion appropriately, and emotion knowledge, the ability to understand one's own and others' emotions as guides to emotion regulation, are deeply integrated in social competence (Halberstadt, Denham, & Dunsmore, 2001; Lemerise & Arsenio, 2000). Moreover, evidence suggests that emotional competencies are integrally related to the development of social competence (Chen & French, 2008; Denham et al., 2003; Spinrad et al., 2006). Thus, emotion regulation serves the development of social competence.

Universal and Individual Developmental Conditions for Emotional and Social Development

Universalities

Universal developmental conditions are partly based on innate biological processes (e.g., maturation) and partly based on universal social processes (e.g., formation of attachment relationships). The biological organism depends on an environment to develop, and this circumstance includes social input that provides an environment in which the neurobiology of social behavior can develop. For instance, in all societies, children typically acquire the rules of conduct of their communities. These rules may differ, and yet universally most children are capable of acquiring and behaving according to the rules of their social worlds (Whiting & Whiting, 1975), although some have impairments that compromise this development. Similarly, children in all societies form emotional attachments with their primary caregivers despite the fact that the means by which attachment is formed and the behaviors that constitute security may differ across cultural contexts (Cole & Tan, 2007).

For the purposes of our chapter, we assume that children have innate capacities for being emotional, for being social, and for engaging in regulatory processes; these capacities permit their agentic motivations to meet their goals for well-being to be modulated by cultural standards for social conduct. From the time the child begins to experience a social environment (including in utero), the specific influences of the child's particular developmental niche begin to transmit cultural influences on the child's development, including the rate of maturation as well as the development of behavioral skills (Harkness & Super, 2002). The socialization processes that transmit cultural standards then have their influences on the biological and behavioral development of the child. For example, executive functions first develop in nonspecific ways during the first years of life. Later they are related to the cognitive and conscious processes of emotion and self-regulation in line with the particular cultural values that are transmitted through socialization processes (for an overview of emotional development in young children, see Denham, 1998).

The development of prosocial behavior is a key aspect of social competence (Eisenberg, 2007). Prosocial behavior, such as empathy and altruism, depends upon the development of the self and the ability to coordinate the needs of the self and others. Evidence suggests that the roots of prosocial development can be perceived once the concept of the self has developed. There is evidence that 2-year-old children are beginning to develop a concept of the self. They are able to differentiate their own and others' needs and to display other-focused as well as self-focused emotions (Bischof-Köhler, 2000). However, Bischof-Köhler (2000) did not differentiate between empathy and prosocial behavior.

Other studies also report that self-recognition has been observed in 18- to 24-month-old children (Lewis & Brooks-Gunn, 1979; Lewis & Ramsay, 2004). Attachment fosters the development of the self-recognition. Securely as compared to insecurely attached children showed better self-recognition (Pipp, Easterbrooks, & Harmon, 1992). As early as 2 years of age, children begin to cooperate with social partners (Tomasello, 1999). Cooperation indicates social competence. Further, the growth of prosocial behavior is linked to the development of empathy; as we noted, any prosocial skills reflect an integration of emotional, cognitive, and behavioral processes. For instance, empathy requires the ability to feel concern for another's distress, to understand at a basic level that the other's distress is distinct from your own, and to engage in socially skilled behaviors such as information seeking, support seeking, or caregiving. Twin studies suggest that the emotional aspects of empathy may have a *hereditary* basis, whereas the behavioral elements do not (Zahn-Waxler, Robinson, & Emde, 1992). Thus, the capacity to express concern for others may be more rooted in biological dispositions, whereas how one behaves toward others may be more influenced by situational context and learning.

Concern for others is not generally discussed as a dimension of children's temperament, but negative emotionality, effortful control, and urgency—the main dimensions of temperament—may influence children's proclivity for feeling concern for others. These temperamental dimensions are believed to have extensive influences on emotional and social development. According to Rothbart and Bates (2006), individual differences in infant temperament can be observed for six dimensions: fearful distress (fearfulness), irritable distress, positive affect, (motor) activity level, attention span (persistence), and rhythmicity. These dimensions reflect negative emotionality (fearfulness and irritability) and a global positive emotionality. Attention span can be observed, for example, as affecting effortful control, which contributes to emotion regulation. A longitudinal study has shown that effortful control, an aspect of temperamental regulation, was a more consistent predictor of empathy (especially for boys) than was impulsivity (Eisenberg et al., 2007).

Individual Differences

Genetically influenced temperamental factors do not fully explain individual differences in social development; rather, they account for a child's preferred response tendencies. However, the development of social competence depends on children's ability to behave according to the standards of their cultural niche, regardless of their temperamental tendencies. For this reason, it is fortunate that environmental factors such as parenting can foster self-regulation in children of diverse temperaments (Eisenberg et al., 2005) and in this way promote socially appropriate behavior. Indeed, children predisposed to react negatively to novelty or limitations, and to be less inclined to engage in effortful control, may be particularly dependent on the quality of caregiving they receive from parents and other adults such as teachers.

Positive effects of warm parenting on self-regulation (inhibitory control, emotion regulation) have been shown in several studies (see meta-analyses by Karreman, van Tuijl, van Aken, & Dekovic, 2006; overview by Grusec & Davidov, 2007). Other studies have shown that attachment is a moderator for relationships between parenting and self-regulation (Kochanska, Aksan, Knaack, & Rhines, 2004). Child temperament can also be a moderator of these relationships (Kochanska, 1997). Recent studies focus on the mutual responsivity between parents and their children as predictors of self-regulation at preschool age (Kochanska, Aksan, Prisco, & Adams, 2008). In general, direct and indirect effects of parenting have to be distinguished (see overview by Grusec & Davidov, 2007). For example, others' self-esteem and self-efficacy beliefs in regulating emotions are positively related to mothers' positive reactions to children's distress and to preschool children's active and successful emotion regulation, while parenting behavior is a mediator (Heikamp, Hoffmann, Suchodoletz, & Trommsdorff, 2009).

Kochanska (1993, 1997) has asserted and demonstrated that the goodness of fit between the child's temperament and the parent's style fosters internalization of standards in children of diverse temperamental tendencies. For example, fearless and fearful children profit most from "sensitive" parenting, that is, parenting that takes into account the child's characteristics (e.g., fearlessness or fearfulness). In case of warm and positive parenting, fearless children are more likely to develop secure attachment relationships and establish a mutually positive orientation that leads to committed compliance from the child; this tendency is more likely despite the fact that fearlessness supports bold, assertive, or impulsive behavior that could be noncompliant. Fearful children profit most from low power assertive parenting. They develop committed compliance, perhaps because low-power parenting helps give children the feeling they are in control of their situations and reduces the need to be fearful and avoidant. These examples of "goodness of fit" between parenting and children's temperament may need to be qualified on the basis of the child's developmental age. Longitudinal studies by Kochanska, Aksan, and Joy (2007) underscore the importance of developmental period. The child's second year appeared to be most sensitive to parents' impact on their children's moral internalization. To summarize, biological and environmental factors influence emotional and social development through direct and indirect processes. Socialization factors, their respective fit with variables of child temperament at various developmental ages, and their mutual interdependencies have to be taken into account. In the next section we discuss environmental influences, especially parents as socialization agents, on children's emotional and social development, taking into account the role of culture.

The Role of Culture-Specific Socialization Conditions in the Development of Emotions and Social Behavior

Components of Socialization and the Developmental Niche

Parenting, including parents' beliefs and behavior, has been studied as an important factor in the socialization of children in a cultural context (e.g., Bornstein, 1991, 2001; Harkness & Super, 2002; Rubin, 1998; Rubin et al., 2006). In parenting, biological and environmental factors also play a role. Parents differ in their behavior on account of their own biological characteristics—for example, different temperaments or a different sensitivity to their children's signals. Further, economic and cultural factors influence parenting goals and behavior as part of the process to achieve an optimal adaptation to the resources and constraints of the environment and the needs of the child (Bornstein & Cheah, 2006).

Parenting, development, and culture have long been topics in anthropological research (e.g., Harkness & Super, 2002). Whiting and Whiting (1975) recommended an ecological approach that partly served as a guiding framework for Trommsdorff and Nauck's (2005) study on the value of children (including socioeconomic and cultural factors). However, it is also important for culturally sensitive work to incorporate bidirectional influences, including how a child's dispositions shape the child's experiences. In his ecological systems theory, Bronfenbrenner (1979) specified the interdependent contextual factors on various levels in human development; however, he did not specifically focus on culture.

In contrast, the theoretical framework of the "developmental niche" proposed by Super and Harkness (1997; Harkness & Super, 2006) clarifies the interface between child development and culture by focusing on the role of parents and their cultural belief systems (parental ethnotheories). The authors point out the importance of studying ethnotheories through their relations to the other components of the developmental niche. The concept of the developmental niche is useful in studying the culturally constructed environment of the child through several lenses of physical and social settings of the child's daily life and through customs, parental practices, and parental ethnotheories. Within the developmental niche, caregivers, including parents, begin to socialize a child's behavior as soon as the infant and caregivers begin to interact. For instance, although infants are not yet expected to engage in self-regulated social behavior, they actively express emotions, and the socialization of emotion thus begins early in life (Cole & Tan, 2006). Caregivers hold culturally specific sets of goals for their children's competence and beliefs about how competence develops (Bornstein & Cheah, 2006; Cole, Tamang, & Shrestha, 2006; Rubin et al., 2006; Trommsdorff & Kornadt, 2003), and these goals likely guide caregivers' choice of practices, consciously or otherwise, as they respond to their children's emotions and emotion-related behavior.

The Role of Parents' Naïve Theories and Parenting in Emotional and Social Development

Parents' naïve theories or ethnotheories include beliefs about the nature of child competence, the means by which children acquire competence, and the appropriate ways that caregivers can foster competence. Their elucidation provides insights into caregivers' socialization goals and their views of the most significant features of the parent–child relationship. Certain theories may be subtle enough to escape the caregiver's awareness and therefore not be readily expressible verbally. Parents' naïve theories are subject to the same distortions as other forms of self-report, as they are also prone to the influences of social desirability, to the imperfections of memory, and to the distortions that risk and psychopathology can introduce when one reports beliefs and practices. It has been asserted that parents' reports about their children's characteristics (e.g., temperament) are influenced by personal biases and therefore not wholly valid (e.g., Kagan, 1998). However, many more factors contribute to inconsistencies about direct observations, which usually are sampled in a single situation, and parental reports, which are based on the broader experience of their children in a variety of situations over time but are subject to self-report biases. Beside the well-known sources of discrepancies between parental self-reports and observed behavior (Denham et al., 2000; Rothbaum & Weisz, 1994), specific methodological factors should be taken into account, for example, the researcher's selection of observed behavior in certain situations or the researcher's influence on parents' behavior in such situations (see Arney, 2004, for an overview on studies comparing direct observations and self-report measures of parenting behavior).

Nonetheless, caregivers' naïve theories or ethnotheories are indices of what parents and other caregivers believe to be the goals of socialization and the strategies for achieving them. These ethnotheories reveal the degree to which parents share universal values and the degree to which they hold culturally specific values. Harkness and Super (2006) posit a hierarchical system of ethnotheories that starts with implicit cultural models (culturally shared values and beliefs, e.g., concerning the relationships among family members', parents, and the child) that influence domain-specific beliefs (children's emotion regulation patterns depend on one's age) and that, in turn, influence explicit ideas about appropriate practices and their role in influencing child outcomes (e.g., the child will mature) (p. 71). They also acknowledge important intervening factors such as whether the child's temperament is regarded as an important consideration. These beliefs finally influence the actual parenting practices (e.g., ignoring the child's distress) and, furthermore, the developmental outcome for the child (e.g., the child does not adequately regulate distress).

The characteristics of parents' naïve theories are valuable information in understanding child development (Goodnow & Collins, 1990). Rubin et al. (2006) further maintain that parents' naïve theories predict child outcomes: "For example, there is emerging evidence that parents' ideas, beliefs, and perceptions concerning the origins of the children's acceptable and unacceptable behavioural and emotional styles, in particular, contribute to, predict, and partially explain the development of adaptive and maladaptive behaviour in childhood" (Rubin et al., 2006, p. 82). More cautious about direct prediction, Harkness and Super (2006) state: "Thus, parental ethnotheories by themselves cannot predict child outcomes, but it would be difficult to understand cultural differences in development without reference to how parents in different cultures think about children" (p. 78).

From our point of view it is crucial, especially in cross-cultural or culture-informed studies, to acquire information on parents' beliefs about adequate developmental pathways to the social and emotional competence of their child, including beliefs about their child's characteristics, about their relationship with their child, and their parenting practices, including the way parents structure the social and physical environment of their child (including peer relations) (see Cole, et al., 2006; Trommsdorff & Friedlmeier, 2010). Such information about parents' naïve theories on their child will help them to understand the cultural specificities versus universals in their child's emotional and social development, since the focus is on the subjective meaning of beliefs and behavior. For example, Cole and colleagues (2004, 2006) found that elders in Brahman and Tamang villages had different criteria for defining child competence, and these differences placed in context observed differences in the socialization of anger and shame in preschool-age children. Similarly, Keller and colleagues (2004) showed video records of German and Cameroonian Nso mothers and infants to the mothers in each nation. When Cameroonian mothers observed the higher degree of *en face* contingent responding between German mothers and infants, they offered to come help German mothers learn how to more easily be close to their infants. Without a means of seeing child behavior and interactions through the eyes of the socialization agent, culturally meaningful information is lost to the scientist. Therefore, we are presently involved in a cross-cultural research project on parents' naïve theories on children's emotion regulation and social development in Germany, the United States, India, Nepal, and South Korea (Trommsdorff, Cole, Mishra, Niraula, & Park, in preparation).

The Role of Cognitive and Emotional Development in the Development of Self-Regulation

In general, internalization of the rules and values of one's parents or society is premised on positive parent–child relationships. Grusec and Goodnow (1994) articulated the preconditions for achieving successful internalization, including open communication and clarity in rules and values, and the child's acceptance of caregivers' messages. This model is useful in explaining the successful intergenerational transmission of values (Albert, Trommsdorff, & Wisnubrata, 2009; Trommsdorff, 2009b). Positive relationships between children and the primary caregivers in their lives foster this transmission. Secure attachment, one indicator of a positive parent–child relationship, has been shown repeatedly to be associated with children's internalization of values that guide their self-regulation (Grusec & Davidov, 2007; Kochanska, 1997). This view includes, of course, the contribution of children to their sociomoral development and the importance of a good fit between parenting style and the children's temperamental dispositions (Kochanska et al., 2007).

Research on emotional and social development has often tended to overlook the important role of culture. Most research has been conducted with European or U.S. samples, mostly in the United States. Recent cross-cultural studies clearly suggest that there are universal aspects of emotion, including the commonality of certain emotions, that are strongly influenced by the basic neurobiology of the human organism, such as fear and disgust (Izard, 1994; Matsumoto, 2001). However, cross-cultural studies also clearly reveal cultural specificity in the relations between the individual and the circumstances that influence the elicitation, expression, and regulation of emotions (e.g., see reviews by Cole & Tan, 2006; Friedlmeier

& Matsumoto, 2007; Kitayama, Mesquita, & Karasawa, 2006; Trommsdorff, 2006). These cultural specificities seem to be related to cultural values, socialization conditions, and, moreover, to the cultural model of self (Trommsdorff, 2009a). In the next section we deal with the role of culture in the development of emotional and social behavior.

The Role of Culture in the Socialization of Emotion, Emotion Regulation, and Social Development

The Role of Culture in Socialization Processes

Caregivers' beliefs, goals, and practices cannot simply be explained by studying their naïve theories. It is more important to understand the *meaning* of the specific naïve theories in the respective cultural context. Parents, for example, are members of a specific culture; the culturally shared values and behavioral practices structure the goals and beliefs of the individual members of a culture (Harkness & Super, 1995). Some parenting actions function as "cultural practices"; these are actions that are shared with others, related to normative expectations, and have a meaning that goes beyond the immediate goals of the action (Miller & Goodnow, 1995). Therefore, childrearing concepts can be seen as a belief system aligned with the values of the society and the individual (Kojima, 1986; Trommsdorff & Friedlmeier, 2004).

Accordingly, culture plays an important role in the socialization process, for example, mediated by parental ethnotheories or naïve theories. In a specific culture, parents may believe that expression of emotions is desirable and that the emotional development of their children should follow this goal. In another cultural context, parents may believe that self-restrained and inhibited expression of emotions is desirable; accordingly, parents may follow this developmental goal and promote related emotion regulation of their children. These differences are observable not only in comparisons among different cultures but also when assessing values, beliefs, and developmental outcomes over time in longitudinal studies. Accordingly, Chen and Chen (2010) report a decrease of shyness in Chinese children over the course of more than a decade, which they associate primarily with peer acceptance (Chen & French, 2008). Obviously, socioeconomic and cultural changes have contributed to a value change, to related changes in socialization conditions, and significant changes in developmental outcomes. Thereby, social competence has adopted a different meaning after a decade of fundamental socioeconomic changes in China.

Cross-cultural studies on emotion have shown that in socialization contexts in which the uniqueness of the self is valued highly open expression of emotions is encouraged by parents, in contrast to contexts in which the individual's relatedness to others is highly valued and in which parents intend to promote self-restraint in children (e.g., see reviews by Cole & Tan, 2006; Trommsdorff, 2006, 2009a). Furthermore, in cultural contexts emphasizing the interdependence of the individual with others, certain emotions are particularly undesirable, such as anger that has the potential to threaten interpersonal harmony (Cole et al., 2006; Cole, Walker, & Lama-Tamang, 2006). Even in case of an angry conflict of interest, Asian mothers pursued a cooperative and trusting relationship with their child, whereas Western mothers engaged in escalating conflicts based on their attribution of negative intentions to their children (Trommsdorff & Kornadt, 2003). Accordingly, Asian mother–children interactions ended peacefully, while German mother–child interactions ended with mothers' and their children being frustrated. In these various cultural climates fostering different value orientations, self-construals, and motivational and cognitive dispositions (e.g., attribution tendencies), diverse developmental paths emerge with respect to emotional and social development.

In cultural contexts characterized by social orientation and relatedness, parents hold culture-specific beliefs about the desirability of modesty and of social behavior that accommodates others (Rothbaum & Trommsdorff, 2007; Trommsdorff & Rothbaum, 2008). These parental beliefs are usually influenced, supported, and mirrored by such other socialization agencies as teachers and the school environment (Trommsdorff, 2009c). Therefore, it is useful to study relevant aspects of the cultural context and other socialization conditions besides the family in order to better understand the factors influencing the parents' belief system and parenting practices (Bornstein, 1991, 2001; Harkness & Super, 1995).

The Role of Culture in Emotional and Social Development

A leading influence on how culture is conceptualized in the psychological literature is the self-construal framework offered by Markus and Kitayama (1991). They postulate that the ways in which an individual views self relative to others are culturally variable and constitute an organizing influence on cognition and emotions that in turn affects social behavior (Markus & Kitayama, 1994). They further underscore psychological motivations for agency and how culture influences value orientations relating to the self's agency and emotions (Kitayama et al., 2006; Kitayama & Uchida, 2005). Although this framework is often applied in differentiating nations, its greatest utility is in understanding that all individuals strive for agency and for relatedness and that cultures vary in the relative value they place on each striving and on the means by which one achieves agency and relatedness.

Rothbaum, Weisz, Pott, Miyake, and Morelli (2000) elaborated on this view in their examination of the culture-specific functional role of attachment. Attachment theory postulates a universal need for autonomy that is supported by satisfaction of the universal need to feel secure. In socialization contexts valuing the interdependence of the self (e.g., Japan), the development of attachment is based on a specific mother–child relationship characterized by a symbiotic relationship (Azuma, 1986; Rothbaum, Pott, Azuma, Miyake, & Weisz, 2000). The assumed universal need of competence underlies a specific kind of agency in Japan—integration in an interdependent relationship that provides assurance (Rothbaum & Trommsdorff, 2007). In contrast, in Western cultures, the need for competence is related to the goal of following the path of independence and separateness. Therefore, depending on the cultural meaning of the assumed basic needs (competence, autonomy, and relatedness) attachment should have different consequences for the child's emotional and social development. Rothbaum, Pott, et al. (2000) integrate research on parenting and the parent–child relationship in lifespan development and suggest culture-specific pathways for emotional and social development. These pathways are related to different cultural models of self—the independent versus the interdependent self. While maintaining harmony is most important in cultures favoring the interdependent model of the self, achieving self-reliance and free expression of one's will is important in cultures favoring the independent model of the self. These values underlie parent–child interactions and the ways in which parents foster emotion regulation and the development of the self and of social competence in their children (Dennis, Cole, Zahn-Waxler, & Mizuta, 2002). In other studies, Japanese mothers responded to their children before they showed distress, while German mothers reacted *after* their children showed distress. These differences in mothers' proactive and reactive sensitivity were related to their children's successful emotion regulation (Trommsdorff & Friedlmeier, 2010; Trommsdorff & Rothbaum, 2008). Accordingly, we next turn to universal and culture-specific aspects of emotion regulation and self-regulation.

Universal and Culture-Specific Conditions of Emotion Regulation

A first step in considering cultural influences on emotion regulation and self-regulation is to address individual differences in infant temperament. Temperament is presumed to reflect innate, biologically based behavioral tendencies, although recent work highlights the fact that the *in utero* environment may influence infant temperament (e.g., Davis et al., 2007). A recent review reveals that there is much more to be known regarding whether or not there are cultural differences in infant temperament (Cole

& Tan, 2006). We assume that infants vary in temperament in all cultural contexts and that a dimension of these individual differences is variability across infants in their tendencies to react negatively to novelty or limitations. Furthermore, we assume that caregivers in all cultures nonetheless strive to promote a culturally specific standard of social conduct in their children, which affects the socialization of emotion and therefore self-regulation. The basis for the development of self, self-efficacy, and self-regulation, however, has to be seen in both biological and environmental factors, especially in parenting and culture-specific socialization conditions (as already specified).

In order for emotions to contribute to culturally appropriate social behavior, they must be regulated. The literature generally regards this regulation as involving the reduction of negative emotions and, less often, the up-regulation or maintenance of positive emotions. However, what is regarded as negative or positive emotion and how different emotions are valued, varies with the specific culture (Mesquita & Fridja, 1992; Mesquita, Frijda, & Scherer, 1997; Russell, 1994; Scherer, 1997). In Western societies, for instance, joy, happiness, and pride are regarded as positive emotions, their expression is highly valued, and parents encourage their expression (see overview by Cole & Tan, 2007). This pattern is consistent with a self-orientation that emphasizes individuality, uniqueness, and achievement. However, in Asian countries caregivers are less comfortable with their children expressing high levels of these emotions. All parents want their children to be secure, but in Asian countries there is less value attached to happiness and pride (Kitayama, 2001; Kitayama, Markus, & Kurokawa, 2000; Trommsdorff & Rothbaum, 2008; Tsai, Miao, Seppala, Fung, & Yeung, 2007), because these are regarded as lacking sensitivity to the needs of others and detracting from the achievement of calmness, which is more highly valued. However, parents in Asian societies may value other positive emotions, such as empathy or peacefulness; a child's being calm may be more valued than a child's being happy (Morelli & Rothbaum, 2007; Mulder, 1992). Furthermore, there is a positive emotion associated with making others feel relieved or peaceful, a topic related to prosociality that is rarely studied. Accordingly, parents in Asian societies are more likely to refrain from praising their children, focusing instead on how to improve their behavior (Miller, 2002, 2003; Rothbaum & Wang, 2010; Trommsdorff & Rothbaum, 2008; Wang, Wiley, & Chiu, 2008). Negative emotions, on the other hand, are also valued differently across cultures. Perhaps the most well understood difference regards negative self-conscious emotions, such as shame and embarrassment. In the United States, shame is regarded as a particularly toxic emotion because of its effects on self-esteem and its association with risk for psychopathology (Ferguson, Stegge, Miller, & Olsen, 1999; Tangney & Fischer, 1995). However, in some Asian societies, shame is a valued emotion and parents encourage it because it demonstrates that the child is learning his or her place in relation to authority and in regretting behavior that compromises interpersonal harmony (Kitayama, 2001; Kitayama, Markus, Matsumoto, & Norasakkunkit, 1997).

Accordingly, from a culture-informed viewpoint, the socialization of emotion fosters patterns of emotion regulation that are organized in regard to how selves best function in their social worlds. This process is related to the emotion focus (self or social), the role of the self, and the respective positive or negative quality of the outcome of emotion regulation for the self and for others. For example, guilt is a self-focused negative emotion in Western cultures, while shame is an other-focused negative emotion in Asian cultures (related to the fear of losing face—a very negative event). Accordingly, in order to avoid shame and self-regard (loss of face), regulatory behavior may already get started before the emotion is experienced— that is, regulation is regarded as most effective *during* the activity (e.g., achievement) in order to avoid a negative outcome in the Asian context. This would be an example of *anticipatory emotion and self-regulation*: investing persistence, effortful control, delay of gratification, etc., should serve the goal to be considered successful. Similarly, expecting positive emotions such as pride to ensue following successful achievement within the Western context would imply the prior investment of similar anticipatory activities of self-regulation. Thus, *emotion* regulation may require certain activities of *self*-regulation.

Culture-Specific Aspects of Emotion Regulation and Social Development

We assume that emotion regulation is related to social development and that both are influenced by cultural values and related socialization practices. First, we give examples for the development of emotion regulation in Asian cultures. Then, we deal with prosocial behavior as an example of social development.

Emotion Regulation

Javanese are traditionally expected to maintain social harmony. Javanese parents are very patient with their children and typically show little irritation over their misbehavior. Only rarely do the children experience inhibition forced on them by their parents. Older siblings learn to yield to the wishes of younger ones. Therefore, Javanese children rarely experience frustration, as they internalize the rules of emotion regulation and prosocial behavior relatively easily. "It is in this atmosphere of warm togetherness that the Javanese learn to express their own desires, to avoid conflict, and at the same time not be disappointed" (Magnis-Suseno, 1997, p 168). In order to maintain social harmony, children have to learn their position in the society, to perform their duties, and to internalize ways of emotion regulation and social competence. Since emotion regulation is related to the experience and the expression of emotions, Javanese "strive to control one's emotions and drives as well as to take an inner attitude of resignation" (p. 193). Here we observe a culture-specific method of emotion regulation that enables Javanese to fulfill their duties in a peaceful, secure (*slamet*), and unfrustrated way: "Outward harmony thus corresponds to an inward condition of *slamet*" (p. 193). In sum, emotion regulation as part of emotional and social competence overlap and indicate maturity, according to the Javanese belief system.

Japanese also focus on harmony as the basic goal of children's emotion regulation and as an indicator of emotional and social competence (Kitayama et al., 2000; Lebra, 1994; Morelli & Rothbaum, 2007; Trommsdorff & Rothbaum, 2008). Caregivers' socialization is therefore characterized by a culture-specific way of anticipating children's needs and emotions and engaging in "proactive sensitive" behavior (Rothbaum & Trommsdorff, 2007; Trommsdorff & Friedlmeier, 2010). Since mothers view a child's expression of negative emotions as an expression of lack of maturity, they do not react by scolding or blaming the child. Thereby they avoid becoming angry themselves, which would be a bad model for imitation; they also avoid negative attributions and a negative self-evaluation of the child by referring to a malleable cause ("a child is only a child"; that is, the child is not yet mature) (Trommsdorff & Kornadt, 2003).

Indian children also seem to regulate their emotions in accordance with the cultural values of harmony and a peaceful mind. When Indian and German preschool children expected a gift in a box but found the box empty, the Indian children soon regulated their disappointment, guided by the positive reactions of their mothers; in contrast, the German children were frustrated and showed negative emotions such as anger for a while until they were given a present by the experimenter. The German mothers often even encouraged their children's anger (unpublished data by Trommsdorff, Mishra, Heikamp, Suchodoletz, & Merkel, 2009).

However, not all Asian societies approach childrearing and the socialization of emotion in the same manner. For instance, Cole and colleagues found that Nepalese Brahman caregivers are more likely to engage in emotionally neutral control of their preschool-age children whereas Nepalese Tamang caregivers engage in more affiliative control. In regard to emotion socialization, the Brahmans tend to ignore child shame and to be responsive to child anger, whereas Tamang ignore or punish child anger but are responsive to child shame (Cole et al., 2006). Conversations with elders in these communities about what constitutes competence in a child reveal that the Tamang prioritize social skills that involve making others feel good, whereas Brahmans prioritize individual achievement, particularly in school. These observations of childrearing and emotion socialization are thus consistent with cultural definitions of competence and likely explain why Brahman children value anger but Tamang children value shame (Cole, Bruschi, & Tamang, 2002; Cole & Tamang, 1998). Importantly, comparative studies within putatively independent or interdependent societies further our ability to understand cultural influences. The socialization of emotion that leads to a child's regulation of emotion and behavior thus relates directly to the child's tendencies toward social behavior.

Prosocial Behavior

The literature indicates that the development of prosocial behavior in children is partly based on heritable genetic influences (e.g., Hastings, Zahn-Waxler, & McShane, 2005) and partly based on environmental influences (e.g., Zahn-Waxler et al., 1992). Psychoevolutionary theorizing underlines the role of emotions (empathy) for prosocial behavior (see Hastings, Utendale, & Sullivan, 2007). Research in Western countries has shown that nonpunitive parenting and other-oriented reasoning that activates the child's understanding of the situation fosters prosocial development (Grusec & Goodnow, 1994). However, parenting styles are complex; they are related to parents' naïve theories and goals, and they vary across contexts. Therefore, the specific meaning of parenting should be assessed—and this is even more necessary in case of cross-cultural comparisons.

Prosocial behavior has been associated with parental warmth and child-centered discipline. Also, warm and sensitive parenting should allow for the development of prosocial behavior. However, sensitivity has a culture-specific meaning (proactive vs. reactive sensitivity; see Rothbaum & Trommsdorff, 2007). Further, it does not necessarily imply warmth. However, when taking into account the role of emotions, a clearer picture may emerge. Cultural values of interdependence would undermine the self–other differentiation that is necessary for the experience of empathy (feeling compassion for the other person), a precondition of prosocial behavior. Thereby, distress may also arise when one vicariously shares the unhappy or negative emotions of another person. Accordingly, the child needs to regulate this distress.

Observational studies of 2- and 5-year-old children in Germany and Japan showed that 2-year-old toddlers in both countries were sometimes overwhelmed by their distress when observing another person in distress. They were looking for the support of their mothers in order to be able to overcome their own distress and to engage in helpful acts. These very young children could not regulate their distressing emotions by themselves. Emotion regulation is therefore a necessary skill in both cultures for empathic prosocial behavior (Trommsdorff, 1995), as suggested by Eisenberg (1995). Five-year-old German children, in contrast to Japanese children, could already regulate distress by themselves. In the case of self-focused distress, children acted less prosocially than in the case of other-focused distress or in the case of empathy.

In our four-culture study on empathy, distress, and prosocial behavior, we found again a significant contribution of other-focused distress and of empathy to prosocial behavior. We also have shown that, among children who were socialized in a cultural context favoring interdependence, more other-focused distress occurred and less ability to "interfere" with the distressed state of another person was observed (Trommsdorff, Friedlmeier, & Mayer, 2007). These results underline that distress, empathy, and prosocial behavior have different meanings, depending on the cultural context.

To summarize, emotion regulation can obviously affect aspects of social development in line with cultural values. Cultural values on interdependence undermine aggression; they also can foster other-oriented distress that needs to be regulated efficiently in order not to undermine prosocial behavior (toward strangers) in young children. The cultural values of independence can foster readiness to face conflicts and engage in anger-based aggression while also fostering prosocial behavior based on empathy.

Summary: A Cultural Model of Emotion, Self-Regulation, and Social Development

The basic components of our cultural model are (1) cultural variations in the goals and practices parents have for socializing emotion, (2) the effects these have on promoting culturally specific patterns of emotion regulation, and (3) the role these effects play in promoting culturally defined prosocial behavior. We draw from the work on self-construal to emphasize the universal motivations in humans to strive for both agency and relatedness, recognizing that the ways in which a balance between these strivings is achieved is culturally variable. Culture, in our view, is defined by shared practices that derive from shared values and beliefs. Self-construal develops through the socialization process, which filters cultural values and beliefs. As children develop, they have the opportunity to internalize cultural values and to use these to evaluate themselves and others with whom they interact. Optimally, in each cultural niche, a child feels securely embedded in family relationships and able to explore and learn about the world beyond the family as part of a striving for efficient functioning or a sense of agency. Depending on the child's self-construal, derived in the process of socialization by adults close to the child, the well-adapted child behaves in culturally appropriate ways to meet personal goals and to maintain good relationships with others.

Ryan and Deci (2000) have assumed that universal needs influence behavior. However, we believe that these universal needs are met differently, depending on the cultural model in which the self develops (Trommsdorff, 2009a). Accordingly, evaluations, motivations, and emotions and emotion regulation develop in culturally variable ways, for example, regulating distress through primary control (changing the environment) or secondary control (changing the self) (Essau & Trommsdorff, 2000; Weisz, Rothbaum, & Blackburn, 1984). All together, the different components underlying the processes of emotion regulation and self-regulation build a pattern that in general fits with the dominant cultural model of the self and allows for optimal culture-specific emotional and social competence.

Outlook and Conclusions

Conclusions for a Culture-Informed Theory on Emotion Development and Social Development

Research on emotion regulation and social development has so far largely neglected the role of culture. On the other hand, culture-informed research on emotion and social behavior has so far rather focused on the cultural and psychological aspects of the self and neglected developmental psychological approaches. A cultural–psychological approach to the development of emotion and social behavior has to take into account the cultural meaning of socialization conditions (such as parenting and kinds of sensitivity), of emotion and emotion regulation, and of desirable social behavior. As we have seen, beliefs of social competence and desirable behavior can change over time (Chen & Chen, 2010; Chen & French, 2008). Therefore, developmental outcomes of emotion regulation and social behavior can only be evaluated as representing emotional and social competence when their respective cultural meanings are taken into account (Friedlmeier & Trommsdorff, 2002).

We do acknowledge the biologically based universals in the development of emotion and social development. Other universals may be related to internal psychological processes in emotion and social development. However, culture specificities cannot be ignored. These can only be understood when taking the perspective of the respective cultural values and the belief system underlying the socialization conditions and developmental outcomes (Cole & Tamang, 1998; Cole & Tan, 2007; Rothbaum, Pott, et al., 2000; Trommsdorff, 2006; 2009a). A culturally-informed view on the development of emotion and social behavior allows us to evaluate the fit between the cultural model and actual developmental outcomes.

Conclusions Regarding Interventions

Emotion regulation and social behavior are influenced by biological and environmental factors and can become relevant in the development of *problematic* developmental paths. For example, in their recent review Rubin, Burgess, and Coplan (2002) argued that behavioral inhibition (e.g., showing signs of reactive anxiety, distress, or disorganization) is related to *emotion dysregulation* that is possibly determined by temperament. The authors claim that behavioral inhibition is a developmental precursor of social reticence, social withdrawal, and anxiety in childhood and adolescence. Behavioral inhibition and social withdrawal are stable variables. Moreover, social withdrawal in mid-childhood predicts negative self-concept, loneliness, peer rejection, and emotion dysregulation such as depression in early adolescence. The physiological basis of behavioral inhibition has been revealed in several studies (e.g., Fox & Calkins, 1993).

We know from past research that environmental factors can play a significant role in changing undesirable behavior. Thus, we can assume that parents will try to determine whether the development of emotion regulation and the self-regulation of their children are congruent with the "normative" (culturally preferred) cultural model. However, differences in the cultural appropriateness (that is, the cultural fit) of developmental outcomes relating to emotions and social behavior can occur (e.g., dysregulation of inhibited children). Therefore, interventions may become necessary that, in turn, require a theoretical basis and input from empirical research. As we noted, very little research directly addresses cultural influences in the socialization of emotion and self-regulation. Therefore, it is not well known when certain forms of inhibited behavior may be culturally acceptable and, if so, whether this shortcoming reduces the possibility that the inhibited behavior will lead to forms of psychopathology. Of special note is recent work by Chen and Chen (2010) in which the authors demonstrate that recently evolving cultural values in China likely account for changing relations between child inhibition and child behavior problem symptoms. In sum, we advocate for an increase in the number of cross-cultural, within-culture, and culturally informed studies of the development of emotion regulation, self-regulation, and social competence.

Acknowledgments

This research was financed by a grant from the German Research Foundation (No. DFG GZ, TR 169/14-2) to Gisela Trommsdorff and by grants from the National Science Foundation (No. 9711519) and the National Institute of Mental Health (No. MH61388) to Pamela M. Cole.

References

Albert, I., Trommsdorff, G., & Wisnubrata, L. (2009). Intergenerational transmission of values in different cultural contexts: A study in Germany and Indonesia. In A. Gari & K. Mylonas (Eds.), *Quod erat demonstrandum: From herodotus' ethnographic journeys to cross-cultural research. Book of selected chapters of the 18th International Congress of the International Association for Cross-Cultural Psychology* (pp. 221–230). Athens, Greece: Pedio Books.

Arney, F. M. (2004). *A comparison of direct observation and self-report measures of parenting behaviour.* Dissertation, University of Adelaide, Australia.

Azuma, H. (1986). Why study child development in Japan? In H. W. Stevenson, H. Azuma, & K. Hakuta (Eds.), *Child development and education in Japan* (pp. 3–12). New York: Freeman.

Bandura, A. (1989). Social cognitive theory. In R. Vasta (Ed.), *Annals of child development: Vol. 6. Six theories of child development* (pp. 1–60). Greenwich, CT: JAI Press.

Bandura, A. (2001). Social cognitive theory: An agentic perspective. *Annual Review of Psychology, 52,* 1–26.

Barbee, A. P. (1990). Interactive coping: The cheering-up process in close relationships. In S. Duck (Ed.), *Personal relationships and social support* (pp. 46–65). London: SAGE.

Barrett, K. C., & Campos, J. J. (1987). Perspectives on emotional development: II. A functionalist approach to emotions. In J. Osofsky (Ed.), *Handbook of infant development* (pp. 555–578). New York: Wiley.

Batson, C. D. (1991). *The altruism question: Toward a social-psychological answer.* Hillsdale, NJ: Erlbaum.

Bischof-Köhler, D. (2000). Empathie, prosoziales Verhalten und Bindungsqualität bei Zweijährigen [Empathy, prosocial behavior, and attachment quality of two year olds]. *Psychologie in Erziehung und Unterricht, 47,* 142–158.

Blair, C. (2002). School readiness: Integrating cognition and emotion in a neurobiological conceptualization of children's functioning at school entry. *American Psychologist, 57,* 111–127.

Bornstein, M. H. (Ed.). (1991). *Cultural approaches to parenting.* Hillsdale, NJ: Erlbaum.

Bornstein, M. H. (2001). Some questions for a science of "culture and parenting" (. . .but certainly not all). *International Society for the Study of Behavioural Development Newsletter, 1,* 1–4.

Bornstein, M. H., & Cheah, C. S. L. (2006). The place of "culture and parenting" in an ecological contextual perspective on developmental science. In K. Rubin & O. B. Chung (Eds.), *Parental beliefs, parenting, and child development in cross-cultural perspective* (pp. 3–33). New York: Psychology Press.

Bronfenbrenner, U. (1979). *The ecology of human development: Experiments by nature and design.* Cambridge, MA: Harvard University Press.

Brownell, C. A., & Kopp, C. B. (Eds.). (2007). *Socioemotional development in the toddler years: Transitions and transformations.* New York: Guilford Press.

Calkins, S. D., & Williford, A. P. (2009). Taming the terrible twos: Self-regulation and school readiness. In O. A. Barbarin & B. H. Wasik (Eds.), *Handbook of child development and early education: Research to practice* (pp. 72–198). New York: Guilford Press.

Chen, X., & Chen, H. (2010). Children's socioemotional functioning and adjustment in the changing Chinese society. In R. K. Silbereisen & X. Chen (Eds.), *Social change and human development: Concepts and results* (pp. 209–226). London: Sage.

Chen, X., & French, D. C. (2008). Children's social competence in cultural context. *Annual Review of Psychology, 59*, 591–616.

Cole, P. M., Bruschi, C. J., & Tamang, B. L. (2002). Cultural differences in children's emotional reactions to difficult situations. *Child Development, 73*(3), 983–996.

Cole, P. M., Dennis, T. A., Martin, S. E., & Hall, S. E. (2008). Emotion regulation and the early development of psychopathology. In M. Vandekerckhove, C. von Scheve, S. Ismer, S. Jung, & S. Kronast (Eds.), *Regulating emotions: Culture, social necessity and biological inheritance* (pp. 171–188). Malden, MA: Blackwell.

Cole, P. M., Martin, S. E., & Dennis, T. A. (2004). Emotion regulation as a scientific construct: Methodological challenges and directions for child development research. *Child Development, 75*, 317–333.

Cole, P. M., & Tamang, B. L. (1998). Nepali children's ideas about emotional displays in hypothetical challenges. *Developmental Psychology, 34*, 640–646.

Cole, P. M., Tamang, B. L., & Shresta, S. (2006). Cultural variations in the socialization of young children's anger and shame. *Child Development, 77*, 1237–1251.

Cole, P. M., & Tan, P. Z. (2006). Capturing the culture in the cultural socialization of emotion. *ISSBD Newsletter, 49*, 5–7.

Cole, P. M., & Tan, P. Z. (2007). Emotion socialization from a cultural perspective. In J. E. Grusec & P. D. Hastings (Eds.), *Handbook of socialization: Theory and research* (pp. 516–542). New York: Guilford Press.

Cole, P. M., Walker, A. R., & Lama-Tamang, M. S. (2006). Emotional aspects of peer relations among children in rural Nepal. In X. Chen, D. C. French, & B. H. Schneider (Eds.), *Peer relationships in cultural context* (pp. 148–169). New York: Cambridge University Press.

Darwin, C. (Ed.). (1859). *On the origin of the species by means of natural selection, or, the preservation of favoured races in the struggle for life.* London: John Murray.

Davis, E. P., Glynn, L. M., Schetter, C. D., Chicz-Demet, A., Sandman, C. A., & Hobel, C. (2007). Prenatal exposure to maternal depression and cortisol influences infant temperament. *Journal of the American Academy of Child and Adolescent Psychiatry, 46*, 737–746.

Denham S. A. (1998). *Emotional development in young children.* New York: Guilford Press.

Denham, S. A., Blair, K. A., DeMulder, E., Levitas, J., Sawyer, K., Auerbach-Major, S., et al. (2003). Preschool emotional competence: Pathway to social competence. *Child Development, 74*, 238–256.

Denham, S. A., Workman, E., Cole, P. M., Weissbrod, C., Kendziora, K. T., & Zahn-Waxler, C. (2000). Prediction of externalizing behavior problems from early to middle childhood: The role of parental socialization and emotion expression. *Development and Psychopathology, 12*, 23–45.

Dennis, T. A., Cole, P. M., Zahn-Waxler, C., & Mizuta, I. (2002). Self in context: Autonomy and relatedness in Japanese and U.S. mother–preschooler dyads. *Child Development, 73*, 1803–1817.

Dodge, K. A., & Pettit, G. S. (2003). A biopsychosocial model of the development of chronic conduct problems in adolescence. *Developmental Psychology, 39*, 349–371.

Eisenberg, N. (1995). Prosocial development: A multifaceted model. In W. M. Kurtines & J. L. Gewirtz (Eds.), *Moral development: An introduction* (pp. 401–429). Boston: Allyn & Bacon.

Eisenberg, N. (2007). Empathy-related responding: Its role in positive development and socialization correlates. In R. K. Silbereisen & R. M. Lerner (Eds.), *Approaches to positive youth development* (pp. 75–91). London: Sage.

Eisenberg, N., & Fabes, R. A. (1990). Empathy: Conceptualization, measurement, and relation to prosocial behavior. *Motivation and Emotion, 14*, 131–149.

Eisenberg, N., Fabes, R. A., & Spinrad, T. L. (2006). Prosocial development. In W. Damon, R. M. Lerner, & N. Eisenberg (Eds.), *Handbook of child psychology. Social, emotional, and personality development* (pp. 646–718). New York: Wiley.

Eisenberg, N., Michalik, N., Spinrad, T. L., Kupfer, A., Liew, J., Reiser, M., et al. (2007). The relations of effortful control and impulsivity to children's sympathy: A longitudinal study. *Cognitive Development, 22*, 544–567.

Eisenberg, N., & Spinrad, T. L. (2004). Emotion-related regulation: Sharpening the definition. *Child Development, 75*, 334–339.

Eisenberg, N., Zhou, Q., Spinrad, T. L., Valiente, C., Fabes, R. A., & Liew, J. (2005). Relations among positive parenting, children's effortful control, and externalizing problems: A three-wave longitudinal study. *Child Development, 76*, 1055–1071.

Ekman, P., Friesen, W. V., & Ellsworth, P. C. (1972). *Emotion in the human face: Guidelines for research and an integration of findings.* New York: Pergamon Press.

Essau, C. A., & Trommsdorff, G. (2000). Primary and secondary control in Iban students. In V. Sutlive & J. Sutlive (Eds.), *The encyclopedia of Iban studies* (Vol. 1, pp. 489–492). Kuching, Malaysia: The Tun Jugah Foundation.

Ferguson, T. J., Stegge, H., Miller, E. R., & Olsen, M. E. (1999). Guilt, shame, and symptoms in children. *Developmental Psychology, 35*, 347–357.

Fox, N. A., & Calkins, S. D. (1993). Pathways to aggression and social withdrawal: Interactions among temperament, attachment, and regulation. In K. H. Rubin & J. B. Asendorpf (Eds.), *Social withdrawal, inhibition, and shyness in childhood* (pp. 81–100). Hillsdale, NJ: Erlbaum.

Friedlmeier, W. (1996). Development of empathy and prosocial behavior in childhood. *Polish Quarterly of Developmental Psychology, 2*, 17–36.

Friedlmeier, W., & Matsumoto, D. (2007). Emotion im Kulturvergleich [Emotion in cross-cultural comparison]. In G. Trommsdorff & H.-J. Kornadt (Eds.),

Enzyklopädie der Psychologie: Themenbereich C. Theorie und Forschung: Serie VII. Kulturvergleichende Psychologie: Band 2. Erleben und Handeln im kulturellen Kontext (pp. 219–281). Göttingen, Germany: Hogrefe.

Friedlmeier, W., & Trommsdorff, G. (2002). Emotionale Kompetenz im Kulturvergleich [Emotional competence in cross-cultural comparison]. In M. von Salisch (Ed.), *Emotionale Kompetenz entwickeln: Grundlagen in Kindheit und Jugend* (pp. 229–262). Stuttgart, Germany: Kohlhammer.

Gallese, V., Fadiga, L., Fogassi, L., & Rizzolatti, G. (1996). Action recognition in the premotor cortex. *Brain, 119,* 593–609.

Garon, N., Bryson, S. E., & Smith, I. M. (2008). Executive function in preschoolers: A review using an integrative framework. *Psychological Bulletin, 134,* 31–60.

Goodnow, J. J., & Collins, W. A. (Eds.). (1990). *Development according to parents: The nature, sources, and consequences of parents' ideas.* Hillsdale, NJ: Erlbaum.

Grusec, J. E., & Davidov, M. (2007). Socialization in the family: The roles of parents. In J. E. Grusec & P. D. Hastings (Eds.), *Handbook of socialization: Theory and research.* (pp. 284–308). New York: Guilford Press.

Grusec, J. E., & Goodnow, J. J. (1994). Impact of parental discipline methods on the child's internalization of values: A reconceptualization of current points of view. *Developmental Psychology, 30,* 4–19.

Halberstadt, A. G., Denham, S. A., & Dunsmore, J. C. (2001). Affective social competence. *Social Development, 10,* 79–119.

Harkness, S., & Super, C. M. (1995). Culture and parenting. In M. H. Bornstein (Ed.), *Handbook of parenting: Vol. 2. Biology and ecology of parenting* (pp. 211–234). Mahwah, NJ: Erlbaum.

Harkness, S., & Super, C. M. (2002). Culture and parenting. In M. H. Bornstein (Ed.), *Handbook of parenting: Vol. 2. Biology and ecology of parenting* (2nd ed., pp. 253–280). Mahwah, NJ: Lawrence Erlbaum Associates.

Harkness, S., & Super, C. M. (2006). Themes and variations: Parental ethnotheories in Western culutres. In K. H. Rubin & O. B. Chung (Eds.), *Parental beliefs, parenting, and child development in cross-cultural perspective* (pp. 61–79). New York: Psychology Press.

Hastings, P. D., Utendale, W. T., & Sullivan, C. (2007). The socialization of prosocial development. In J. E. Grusec & P. D. Hastings (Eds.), *Handbook of socialization: Theory and research* (pp. 638–664). New York: Guilford Press.

Hastings, P. D., Zahn-Waxler, C., & McShane, K. (2005). We are, by nature, moral creatures: Biological bases of concern for others. In M. Killen & J. Smetana (Eds.), *Handbook of moral development* (pp. 483–516). Hillsdale, NJ: Erlbaum.

Heikamp, T., Hoffmann, N., Suchodoletz, A., & Trommsdorff, G. (2009, July). Maternal self-efficacy beliefs and the development of their children's emotion regulation. In T. Heikamp & G. Trommsdorff (Chairs), *Coping successfully with emotional experiences: Antecendents, cognitive processes, and development.* Symposium conducted at the 11th European Congress of Psychology, Oslo, Norway.

Holodynski, M., & Friedlmeier, W. (Eds.). (2006). *Development of emotions and emotion regulation*. New York: Springer.

Izard, C. E. (1994). Intersystem connections. In P. Ekman & R. J. Davidson (Eds.), *The nature of emotion: Fundamental questions* (pp. 356–361). New York: Oxford University Press.

Izard, C. E., Ackerman, B. P., Schoff, K. M., & Fine, S. E. (2000). Self-organization of discrete emotions, emotion patterns, and emotion-cognition relations. In M. D. Lewis, & I. Granic (Eds.), *Emotion, development, and self-organization: Dynamic systems approaches to emotional development* (pp. 15–36). New York: Cambridge University Press.

Kagan, J. (1998). *Three seductive ideas*. Cambridge: Harvard University Press.

Karreman, A., van Tuijl, C., van Aken, M. A. G., & Dekovic, M. (2006). Parenting and self-regulation in preschoolers: A meta-analysis. *Infant and Child Development, 15*, 561–579.

Keller, H., Lohaus, A., Kuensemueller, P., Abels, M., Yovsi, R. D., Voelker, S., et al. (2004). The bio-culture of parenting: Evidence from five cultural communities. *Parenting: Science and Practice, 4*, 25–50.

Kitayama, S. (2001). Culture and emotion. In N. J. Smelser & P. B. Baltes (Eds.), *International encyclopedia of the social and behavioral sciences* (pp. 3134–3139). Oxford, UK: Elsevier.

Kitayama, S., Markus, H. R., & Kurokawa, M. (2000). Culture, emotion, and well-being: Good feelings in Japan and the United States. *Cognition Emotion, 14*, 93–124.

Kitayama, S., Markus, H. R., Matsumoto, H., & Norasakkunkit, V. (1997). Individual and collective processes in the construction of the self: Self-enhancement in the United States and self-criticism in Japan. *Journal of Personality and Social Psychology, 72*, 1245–1267.

Kitayama, S., Mesquita, B., & Karasawa, M. (2006). Cultural affordances and emotional experience: Socially engaging and disengaging emotions in Japan and the United States. *Journal of Personality and Social Psychology, 91*, 890–903.

Kitayama, S., & Uchida, Y. (2005). Interdependent agency: An alternative system for action. In R. M. Sorrentino, D. Cohen, J. M. Olson, & M. P. Zanna (Eds.), *Cultural and social behavior: The Ontario symposium* (Vol. 10, pp. 137–164). Mahwah, NJ: Erlbaum.

Kochanska, G. (1993). Toward a synthesis of parental socialization and child temperament in early development of conscience. *Child Development, 64*, 325–347.

Kochanska, G. (1997). Multiple pathways to conscience for children with different temperaments: From toddlerhood to age 5. *Developmental Psychology, 33*, 228–240.

Kochanska, G., Aksan, N., & Joy, M. E. (2007). Children's fearfulness as a moderator of parenting in early socialization: Two longitudinal studies. *Developmental Psychology, 43*, 222–237.

Kochanska, G., Aksan, N., Knaack, A., & Rhines, H. M. (2004). Maternal parenting and children's conscience: Early security as moderator. *Child Development, 75*, 1229–1242.

Kochanska, G., Aksan, N., Prisco, T. R., & Adams, E. E. (2008). Mother–child and father–child mutually responsive orientation in the first 2 years and children's outcomes at preschool age: Mechanisms of influence. *Child Development, 79,* 30–44.

Kojima, H. (1986). Child rearing concepts as a belief-value system of the society and the individual. In H. W. Stevenson & H. Azuma (Eds.), *Child development and education in Japan: A series of books in psychology* (pp. 39–54). New York: Freeman.

Kornadt, H.-J. (2002). Biology, culture, and child rearing: The development of social motives. In H. Keller, Y. H. Poortinga, & A. Schölmerich (Eds.), *Between culture and biology: Perspectives on ontogenetic development* (pp. 191–211). New York: Cambridge University Press.

Kornadt, H.-J. (2007). Motivation im kulturellen Kontext [Motivation in cultural context]. In G. Trommsdorff & H.-J. Kornadt (Eds.), *Enzyklopädie der Psychologie: Themenbereich C. Theorie und Forschung: Serie VII Kulturvergleichende Psychologie. Band 2: Erleben und Handeln im kulturellen Kontext* (pp. 283–376). Göttingen, Germany: Hogrefe.

Kopp, C. B. (1982). Antecedents of self-regulation: A developmental perspective. *Developmental Psychology, 18,* 199–214.

Lebra, T. S. (1994). Mother and child in Japanese socialization: A Japan–U.S. comparison. In P. M. Greenfield & R. R. Cocking (Eds.), *Cross-cultural roots of minority child development* (pp. 259–274). Hillsdale, NJ: Erlbaum.

Lemerise, E. A., & Arsenio, W. F. (2000). An integrated model of emotion processes and cognition in social information processing. *Child Development, 71,* 107–118.

Lewis, M., & Brooks-Gunn, J. (1979). *Social cognition and the acquisition of self.* New York: Plenum Press.

Lewis, M., & Ramsay, D. (2004). Development of self-recognition, personal pronoun use, and pretend play during the 2nd year. *Child Development, 75,* 1821–1831.

Magnis-Suseno, F. (1997). *Javanese ethics and world view: The Javanese idea of the good life.* Jakarta: Gramedia Pustaka Utama.

Markus, H. R., & Kitayama, S. (1991). Culture and the self: Implications for cognition, emotion, and motivation. *Psychological Review, 98,* 224–253.

Markus, H. R., & Kitayama, S. (1994). The cultural construction of self and emotion: Implications for social behavior. In S. Kitayama & H. R. Markus (Eds.), *Emotion and culture: Empirical studies of mutual influence* (pp. 89–130). Washington, DC: American Psychological Association.

Matsumoto, D. R. (Ed.). (2001). *The handbook of culture and psychology.* New York: Oxford University Press.

Mesquita, B., & Frijda, N. H. (1992). Cultural variations in emotions: A review. *Psychological Bulletin, 112,* 179–204.

Mesquita, B., Frijda, N. H., & Scherer, K. R. (1997). Culture and emotion. In J. E. Berry, P. B. Dasen, & T. S. Saraswathi (Eds.), *Handbook of cross-cultural psychology: Vol. 2. Basic processes and developmental psychology* (pp. 255–297). Boston: Allyn & Bacon.

Miller, J. G. (2002). Integrating cultural, psychological and biological perspectives in understanding child development. In H. Keller, Y. H. Poortinga, & A. Schölmerich (Eds.), *Between culture and biology: Perspectives on ontogenetic development* (pp. 136–156). New York: Cambridge University Press.

Miller, J. (2003). Culture and agency: Implications for psychological theories of motivation and social development. In V. Murphy-Berman & J. Berman (Eds.), *Nebraska Symposium on Motivation: Vol. 49. Cross-cultural difference in perspectives on the self* (pp. 59–99). Lincoln: University of Nebraska Press.

Miller, P. J., & Goodnow, J. J. (1995). Cultural practices: Toward an integration of culture and development. In J. J. Goodnow & P. J. Miller (Eds.), *Cultural practices as contexts for development. New directions for child development* (pp. 5–16). San Francisco: Jossey-Bass.

Morelli, G. A., & Rothbaum, F. (2007). Situating the child in context: Attachment relationships and self-regulation in different cultures. In S. Kitayama & D. Cohen (Eds.), *Handbook of cultural psychology.* (pp. 500–527). New York: Guilford Press.

Mulder, N. (1992). *Individual and society in Java: A cultural analysis* (2nd ed.). Yogyakarta, Indonesia: Gadjah Mada University Press.

Pipp, S., Easterbrooks, M. A., & Harmon, R. J. (1992). The relation between attachment and knowledge of self and mother in one- to three-year-old infants. *Child Development, 63,* 738–750.

Posner, M. I., & Rothbart, M. K. (2007). Research on attention networks as a model for the integration of psychological science. *Annual Review of Psychology, 58,* 1–23.

Rizzolatti, G., & Fabbri-Destro, M. (2008). The mirror system and its role in social cognition. *Current Opinion in Neurobiology, 18,* 179–184.

Rothbart, M. K., & Bates, J. E. (2006). Temperament. In W. Damon, R. M. Lerner, & N. Eisenberg (Eds.), *Handbook of child psychology: Social, emotional, and personality development* (Vol. 3, pp. 99–166). New York: Wiley.

Rothbaum, F., Pott, M., Azuma, H., Miyake, K., & Weisz, J. (2000). The development of close relationships in Japan and the United States: Paths of symbiotic harmony and generative tension. *Child Development, 71,* 1121–1142.

Rothbaum, F., & Trommsdorff, G. (2007). Do roots and wings oppose or complement one another?: The socialization of autonomy and relatedness in cultural context. In J. E. Grusec & P. D. Hastings (Eds.), *The handbook of socialization: Theory and research* (pp. 461–489). New York: Guilford Press.

Rothbaum, F., & Wang, Y. Z. (2010). Fostering the child's malleable views of the self and the world: Caregiving practices in East Asian and European-American communities. In B. Mayer & H.-J. Kornadt (Eds.), *Psychologie-Kultur-Gesellschaft* (pp. 101–120). Wiesbaden: VS Verlag.

Rothbaum, F., & Weisz, J. R. (1994). Parental caregiving and child externalizing behavior in nonclinical samples: A meta-analysis. *Psychological Bulletin, 116,* 55–74.

Rothbaum, F., Weisz, J., Pott, M., Miyake, K., & Morelli, G. (2000). Attachment and culture: Security in the United States and Japan. *American Psychologist, 55,* 1093–1104.

Rubin, K. H. (1998). Social and emotional development: A cross-cultural perspective. *Developmental Psychology, 34*, 611–615.

Rubin, K. H., Bukowski, W. M., & Parker, J. G. (1998). Peer interactions, relationships, and groups. In W. Damon, R. M. Lerner, & N. Eisenberg (Eds.), *Handbook of child psychology: Vol. 3 Social, emotional, and personality development* (pp. 571–645). New York: Wiley.

Rubin, K. H., Burgess, K., & Coplan, R. J. (2002). Social inhibition and withdrawal in childhood. In P. K. Smith & C. Hart (Eds.), *Handbook of childhood social development* (pp. 329–352). London: Blackwell.

Rubin, K. H., Hemphill, S. A., Chen, X., Hastings, P., Sanson, A., LoCoco, A., et al. (2006). Parenting beliefs and behaviors: Initial findings from the International Consortium for the Study of Social and Emotional Development (ICSSED). In K. H. Rubin & O. B. Chung (Eds.), *Parental beliefs, parenting, and child development in cross-cultural perspective* (pp. 81–103). New York: Psychology Press.

Russell, J. A. (1994). Is there universal recognition of emotion from facial expression? A review of cross-cultural studies. *Psychological Bulletin, 115*, 102–141.

Ryan, R. M., & Deci, E. L. (2000). The darker and brighter side of human existence: Basic psychological needs as a unifying concept. *Psychological Inquiry, 11*, 319–338.

Saarni, C. (1999). *The development of emotional competence.* New York: Guilford Press.

Scherer, K. R. (1997). The role of culture in emotion-antecedent appraisal. *Journal of Personality and Social Psychology, 73*, 902–922.

Spinrad, T. L., Eisenberg, N., Cumberland, A., Fabes, R. A., Valiente, C., Shepard, S. A., et al. (2006). Relation of emotion-related regulation to children's social competence: A longitudinal study. *Emotion, 6*(3), 498–510.

Sroufe, L. A. (1996). *Emotional development. The organization of emotional life in the early years.* New York: Cambridge University Press.

Super, C. M., & Harkness, S. (1997). The cultural structuring of child development. In J. W. Berry, P. R. Dasen, & T. S. Saraswathi (Eds.), *Handbook of cross-cultural psychology: Vol. 2. Basic processes and human development* (2nd ed., pp. 1–39). Boston: Allyn & Bacon.

Tangney, J. P., & Fischer, K. W. (1995). *Self-conscious emotions: The psychology of shame, guilt, embarrassment, and pride.* New York: Guilford Press.

Thompson, R. A. (1994). Emotion regulation: A theme in search of definition. In N. A. Fox (Ed.), *The development of emotion regulation: Biological and behavioural considerations. Monographs of the Society for Research in Child Development* (Vol. 59, Issue 2–3, Series 240, pp. 25–52). Chicago: University of Chicago Press.

Tomasello, M. (1999). Having intentions, understanding intentions, and understanding communicative intentions. In P. D. Zelazo, J. W. Astington, & D. R. Olson (Eds.), *Developing theories of intention: Social understanding and self-control* (pp. 63–75). Mahwah, NJ: Erlbaum.

Tomasello, M., Carpenter, M., Call, J., Behne, T., & Moll, H. (2005). Understanding and sharing intentions: The ontogeny and phylogeny of cultural cognition. *Behavioral and Brain Sciences, 28,* 675–735.

Trommsdorff, G. (1995). Person–context relations as developmental conditions for empathy and prosocial action: A cross-cultural analysis. In T. A. Kindermann & J. Valsiner (Eds.), *Development of person–context relations* (pp. 113–146). Hillsdale, NJ: Erlbaum.

Trommsdorff, G. (2006). Development of emotions as organized by culture. *ISSBD Newsletter, 49,* 1–4.

Trommsdorff, G. (2007). Entwicklung im kulturellen Kontext [Development in cultural context]. In G. Trommsdorff & H.-J. Kornadt (Eds.), *Enzyklopädie der Psychologie: Themenbereich C Theorie und Forschung, Serie VII Kulturvergleichende Psychologie. Band 2: Kulturelle Determinanten des Erlebens und Verhaltens* (pp. 435–519). Göttingen, Germany: Hogrefe.

Trommsdorff, G. (2009a). Culture and development of self-regulation. *Social and Personality Psychology Compass, 2,* 1–15.

Trommsdorff, G. (2009b). Intergenerational relations and cultural transmission. In U. Schönpflug (Ed.), *Cultural transmission: Psychological, developmental, social, and methodological aspects* (pp. 126–160). Cambridge: Cambridge University Press.

Trommsdorff, G. (2009c). Indicators for quality of life and working life in Germany and Japan: A culture–psychological perspective. In G. Széll, D. Ehrig, U. Staroske, & U. Széll (Eds.), *Quality of life and working life in comparison* (pp. 377–385). Bern, Switzerland: Peter Lang Publishing Group.

Trommsdorff, G., Cole, P. M., Mishra, R. C. Niraula, R. R., & Park, Y-S. (in preparation). *Cross-cultural study on parents' naïve theories regarding development of emotions regulation and social behavior.* Unpublished manuscript, University of Konstanz, Konstanz, Germany.

Trommsdorff, G., & Friedlmeier, W. (2004). Zum Verhältnis zwischen Kultur und Individuum aus der Perspektive der kulturvergleichenden Psychologie. In A. Assmann, U. Gaier, & G. Trommsdorff (Eds.), *Positionen der Kulturanthropologie* (pp. 358–386). Frankfurt, Germany: Suhrkamp.

Trommsdorff, G., & Friedlmeier, W. (2010). Preschool girls' distress and mothers' sensitivity in Japan and Germany. *European Journal of Developmental Psychology, 7,* 350–370.

Trommsdorff, G., Friedlmeier, W., & Mayer, B. (2007). Sympathy, distress, and prosocial behavior of preschool children in four cultures. *International Journal of Behavioral Development, 31,* 284–293.

Trommsdorff, G., & Kornadt, H.-J. (2003). Parent–child relations in cross-cultural perspective. In L. Kuczynski (Ed.), *Handbook of dynamics in parent–child relations* (pp. 271–306). Thousand Oaks, CA: Sage.

Trommsdorff, G., Mishra, R. C., Heilkamp, T., von Suchodoletz, A., & Merkel, F. (2009). [Emotion regulation of Indian and German preschool children]. Unpublished raw data, University of Konstanz, Konstanz, Germany.

Trommsdorff, G., & Nauck, B. (Eds.). (2005). *The value of children in cross-cultural perspective. Case studies from eight societies.* Lengerich, Germany: Pabst Science.

Trommsdorff, G., & Rothbaum, F. (2008). Development of emotion regulation in cultural context. In S. Ismer, S. Jung, S. Kronast, C. v. Scheve, & M. Vande-kerckhove (Eds.), *Regulating emotions: Social necessity and biological inheritance* (pp. 85–120). London and New York: Blackwell.

Tsai, J. L., Miao, F. F., Seppala, E., Fung, H. H., & Yeung, D. Y. (2007). Influence and adjustment goals: Sources of cultural differences in ideal affect. *Journal of Personality and Social Psychology, 92*(6), 1102–1117.

Underwood, B., & Moore, B. (1982). Perspective-taking and altruism. *Psychological Bulletin, 91*, 143–173.

Wang, Y. Z., Wiley, A. R., & Chiu, C.-Y. (2008). Independence-supportive praise versus interdependence-promoting praise. *International Journal of Behavioral Development, 32*, 13–20.

Weisz, J. R., Rothbaum, F. M., & Blackburn, T. C. (1984). Standing out and standing in: The psychology of control in America and Japan. *American Psychologist, 39*, 955–969.

Whiting, B. B., & Whiting, J. W. M. (1975). *Children of six cultures: A psychocultural analysis.* Cambridge, MA: Harvard University Press.

Zahn-Waxler, C., & Robinson, J. (1995). Empathy and guilt: Early origins of feelings of responsibility. In J. P. Tangney & K. W. Fischer (Eds.), *Self-conscious emotions: The psychology of shame, guilt, embarrassment, and pride* (pp. 143–173). New York: Guilford Press.

Zahn-Waxler, C., Robinson, J. L., & Emde, R. N. (1992). The development of empathy in twins. *Developmental Psychology, 28*, 1038–1047.

CHAPTER 7

Different Faces of Autonomy

HEIDI KELLER *and* HILTRUD OTTO

Autonomy is regarded as a basic human need (Angyal, 1951; Bakan, 1966; Deci & Ryan, 1991) and thus as a universal developmental goal. It is defined as the psychological capacity to control one's life and one's actions and limit the role of other individuals accordingly. It is based on the philosophy of the right of the individual to self-determination and self-governance through free volition. Autonomy is seen as the expression of agency (Bandura, 1989), that is, the general competence to master one's life in one's own, self-defined way. The self has stable boundaries that are regarded as a necessary precondition for health and well-being (Chirkov, Ryan, Kim, & Kaplan, 2003; Kăgitcibaşi, 2005). From cultural and cross-cultural perspectives, autonomy has been described as expressing the Western ideal of the separate and independent self (Markus & Kitayama, 1991). This conception is often contrasted with a relational cultural orientation in which relatedness is the organizer of development toward an interdependent self, invoking hierarchy and family cohesion. The interdependent self is largely prevalent in the non-Western majority world. Interdependent individuals view responsiveness to the needs of others as a fundamental commitment, whereas independent individuals maintain a balance between prosocial concerns and their own individual freedom to satisfy the concerns by choosing among diverse options (Miller, 1994).

There has been a long-standing debate in the literature as to whether autonomy and relatedness are mutually exclusive, implying that the interdependent self is not considered as being fully agentic (Iyengar & Lepper,

164

1999). This debate, however, can be regarded as a thing of the past, since the coexistence of autonomy and relatedness has been conceptualized theoretically and demonstrated empirically (Deci & Ryan, 1991; Kăgitcibaşi, 1996; Keller, Demuth, & Yovsi, 2008; Kuhl & Keller, 2008). Nonetheless, different proponents hold divergent views on the definition and meaning of autonomy.

Kăgitcibaşi (1995, 1996) was among the first researchers to make a strong case for combining autonomy and relatedness. She proposed two independent dimensions that underlie the independent and interdependent self, namely, the dimension of interpersonal distance, with the polarities of relatedness and separateness, and the dimension of agency, with the polarities of autonomy and heteronomy. The autonomy–heteronomy dimension is defined in broad Piagetian terms of autonomous or heteronomous morality (1948), with heteronomy representing being subject to another's rule and autonomy representing the state of self-governance. Through the combinations possible in a four-field schema, she differentiates four self-concepts: the independent (autonomous and separate), the interdependent (heteronomous and related), the autonomous–related combination (high in both autonomy and relatedness) and the heteronomous–separated combination (which is not further elaborated, but rather regarded as pathological). However, Kăgitcibaşi's (1996) model contains an implicit value dimension: following Piaget's understanding, heteronomy is viewed as a less mature form of morality, with the higher developmental achievement being autonomous morality. In this sense, the interdependent self as heteronomous and relational would not qualify as agentic and volitional. The concept of autonomy is considered as essentially the same within this framework, regardless of its combination with separateness or relatedness.

There are other approaches that propose to conceptualize various modes of agency and that posit interdependence as equally agentic. In this sense, Kitayama and Ushida (2003) differentiate between independent and interdependent agency. Independent agency, in line with the independent self, defines agency as the expression of personal desires, wishes, and intentions as separate from those of others. Others are made meaningful only in reference to the person's inner attributes, such as his or her own goals, wishes, and desires, thus representing the Western conception of autonomy. Interdependent agency, in line with the interdependent self, defines agency as individuals actively referencing others "to affirm their place in the social order" (Yeh, Bedford, & Yang, 2009, p. 214). The goals, desires, and needs of others are often not separable from one's own. Markus and Kitayama (2003) proposed a different terminology for these two models of agency, namely, disjoint (independent) and conjoint (interdependent) agency. These two models of agency are the key modes of action and thought that best capture cultural differences, especially between European American and

East Asian individuals. Similar distinctions were made by Hobfoll and colleagues (Hobfoll, Schroder, Wells, & Malek, 2002) as self-mastery versus
communal mastery, by Gore and Cross (2006) as relationally autonomous
reasons and personally autonomous reasons, and by Yeh und Yang (2006)
as individuating and relating autonomy.

Rudy and colleagues (Rudy, Sheldon, Awong, & Tan, 2007) have a
slightly different perspective with their conception of inclusive versus individual autonomy. They draw on cross-cultural theories and self-determination
theory, arguing that these two latter frameworks emphasize different
aspects. Cross-cultural research focuses on the person who is behaving,
that is, the independent or interdependent self, whereas self-determination
theory focuses on the motivational basis for behavior (autonomous or controlled). Rudy and colleagues (2007) assume that a person who acts may
feel either independent and distinct from others or interdependent and
connected to important others, though his or her motivational basis can
range from controlled to autonomous motivation. Feelings of behavioral
autonomy and feelings of being an independent self thus do not necessarily
have to converge.

All the previous conceptions share the goal of differentiating between
two modes of agency or autonomy, namely, independent (personal, individual, self-determined) and interdependent (relational, communal, inclusive);
they all refer to psychological dimensions as defined beforehand–that is,
wishes, intentions, or volition—and thus to the reflexive individual focusing on inner states and the mental way of being.

All of these approaches generally describe psychological autonomy,
although they differ with respect to the locus of control and the point of
reference. The locus of control can be individual (involving independent
agency, disjointed agency, individual autonomy, individuating autonomy,
self-mastery, personally autonomous reasons) or communal (involving
interdependent agency, conjoint agency, inclusive autonomy, relating autonomy, communal mastery, relationally autonomous reasons). The point of
reference—that is, whom the concerns of autonomy are directed toward—
can be the individual (self) or the communal agent (others). We prefer to
label these conceptions as *individual psychological autonomy* and *communal psychological autonomy*. Individual psychological autonomy refers
to personal desires, wishes, and intentions; as such, individual psychological autonomy emphasizes the self-contained and separated individual with
stable ego boundaries; *communal psychological autonomy*, on the other
hand, refers to the desires, wishes, and intentions of a social unit that need
to be addressed in order to keep the unit healthy and functioning. This
characterization does not imply that the goals, desires, and needs of others are necessarily different from one's own—they may coincide or not.
Communal psychological autonomy is not imposed or controlled from the

outside (Rudy et al., 2007) but rather self-selected and self-determined. Therefore one's own volition is also central in determining communal psychological autonomy.

Individual psychological autonomy can be defined as the self-centered feeling of having control and being in control of all available choices (Heckhausen & Schulz, 1995). Communal psychological autonomy can be regarded as a moral feeling of obligation and respect that is embedded in a hierarchical social system, usually the age and gender hierarchy of the family. Individual psychological autonomy is committed to the obligation to optimize self-development and the realization of one's own wishes and needs; in this context, adopting the needs of others is regarded as rumination or infiltration of external control (Ryan, Kuhl, & Deci, 1997), which may potentially threaten the self. Communal psychological autonomy, in contrast, culminates in the maintenance and care of the communal agent, revealing the understanding of a mature way of being (Killen, 1997). Well-being can only be achieved when one's feeling of obligation is met and satisfied. The primary responsibility for individual psychological autonomy is the development and protection of the self, while the primary responsibility for communal psychological autonomy is the support and protection of the communal system.

Both modes of autonomy may be regarded as universal capacities in that both refer to the same mental processes and both are based on reflective and self-reflective ways of being. They may coexist within individuals but may be differently emphasized, depending on prevailing cultural conceptions of the self. Action is implicitly contained in psychological autonomy. However, the action component is less pronounced than the reflection component in social discourses. This phenomenon can be seen, for example, in psychological theories where the intention is emphasized more strongly than the effect of an action (e.g., Piaget, 1948) or the mode of argumentation more relevant than the behavior (e.g., Kohlberg, Levine, & Hewer, 1983). In our conceptualization, we seek to capture the action component as a separate dimension of autonomy. Action autonomy represents the individual's capacity to act individually in a self-responsible and self-controlled way. This capacity comprises the planning and performance of an action (Bratman, 1987; Heckhausen & Heckhausen, 2006) under the control of the acting individual. Action autonomy becomes a central developmental task during early childhood. Whether in the service of the self or the social unit, it is always based on individual responsibility. Also, action autonomy is considered to be a universal human propensity. While psychological autonomy refers to the reflection of individual choices and control, action autonomy refers to the performance and control of individual actions, which may either be in the service of the individual or the social unit. Figure 7.1 depicts the conceptions and interrelationships of action autonomy and psychological autonomy.

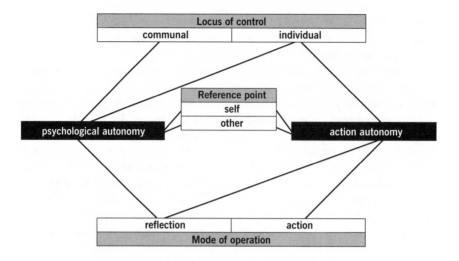

FIGURE 7.1. Psychological autonomy and action autonomy.

As Figure 7.1 shows, psychological autonomy can be controlled by the individual (individual psychological autonomy) or the communal system (communal psychological autonomy); in contrast, action autonomy is always controlled by the individual. Both components of autonomy may refer to either the individual self or to others. They differ again with respect to the mode of operation in that psychological autonomy always includes reflection while action autonomy may be based on reflective processes but can also consist of a nonreflective action.

So far, conceptions of autonomy are not really linked to particular developmental stages, although most of the empirical research concerning autonomy addresses adolescents with the assumption that during adolescence the development of autonomy and independence is a fundamental and universal task (Kăgitcibaşi, 1995, 1996; Stewart, Bond, Deeds, & Chung, 1999). We deal with a different developmental phase and developmental task, that is, parental socialization strategies during infancy. Early socialization strategies are especially prone to be informative about the cultural conceptions of autonomy, because parents embody their developmental goals in their ethnotheories and pursue them through their actions. Parental socialization strategies vary across cultures and can be shown to vary in the emphasis placed on either psychological or action autonomy. In the remainder of this chapter, we present two socialization scenarios that emphasize action autonomy and psychological autonomy (particularly individual psychological autonomy) differently.

Environmental Settings for the Development of Autonomy

We have argued that autonomy is a necessary prerequisite for becoming competent in the environment in which one lives. However, human environments vary greatly; offering different ecocultural constraints and opportunities and requiring different adaptations to cope with the particular challenges (Keller & Greenfield, 2000). In this chapter, we discuss two prototypical environments that differ markedly with respect to the conception of autonomy most suited to living and thriving in that environment. One prototypical environment is represented by the rural agrarian subsistence-based economy, which encourages cooperation among the members of the social unit. The other prototype is represented in the postindustrial urban lifestyle, where competition among relatively anonymous individuals for the publicly available resources is crucial for successful living.

These two contexts differ dramatically in terms of their sociodemographic characteristics. The agrarian subsistence-based environment is associated with low levels of formal education, the early onset of reproduction, and large numbers of children. The (predominantly Western) urban lifestyle of intense competitiveness is associated with high levels of formal education, a comparatively late beginning of reproduction, and small numbers of offspring.

We use North West Cameroonian Nso mothers to represent the subsistence-based agrarian prototype. Nso women typically have their first baby in their late teens and usually have three to eight children (Keller, 2007; Lamm, 2008; Otto, 2008; Yovsi, 2003). The mean fertility rate in Cameroon is 4.3 children per woman (The World Fact Book, 2009). Nso families are patrilineal and patrilocal and strictly hierarchically organized. The Nso live together in extended families, with the oldest male being the family head, and their livelihood is one of subsistence-based farming in which women do the bulk of the farm work.

Nso women normally work until the moment of childbirth and then resume their daily routines (i.e., going to the fields, doing household chores, and selling crops) soon afterward. Since Nso babies grow up in extended families, they have many different caretakers from early on (Lamm, 2008). Usually Nso mothers breastfeed their babies for about 2 years (Yovsi & Keller, 2007); while they are nursing, babies are usually in close proximity to their mothers—even when cared for by others. However, Nso mothers are often not the main and favorite caretaker of their babies (Otto, 2008), and fathers are rarely involved in early childcare issues. Nso babies spend much of the daytime being carried on the backs of their mothers, grandmothers, or sibling caretakers; during the night, they sleep with their mothers and other family members and are able to breastfeed on demand without disturbing their mothers' sleep.

We use middle-class Germans to represent the urban postindustrial (Western) prototype. Middle-class German mothers plan for their first child during their late twenties once they have finished their higher education and settled into their respective careers (Statistisches Bundesamt: Geburten in Deutschland, Stand 2007). They prefer to enjoy their independence, typically enjoying an active nightlife and traveling extensively before starting a family. In an interview about family planning, an 18-year-old German university student explained that she first wants to work and to travel a lot later and then to be able to provide her children with the kind of lifestyle that she was accustomed to as a child (P2; Döge & Keller, 2009). The first child is often the only one in a German family, with women having a mean fertility rate of 1.4 (Statistisches Bundesamt, 2007). Since this number represents the country's mean fertility rate, middle-class families may actually can be expected to have even fewer children. Middle-class mothers usually take a maternity leave of up to 12 months. With the advent of relatively new government-supported programs, fathers can also take paternal leave. However, fathers still take less care of their infant children than mothers do; only 13% of German fathers take a paternal leave of 12 months (Drucksache des Deutschen Bundestages, 2008). Babies spend their first years mainly with their mothers during the day, and only 18% of children younger than 3 years old attend public daycare centers or are cared for by nonfamily members. Only by age 3 do the majority of children attend daycare regularly. Typically, babies have their own room in which to sleep early on, but of often, because of nocturnal protests, parents decide to keep the infant's bed or crib in the parents' bedroom. About half of German mothers breastfeed their infants for the first 3–6 months and start feeding the baby with solid food from then on (Baumgarten, 2004). During a typical day, babies interact most often with their mothers and less frequently with their fathers, siblings, and grandparents.

In order to ensure competence in mastering such diverse living conditions, humans have developed adaptive frames of mind that operate on conscious as well as nonconscious levels of information processing. These frames of mind are cultural models that express norms, values, and beliefs that are then translated into actual behavior, for example, parenting behavior as it affects the development of autonomy. It appears obvious that two totally different conceptions of autonomy are necessary in order to become competent in these two extremely different environments. In the following section, the divergent behavioral strategies of parents that promote these very different modes of autonomy in early infancy are discussed.

Behavioral Contexts for the Development
of Autonomy: Proximal and Distal Parenting

Parents, along with the other caretakers in the two environments that we have previously described, employ extremely different behavioral strategies when interacting with small babies. These differences can be captured in the Component Model of Parenting (Keller, 2000, 2007; Keller, Hentschel, et al., 2004), which considers not only universal propensities but also the cultural idiosyncrasies of parent–infant interactions. Although German middle-class mothers and Cameroonian Nso mothers use much the same parenting systems and interactional mechanisms when caring for infants and small children, they vary in the relative emphasis they place on them in general, as well as on particular aspects of them.

The behavioral parenting strategy of German middle-class mothers uses a distal (as opposed to proximal) parenting style, focusing on verbal exchanges, object play, and face-to-face contact within the context of exclusive attention. The baby, as the central object and center of attention, typically lies on his or her back on a blanket or bed with little or no body contact with the interacting partner; the mother leans over the baby, establishing face-to-face contact and utilizing object stimulation in ongoing verbal conversations. During the day babies are often put in baby carriers or buggies, while during the night they are supposed to sleep in their own bed. In general, parents support their children's inclination to entertain themselves or to engage in activities on their own as well as to choose the activities they "want" to perform with their parents; the physical contact between the infant and caretaker is often limited. Figures 7.2–7.4 illustrate typical everyday situations in German middle-class families with small children. Figure 7.2 shows a mother interacting with her 3-month-old baby in the typical face-to-face position, her attention focused exclusively on the baby. Figure 7.3 shows a one-and-a-half-year old baby lying in her own bed. Figure 7.4 shows a mother with her 6-month-old baby playing with various toys, the mother, again, exclusively focused on the child in the typical face-to-face position.

The rural Nso caregivers use a proximal parenting style with an emphasis on primary care, physical closeness, and body stimulation in the context of shared attention (Keller, 2007; Keller, Kärtner, Borke, Yovsi, & Kleis, 2005; Keller, Kuensemueller, et al. 2005). Typically, Nso mothers try to get their babies used to many different caretakers from early on, since this practice enables them to pursue their own work in an environment where free time is an unaffordable luxury (Otto, 2008). Hence, various people carry the babies around, typically wrapped in a piece of cloth, on their back. However, the multiple caretakers have a keen sense of the needs of the baby—even children between 4 and 8 years of age say that they feel

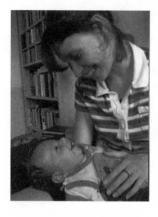

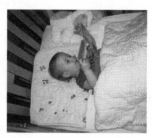

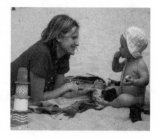

FIGURE 7.2. German mother with her 3-month-old baby in face-to-face position. Copyright 2010 by the Department of Culture and Development, University of Osnabrück. Reprinted by permission.

FIGURE 7.3. German 18-month-old child in her own bed "reading" a book. Copyright 2010 by the Department of Culture and Development, University of Osnabrück. Reprinted by permission.

FIGURE 7.4. German mother with her 6-month-old child, playing in face-to-face position. Copyright 2010 by the Department of Culture and Development, University of Osnabrück. Reprinted by permission.

competent to care for a baby, and some 70% of the caretakers believed themselves to be the best babysitter for a baby (Lamm, 2008). Sibling caregivers have similar opinions to their mothers on what constitutes good care for a small baby, and they act accordingly (Lamm, 2008). Like Nso mothers, the sibling caregivers focus on body contact and primary care in their caregiving strategies.

Typical everyday experiences of Cameroonian Nso babies are depicted in Figures 7.5–7.7. Figure 7.5 shows a group of Nso children, among them a 4-month-old baby being carried on the back of a sibling caretaker. Figure 7.6 shows a proud Nso mother showing off the perfect bodily control that her 3-month-old daughter has already achieved. Finally, Figure 7.7 shows a sibling caretaker stimulating a 3-month-old baby motorically by tossing her up and down.

It becomes evident from looking at the photographs that the German mothers' distal interaction style, combined with exclusive attention, helps to foster a sense of individuality, early agency, and self-efficacy in the babies, which can be regarded as a necessary prerequisite for the development of individual psychological autonomy. Correspondingly, the Cameroonian Nso mothers' proximal interaction style, with its focus on motor stimulation, accelerates their infants' motor development, thereby help-

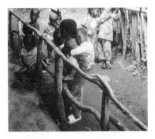

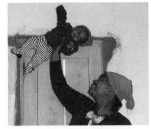

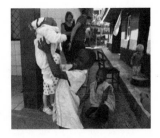

FIGURE 7.5. Older sibling carries a 4-month-old Nso baby. Copyright 2010 by the Department of Culture and Development, University of Osnabrück. Reprinted by permission.

FIGURE 7.6. Nso mother lifts her 3-month-old daughter up in the air. Copyright 2010 by the Department of Culture and Development, University of Osnabrück. Reprinted by permission.

FIGURE 7.7. Nso sibling caretaker tosses a 3-month-old baby up and down. Copyright 2010 by the Department of Culture and Development, University of Osnabrück. Reprinted by permission.

ing to promote early action autonomy. At the same time, shared attention mechanisms and multiple caregiver arrangements make the babies aware of the larger social community and facilitate the development of a communal sense of self.

Narrative Envelopes for the Development of Autonomy: Mother–Infant Dialogues

Verbal/vocal dialogues with infants are another parenting system that is saturated with cultural meaning. In a microanalytic study of the vocal/verbal communication patterns used in mother–infant communication during the first 3 months, Keller and colleagues (Keller, Otto, Lamm, Yovsi, & Kärtner, 2008) found that German middle-class mothers use a diachronous dialogue structure, where the Cameroonian Nso mothers follow a synchronous dialogue structure.

The diachronous style of German middle-class mothers is responsive to the infants' communicative initiatives in that the mothers react to the infants' vocal signals by using an alternating turn-taking style of communication (Keller, 2007; Keller et al., 2006); this responsive communication style helps infants develop a feeling of their own agency in interactional situations. In contrast, the synchronous style found in Cameroonian mother–infant communication is characterized by overlapping vocalizations/verbalizations in which mothers often start talking simultaneously when their babies vocalize; this co-action mode can be assumed to foster the experience of synchrony and harmony between interaction partners (Keller, Otto, et al., 2008), and this overlapping communication style helps babies to perceive themselves as part of a social action, thereby supporting the development of a communal self.

Additionally, Demuth (2008) analyzed the discursive practices of mothers and their 3-month-old infants qualitatively and found that German middle-class mothers use mainly cooperative discourse patterns. They treat the child as a quasi-equal interaction partner, granting him or her a high degree of psychological autonomy by negotiating everything with the child: "Do we wanna do gymnastics once more? Do we both wanna do gymnastics once more?" (Muenster17). And though the preverbal 3-month-olds are unable to answer their mothers, the mothers ask for their children's preferences and individual wishes: "Is it better like this? Not yet? Better like this?" (Muenster06).

In contrast, the Cameroonian Nso mothers use a hierarchical discourse structure where the child has to obey and comply: "Don't cry again! We don't cry in Mbah! Stop fast!" (Nso09) or "You should be dancing! He? You should keep quiet!" (Nso06). By instructing the child to stop crying, the Nso mothers also convey the wider social norms of behavior, that is, to keep quiet. The Nso mothers use directives frequently, demanding and teaching proper demeanor in their children, which consists mainly of keeping quiet.

It is obvious that both the German middle-class mothers and the Cameroonian Nso mothers inculcate autonomy in their dialogues with the 3-month-old infants—but regarding very different domains. In brief, German mothers stress self-expression, whereas Nso mothers stress self-regulation.

German middle-class mothers embrace and further encourage what their child does and wishes; thereby their children learn to put forward their own views and to choose what they want to do. German children are supposed to develop their own mind, to discuss matters, to reflect on their experiences, and very largely to make their own decisions. Parents generally do not want their children to "blindly" obey their directives, and they generally consider mature forms of social regulation to be subject to voluntary, not mandatory, compliance (Keller, Yovsi, et al., 2004). Figure 7.8 shows a German middle class mother negotiating with her 19-month-old toddler on a compliance task. Thus, early mother–infant interactions convey the importance of individual psychological autonomy.

In the Nso culture, mothers know what is best for their children. Hence, the mothers monitor, direct, and control the child's activities by taking the lead in interactional situations, even verbally. Nso children are not granted much individual psychological autonomy; clear directives teach children from early on how they are expected to behave. Nso children should read-

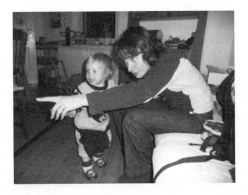

FIGURE 7.8. German mother and her son negotiating over a compliance issue. Copyright 2010 by the Department of Culture and Development, University of Osnabrück. Reprinted by permission.

ily understand from the situational context how to behave—without negotiations or questions. Consequently Nso toddlers comply easily when, for example, they are asked to fetch objects during a compliance task (Keller, Yovsi, et al., 2004). Therefore, their autonomy is more or less based on concrete actions. Thus, for example, children are expected to run errands, implying that they can move around unattended in the community. Similarly, they are allowed to handle household equipment to learn how to use it; even 1-year olds may be seen handling large, sharp knives, as illustrated in Figure. 7.9.

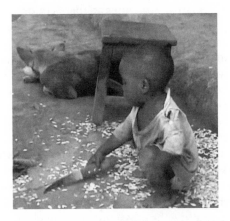

FIGURE 7.9. A 1-year-old Nso boy handling a large knife. Copyright 2010 by the Department of Culture and Development, University of Osnabrück. Reprinted by permission.

Socialization Goals as They Relate
to Different Types of Autonomy

Parental behavior is affected by conscious and/or unconscious parenting goals that largely define desirable developmental outcomes. In the two prototypical environments that we have discussed, parenting goals and beliefs differ substantially.

German middle-class mothers believe that every child has his or her own character and personality and that should be accepted by all: "An ideal child for me is when they, yes, when they develop, when they have their own personality. . . . They form their own personality" (D17). The ideal state of mind of a child is being happy ("I believe a child is ideal when it has the feeling for him- or herself to be happy [D10]"), having his or her own opinion ("They do not need to do what they are told [D17]") and being curious and inquisitive ("Thirst of knowledge—is this how it is called? I would like that" [D15]).

A good mother is supposed to have an intimate, close relationship with her child and yet grant that child personal freedom: "A good mother for me is loving, in any case. This very important . . . having time for the children . . . to give the security, yet nevertheless grant freedom to some degree" (D1).

The values that these mothers emphasize refer to respecting others as individual agents: "To respect the other one the way he or she is . . . because that . . . is important for living together in life and for . . . development towards a self-confident individual, who can master later in life his life independently" (D10).

In sum, the German mothers want their children to grow up in an atmosphere of psychological closeness and individual freedom. Respect for others is based on equality and deliberate choice. Becoming an independent and self-assured individual is a primary socialization goal. Parental aspirations are transmitted in discourses that center around the reflection of their own and others' state of mind—but from an individual perspective. Psychological autonomy is therefore the armamentarium to achieve these goals.

Rural Cameroonian Nso mothers want to instill into their children respect for others, obedience, and social harmony as early as possible (Keller, Lamm, et al., 2006). Whereas the German middle-class mothers stress the individuality of each child's personality, the Nso mothers have a clear image of a good/ideal child: "A good child is one who when you are leaving the house, you give him assignments, he cleans the dishes, cleans the dresses. When he stays he will do all these things" (KR3). Mothers conform in their views: "A good child is one who works hard in the house, helps you in everything, does anything you ask him or her to do" (KR17), or "Even no matter where you send the child, it will not be angry and go on the errand. Even when you ask the child to go to the farm and bring anything . . . and you ask for him to bring to the farm, he doesn't have any problem. Is never angry, no matter what you ask her to do, she'll do" (KR7). However, the Cameroonian mothers want their children to perform actions in a self-responsible way not just in a work-based setting but also in the broader social context: "A good child, . . . if she goes out, she cannot talk carelessly to an elderly person" (K18); "a good child is one who greets people. And when you come to the house and say the parents are not there, it should welcome you very well. Anywhere the child goes, it behaves well. You know that it's a good child" (KR2).

A responsible mother therefore educates her children to develop these competencies and attitudes, since "when you see the way the children behave, it reflects the way the mother teaches them" (KR2). Accordingly, a good mother is one who teaches her children in both domains (house-/farmwork and proper demeanor) well: "I can teach my children that they should always greet people when they meet them. . . . And that they should be hard-working in the house. And anywhere they go, they have to work there" (KR2).

The virtues that Nso children should learn are based on religion: "I want them to grow up with good manners . . . in a Godly manner. And anything you do, you know you have to pray and put it in God's hands first. You have to pray for it. And know that it is God who gives force (strength) to human beings to do anything that you have to do" (KR21).

In sum, the Nso mothers want their children to grow up as respectful and obedient children who demonstrate their good manners to the social community. Religion is the foundation of life; within this social climate Nso children are expected to support and help the mothers with household chores and babysitting. In order to perform these chores sufficiently and independently, action competence is the armamentarium to be able to fulfill the role expectations.

Socialization Strategies as Avenues toward Psychological Autonomy and Action Autonomy

Parental socialization strategies differ between the urban German and the rural Cameroonian socialization context. These differences in socialization strategies entail profound consequences for the development of autonomy in infants. Although both conceptions of autonomy discussed in this chapter can be regarded as universal human needs, psychological autonomy and action autonomy are emphasized differently in the two contexts. German middle-class parents nurture individual psychological autonomy from their infants' earliest days of life. A focus on distal interactive behaviors and parent–infant dialogues focusing on the individual psychological experiences of the infant allow infants to develop a sense of autonomous agency and self-efficacy almost from birth.

Cameroonian Nso mothers foster the development of communal psychological autonomy with the early expression of action autonomy. Babies experience a proximal interaction style with simultaneous communication patterns; thereby, they develop a symbiotic sense of self. The developmental goals for the child are geared toward social integration and teaching the child its basic social roles. These goals require the self-responsible performance of actions. The vigorous motor stimulation, in particular, leads to accelerated motor development that enables children to perform required chores early on. The rural village child is expected to develop action competence with respect to the social communal system, which includes such tasks as self-responsible care for younger siblings, fetching firewood and water, and selling products that have been produced at home (e.g., food items).

Western middle-class children also develop action competence, but mainly in relation to the individual self. They are supported in their natural desire to be self-assertive, to perform self-directed actions, and to exert control over the environment (e.g., to act in their own self-interest both with other children and with their parents). Accordingly, children from very early on insist on their right to do things on their own when they limit their parents' tendencies to help them (e.g. they may want to build their own piles of blocks without their mother's help or may want to turn pages in children's books before their father has finished reading them).

The life of German children is dominated by the philosophical concept "I am what I am, I am my own special creation," a theme that has been incorporated into various pieces of music since the 1980s (beginning in 1983, by Jerry Herman). The contrasting philosophy, "I am because we are," is a common saying in rural sub-Saharan African villages. Both philosophies of life reflect the underlying cultural models and highlight the prevailing conceptions of autonomy.

The Learning Contexts of Different Conceptions of Autonomy

Early cultural messages are appropriated and instantiated in the learning environments of children. The skills that Cameroonian Nso children need most are subsistence survival skills. These skills are acquired through the informal practices of observation and imitation. This popular learning mode in rural families has also been described as characteristic of rural

Mexican Mayan children, specifically, participation in everyday activities through observation and imitation (Greenfield, 2004; Maynard, 2002; Morelli, Rogoff, & Angelillo, 2003). Children are not verbally instructed how to use a plow or prepare a meal. Instead, they are supposed to watch closely what elders do and to start acting themselves when they feel confident enough to master the task. Peer group interactions, in particular, are an important medium for cultural teaching and learning, since children of different ages spend a lot of time together. Sometimes such peer groups roam around, sometimes they do household chores such as washing clothes and bathing themselves at the same time (see Figure 7.10). These everyday activities are learning scenarios in which the young ones watch the elders closely (see Figure 7.11), and the elders thereby tutor the young ones, even if inadvertently (see Maynard, 2002, for a discussion of cultural teaching and learning among Mexican Mayan children). In these environments there is no separation between knowing and doing; instead, the activity itself and the context in which it takes place are sufficient for children to learn a new task without reflecting upon the task, the performance, and the acting individual. This action-based apprenticeship model (Greenfield, Maynard, & Childs, 2000; Keller, 2007) leads to a high level of action autonomy.

The majority of German middle-class children learn particular skills in particular teaching environments (e.g., in nursery school, music classes,

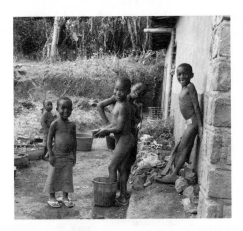

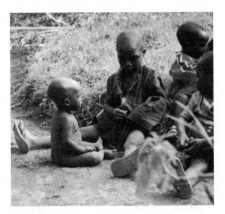

FIGURE 7.10. Nso peer group washing dresses and taking a bath. Copyright 2010 by the Department of Culture and Development, University of Osnabrück. Reprinted by permission.

FIGURE 7.11. Nso child watching older children closely. Copyright 2010 by the Department of Culture and Development, University of Osnabrück. Reprinted by permission.

science training, and other settings). Education is based very much on cognitive abilities and technological intelligence (Mundy-Castle, 1974; Neisser et al., 1996). Learning is mainly embodied in verbal discourses. Children are expected to play an active role in the learning process. Teachers provide information, and the children ask questions and discuss and negotiate the information with the teacher (Nucci, Saxe, & Turiel, 2000). Thus, formal learning environments mirror the mode of social exchange and interaction in the family. Children experience a separation between knowing and doing, since knowing and reflecting on knowledge are emphasized more than actually doing (Brown, Collins, & Duguid, 1989). Choices are important ingredients in learning, which may be enacted at various levels within the learning process (e.g., children may decide which animal they wish to portray in a nursery school skit—see Figures 7.12 and 7.13). Thereby, the educational settings as well as the socialization practices in the family primarily foster psychological autonomy.

Compared to the Cameroonian Nso children, German middle-class children are bombarded with choices, and although many of these choices deal with actions, they require the child to reflect about preferences, competencies, and future consequences. In the end, these actions are aimed at the development of personal talents and individuality and finally rely on and support individual psychological autonomy. These actions may be socially induced, but they are nevertheless in the service of the individual. Cameroonian Nso children feel obligated to perform tasks exactly in the ways that are expected to. Individualized manifestations of freedom or independence are not cherished, but, rather, the normative way of doing things in the community is closely controlled and supervised.

Thus, these two very different conceptions of autonomy have pervasive effects on children's learning and development in the two societies.

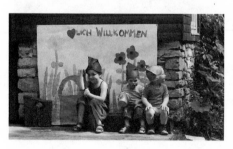

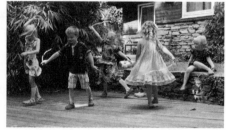

FIGURE 7.12. German children dressed up as dwarfs.

FIGURE 7.13. German children playing.

Conclusion

Humans are uniquely afforded a wide universal repertoire of learning propensities and modes of information processing. However, specific cultural contexts predispose one toward developing certain skills in order to become a competent and successful member of one's native community. We have presented conceptions of autonomy that differentiate between psychological autonomy and action autonomy as parts of this universal repertoire. Psychological autonomy can be in the service of the individual or the social unit of which the individual is a part. It is based on the reflective capacity of the human mind. Action autonomy defines the capacity for the individually responsible performance of actions. This performance can be in the service of the self or the social unit—yet it is not socially imbued.

We have presented two very different prototypical environments that emphasize individual psychological autonomy and action autonomy in very different ways. Parents support their children's development and education in line with these cultural models. Children construct and co-construct their development along different pathways, acquiring and putting into practice different socioemotional and cognitive skills along different time lines (Keller, 2007). There are a multiplicity of cultural contexts that present sociodemographic as well as sociocultural combinations and mixtures of these prototypes. Urban educated middle-class families in traditionally interdependent societies that have been described as autonomous-related by Kăgitcibași (1997) would represent an interesting arena for further study, as would migrants who must often negotiate the change from environments emphasizing on action autonomy to one where the public appreciates psychological autonomy.

Basically, parental socialization strategies aim at supporting their children's development into, ultimately, competent and responsible adults. Differentially focusing on psychological autonomy versus action autonomy also entails different conceptions of responsibility. Children raised with the goal of psychological autonomy foremost in mind are geared toward being responsible for themselves primarily, and they define responsibility for others from their own point of view. Conversely, children raised with the goal of early action autonomy are geared toward being responsible for others, and they define responsibilities chiefly in terms of the communal point of view. Parents who assign their children opportunities for autonomous choice and decision making thereby provide them with the reflective psychological tools that are necessary for success in a world that is characterized by competition. In contrast, action autonomy takes on greater ugency in contexts where children have to grow up fast in order to handle the demands of communal responsibilities. Parents who emphasize action autonomy enable their children to take on social responsibilities early in a world mainly characterized by cooperative efforts.

Of course, in today's world Western middle-class children also acquire action autonomy, and rural children in non-Western societies also acquire psychological autonomy. In this chapter, we highlighted the culturally dominant modes of childrearing in two distinctively different environments. Much more conceptual and empirical work is needed to more fully understand the multiple combinations that are possible and desirable in shaping future childrearing practices.

References

Angyal, A. (1951). A theoretical model for personality studies. *Journal of Personality, 20,* 131–142.

Bakan, D. (1966). *The duality of human existence: Isolation and communication in Western man.* Chicago: Rand McNally.

Bandura, A. (1989). Human agency in social cognitive theory. *American Psychologist, 44,* 1175–1184.

Baumgarten, K. (2004). Tagungsbericht zum Internationalen Symposium Zehn Jahre Nationale Stillkommission in Deutschland [Conference proceedings on the occasion of the 10th anniversary of the National Breastfeeding Committee]. *Deutsche Hebammen-Zeitschrift, 12,* 2004. Retrieved December 30, 2009, from *www.viktoria11.de/artikel/Still-Symposium_Berlin.html.*

Bratman, M. E. (1987). *Intentions, plans, and practical reason.* Cambridge, MA: Harvard University Press.

Brown, J. S., Collins, A., & Duguid, P. (1989). Situated cognition and the culture of learning. *Educational Researcher, 18,* 32–42.

Chirkov, V., Ryan, R. M., Kim, Y., & Kaplan, U. (2003). Differentiating autonomy from individualism and independence: A self-determination theory perspective on internalization of cultural orientations and well-being. *Journal of Personality and Social Psychology, 84*(1), 97–110.

Deci, E. L., & Ryan, R. M. (1991). A motivational approach to self: Integration in personality. In E. Dienstbier (Ed.), *Nebraska Symposium on Motivation 1990* (pp. 237–288). Lincoln: University of Nebraska.

Demuth, C. (2008). *Talking to infants: How culture is instantiated in early mother–infant interactions: The case of Cameroonian farming Nso and North German middle-class families.* Doctoral thesis, University of Osnabrück, Faculty of Human Sciences, Department of Culture & Psychology, Osnabrück, Germany.

Döge, P., & Keller, H. (2009). *Haus, Hof, Hund, mind. 2 Kinder—Die Rolle des Sozialisationskontextes bei der Familienplanung ost- und westdeutscher Studierender [House, coutyard, dog, and at least two kids—the influence of socialization contexts for family planning of East- and West-German students].* Manuscript submitted for publication.

Drucksache des Deutschen Bundestages. (October 30, 2008). *Bericht über die Aus-*

wirkungen des Bundeselterngeld- und Elternzeitgesetzes sowie über die gege-benenfalls notwendige Weiterentwicklung [Report on the effects of laws for child credit and parental leave and their possible enhancements]. Retrieved September 30, 2009, from *dip21.bundestag.de/dip21/btd/16/107/1610770. pdf.*

Gore, J. S., & Cross, S. E. (2006). Pursuing goals for us: Relationally autonomous reasons in long-term goal pursuit, *Journal of Personality and Social Psychology, 90,* 848–861.

Greenfield, P. M. (2004). *Weaving generations together. Evolving creativity in the Maya of Chiapas.* Santa Fe, NM: Sar Press.

Greenfield, P. M., Maynard, A. E., & Childs, C. P. (2000). History, culture, learning and development. *Cross-Cultural Research, 34,* 351–374.

Heckhausen, J., & Heckhausen, H. (Eds.). (2006). *Motivation und Handeln* [Motivation and action]. Heidelberg, Germany: Springer Medizin.

Heckhausen, J., & Schulz, R. (1995). A life-span theory of control. *Psychological Review, 102*(2), 284–304.

Hobfoll, S. E., Schroder, K. E. E., Wells, M., & Malek, M. (2002). Communal versus individualistic construction of sense of mastery in facing life challenges. *Journal of Social and Clinical Psychology, 21,* 362–399.

Iyengar, S. S., & Lepper, M. R. (1999). Rethinking the role of choice: A cultural perspective on intrinsic motivation. *Journal of Personality and Social Psychology, 76,* 349–366.

Kăgitcibaşi, C. (1995). Individualism and collectivism. In J. W. Berry, M. H. Segall, & C. Kăgitcibaşi (Eds.), *Handbook of cross-cultural psychology: Vol. 3. Social behavior and applications* (2nd ed., pp. 1–49). Boston: Allyn & Bacon.

Kăgitcibaşi, C. (1996). The autonomous–relational self: a new synthesis. *European Psychologist, 1*(3), 180–186.

Kăgitcibaşi, C. (2005). Autonomy and relatedness in cultural context: Implications for self and family. *Journal of Cross-Cultural Psychology, 36,* 403–422.

Keller, H. (2000). Human parent–child relationships from an evolutionary perspective. *American Behavioral Scientist, 43*(6), 957–969.

Keller, H. (2007). *Cultures of infancy.* Mahwah, NJ: Erlbaum.

Keller, H., Demuth, C., & Yovsi, R. D. (2008). The multi-voicedness of independence and interdependence—the case of Cameroonian Nso. *Culture and Psychology, 14*(1), 115–144.

Keller, H., & Greenfield, P. M. (2000). History and future of development in cross-cultural psychology. In C. Kăgitcibaşi & Y. H. Poortinga (Eds.). *Journal of Cross-Cultural Psychology, 31*(1), 52–62.

Keller, H., Hentschel, E., Yovsi, R. D., Abels, M., Lamm, B., & Haas, V. (2004). The psycholinguistic embodiment of parental ethnotheories. A new avenue to understand cultural differences in parenting. *Culture and Psychology, 10*(3), 293–330.

Keller, H., Kärtner, J., Borke, J., Yovsi, R. D., & Kleis, A. (2005). Parenting styles and the development of the categorial self. A longitudinal study on mirror self recognition in Cameroonian Nso farming and German families. *International Journal of Behavioral Development, 29*(6), 496–504.

Keller, H., Kuensemueller, P., Abels, M., Voelker, S., Yovsi, R. D., Jensen, H., et al.

(2005). *Parenting, culture, and development. A comparative study.* San José, CR: Universidad de Costa Rica, Instituto de Investigaciones Psychologicas.

Keller, H., Lamm, B., Abels, M., Yovsi, R. D., Borke, J., Jensen, H., et al. (2006). Cultural models, socialization goals, and parenting ethnotheories. A multi-cultural analysis. *Journal of Cross-Cultural Psychology, 37*(2), 155–172.

Keller, H., Otto, H., Lamm, B., Yovsi, R. D., & Kärtner, J. (2008). The timing of verbal/vocal communications between mothers and their infants: A longitudinal cross-cultural comparison. *Infant Behavior and Development, 31*, 217–226.

Keller, H., Yovsi, R. D., Borke, J., Kärtner, J., Jensen, H., & Papaligoura, Z. (2004). Developmental consequences of early parenting experiences: Self regulation and self recognition in three cultural communities. *Child Development, 75*(6), 1745–1760.

Killen, M. (1997). Commentary: Culture, self, and development: Are cultural templates useful or stereotypic? *Developmental Review, 17*, 239–249.

Kitayama, S., & Uchida, Y. (2003). Explicit self-criticism and implicit self-regard: Evaluating self and friend in two cultures. *Journal of Experimental Social Psychology, 39*, 476–482.

Kohlberg, L., Levine, C., & Hewer, A. (1983). *Moral stages: A current formulation and a response to critics.* Basel, New York: Karger.

Kuhl, J., & Keller, H. (2008). Affect-regulation, self-development and parenting: A functional-design approach to cross-cultural differences. In R. Sorrentino & S. Yamaguchi (Eds.), *The handbook of motivation and cognition across cultures* (pp. 19–47). New York: Elsevier.

Lamm, B. (2008). *Children's ideas about infant care: A comparison of rural Nso children from Cameroon and German middle class children.* Dissertation, Faculty of Human Sciences, Institute of Psychology at the University of Osnabrück, Osnabrück, Germany.

Markus, H. R., & Kitayama, S. (1991). Culture and the self. Implications for cognition, emotion and motivation. *Psychological Review, 98*, 224–253.

Markus, H. R., & Kitayama, S. (2003). Culture, self, and the reality of the social. *Psychological Inquiry, 14*, 277–283.

Maynard, A. E. (2002). Cultural teaching. The development of teaching skills in Maya sibling interactions. *Child Development, 73*(3), 969–983.

Miller, J. G. (1994). Cultural diversity in the morality of caring: Individually oriented versus duty-based interpersonal moral codes. *Cross-Cultural Research, 28*, 3–39.

Morelli, G. A., Rogoff, B., & Angelillo, C. (2003). Cultural variation in young children's access to work or involvement in specialized child-focused activities. *International Journal of Behavioral Development, 27*, 264–274.

Mundy-Castle, A. C. (1974). Social and technological intelligence in Western and non-Western cultures. *Universitas, 4*, 46–52.

Neisser, U., Boodoo, G., Bouchard, T. J., Boykin, A. W., Brody, N., Ceci, S. J., et al. (1996). Intelligence: Knowns and unknowns. *American Psychologist, 51*, 77–101.

Nucci, L., Saxe, G., & Turiel, E. (2000). *Culture, thought and development.* Mahwah, NJ: Erlbaum.

Otto, H. (2008). *Culture-specific attachment strategies in the Cameroonian Nso: Cultural solutions to a universal developmental task.* Doctoral dissertation, University of Osnabrück, Osnabrück, Germany.

Piaget, J. (1948). *The moral judgment of the child.* Glencoe, IL: Free Press.

Rudy, D., Sheldon, K. M., Awong, T., & Tan, H. H. (2007). Autonomy, culture, and well-being: The benefits of inclusive autonomy. *Journal of Research in Personality, 41,* 983–1007.

Ryan, R. M., Kuhl, J., & Deci, E. L. (1997). Nature and autonomy: An organizational view of social and neurobiological aspects of self-regulation in behavior and development. *Development and Psychopathology, 9,* 701–728.

Statistisches Bundesamt. (2007). *Geburten in Deutschland [Birth rates in Germany].* Retrieved September 30, 2009, from *www.destatis.de/jetspeed/portal/cms/Sites/destatis/Internet/DE/Content/Publikationen/Fachveroeffentlichungen/Bevoelkerung/BroschuereGeburtenDeutschland.psml*

Stewart, S. M., Bond, M. H., Deeds, O., & Chung, S. F. (1999). Intergenerational patterns of values and autonomy expectations in cultures of relatedness and separateness. *Journal of Cross-Cultural Psychology, 30*(5), 575–593.

The World Fact Book. (2009). *Cameroon.* Retrieved September 30, 2009, from *www.cia.gov/library/publications/the-world-factbook/geos/cm.html.*

Yeh, K.-H., Bedford, O., & Yang, Y.-J. (2009). A cross-cultural comparison of the coexistence and domain superiority of individuating and relating autonomy. *International Journal of Psychology, 44*(3), 213–221.

Yeh, K.-H., & Yang Y.-J. (2006). Construct validation of individuating and relating autonomy orientations in culturally Chinese adolescents. *Asian Journal of Social Psychology, 9,* 148–160.

Yovsi, R. D. (2003). *An investigation of breastfeeding and mother–infant interactions in the face of cultural taboos and belief systems: The case of Nso and Fulani mothers and their infants of 3–5 months of age in Mbvem, subdivision of the Northwest province of Cameroon.* Münster, Germany: Lit.

Yovsi, R. D., & Keller, H. (2007). The architecture of cosleeping among wage-earning and subsistence farming Cameroonian Nso families. *Ethos, 35*(1), 65-84.

CHAPTER 8

Ethnic/Racial Identity
and Peer Relationships across
Elementary, Middle, and High Schools

TIFFANY YIP *and* SARA DOUGLASS

While there has been much research attention on the family as an important and proximal socializing context for youths as they negotiate the
process of ethnic and racial identity formation in the United States (Hughes
et al., 2006; Umana-Taylor, Bhanot, & Shin, 2006), peer interactions have
also been found to be proximal and influential for the development of a
sense of self (Hartup, 1999; Hartup, Campbell, & Muncer, 1998; Rubin et
al., 2006). Moreover, because peer interactions may be more voluntary as
compared to family-based interactions, they provide an interesting view of
the bidirectional association between peer relationships and ethnic identity
development. Recognizing that peer interactions occur in a variety of forms
and settings, in this chapter we review literature that encompasses a broad
definition of peer interactions, including experiences of discrimination,
friendship choices, and racial composition of school settings. The review
includes research conducted among elementary, middle, and high school
students to outline how peer interactions and ethnic identity are related
during the period from childhood to adolescence. In addition, we review
literature on African Americans, Latinos, Asian Americans, and European
Americans, where available.

186

To begin, we define ethnic and racial identity. There are many areas in the research literature where the distinction between these two terms is blurred (Phinney & Kohatsu, 1997), especially in the case where multiple groups are considered in a single study. Sometimes the use of "racial" versus "ethnic" identity depends on the group investigated, such that "racial identity" is more prevalent in research on African and European Americans (e.g., Sellers, Rowley, Chavous, Shelton, & Smith, 1997) while "ethnic identity" seems more popular among Latino and Asian samples (e.g., Phinney, 1992). In other cases, the instrument used to assess identity seems to lead to a propensity to use "racial" versus "ethnic" (e.g., Phinney, 1992; Sellers et al., 1997). Nevertheless, racial identity has been defined as "the significance and qualitative meaning that individuals attribute to their membership within the . . . racial group within their self-concepts" (Sellers, Smith, Shelton, Rowley, & Chavous, 1998, p. 23), whereas ethnic identity has been defined as "the accurate and consistent use of an ethnic label, based on the perception and conception of themselves as belonging to an ethnic group" (Rotheram & Phinney, 1987, p. 17) and as "a social identity based on the culture of one's ancestors' national or tribal group(s), as modified by the demands of the culture in which one's group currently resides" (Helms, 1994, p. 293). Since the current chapter incorporates research spanning various racial and ethnic groups across more than one developmental period, it seems most appropriate to use the broader term "racial/ethnic identity."

Racial/Ethnic Identity Development

Scholars, beginning with the Clarks, have recognized the importance of examining racial/ethnic identity, beginning in childhood (Clark & Clark, 1939). Since the seminal doll studies, theories and research on racial/ethnic identity over the developmental lifespan have continued to grow. Although each of the perspectives on ethnic/racial identity development espouses slightly different approaches to the study of identity development, they all share in common the idea that identity changes over time, and thus the importance of examining the construct over time (e.g., Cross & Fhagen-Smith, 1996; Helms, 1990). For example, based on Erikson's theory of identity development, Phinney (1992) developed one of the most widely cited models of ethnic identity development. In this model, the exploration of and search for one's identity begins during adolescence and culminates in young adulthood. Moreover, peer and familial interactions during this period seem to be especially influential in the eventual attainment of a clear sense of ethnic self (Hill, Bromell, Tyson, & Flint, 2007; Phinney, Romero, Nava, & Huang, 2001). The current chapter focuses on peer influences in this framework.

The Importance of Peer Relationships

Examining the association between ethnic identity and peer relationships seems to be an especially ripe area for attention since there is much research evidence to show a naturally occurring association between the two (Hamm, 2000; Hamm, Brown, & Heck, 2005; Quillian & Campbell, 2003). Indeed, research on the association between peer group affiliation and ethnic identity finds that having a stronger ethnic identity is associated with a higher probability of belonging to peer groups based on ethnic group membership (Brown, Herman, Hamm, & Heck, 2008). Moreover, the importance of peers for ethnic identity development remains throughout the elementary, middle, and high school periods. As such, the following sections review literature from each of these contexts. For the purposes of this review, these contexts are defined as follows: elementary school includes kindergarten through fifth grade, middle school includes sixth through eighth grade, and high school includes ninth through twelfth grade. We recognize that the adopted parameters of these contexts are not uniform across school districts in the United States, and thus this review may not cover the entire range of youths' experiences. These parameters do, however, provide a useful and meaningful framework for the available literature.

From a developmental perspective, it is also important to consider the influence of peers over time, because the demographics of school racial/ethnic composition generally increase; often this increase is attributable to a public school system that merges smaller, more homogeneous, schools into larger, more heterogeneous, schools as youths transition from elementary through high school (Frankenberg & Orfield, 2007; Orfield, 2001). In an attempt to synthesize all the available literature in this area, the chapter includes the available research on African Americans, Latinos, Asian Americans, and European Americans, recognizing that not all of these groups are represented equally across the elementary, middle, and high school contexts.

The Contact Hypothesis

In examining the influence of peer interactions on racial/ethnic identity development, we draw upon *intergroup contact theory* that suggests that under certain conditions the more intergroup contact individuals have, the more likely they are to feel positive toward outgroup members (Pettigrew, 1998). Indeed, research has shown that positive interactions with different-race individuals has been associated with such outcomes as reductions in prejudice (Molina & Wittig, 2006), increases in a sense of common identity (Nier et al., 2001), and personal closeness (Tropp, 2007). In a meta-analytic review of studies that have examined the contact hypothesis, Pettigrew and Tropp (2006) reported that intergroup contact has a positive impact in reducing prejudice toward the members of the general outgroup and not just specific members with whom an individual has had interactions. Further, research among youths also finds benefits attributable to increased intergroup contact. For example, it has been observed that intergroup contact is associated with reporting that race-based exclusion is wrong and unfair (Crystal, Killen, & Ruck, 2008) as well as fewer reports of peer victimization (Graham, 2006). In one of the few studies examining the association between racial identity and intergroup contact, Lee and his colleagues found that, among Koreans living in China, those who reported more social interactions with Chinese reported lower levels of ethnic identity when discrimination was frequent (Lee, Noh, Yoo, & Doh, 2007). Together, theory and research suggest that intergroup contact may have important implications for identity development.

Intragroup Contact and Racial/Ethnic Identity

Although the contact hypothesis focuses primarily on the effects of intergroup contact, research has also examined the very important influence of intragroup interactions on youths' development. As Pettigrew (1998) writes, "Optimal intergroup contact provides insight about ingroups as well as outgroups" (p. 72). Indeed, research suggests that both ingroup and outgroup contacts influence the development of racial identity (Alba & Nee, 2003; Portes & Rumbaut, 2001). For example, in a study of African American adolescents, Rowley and colleagues (Rowley, Burchinal, Roberts, & Zeisel, 2008) found that same-race friendships were associated with increased reports of racial discrimination. Although same-race friends were not linked to racial identity explicitly in that study, recent research suggests that discrimination is a form of social interaction that may then lead to the exploration of and commitment to one's identity (Seaton, Yip, & Sellers, 2009). Specifically, nigrescence theory (a five-phase developmental theory of acquisition of black identification, propounded by William E. Cross, Jr.) suggests that experiences of racial discrimination may serve as encounters that cause individuals to rethink the role of race in their lives, a process that can occur anywhere during the developmental lifespan (Cross & Fhagen-Smith, 2001). In research that considers ethnic identity as an outcome, researchers found that having a stronger sense of ethnic identification was associated with more ingroup peer interaction (Phinney et al., 2001). In retrospective research on African American college students attending predominantly white high schools, having positive same-race peer relationships was associated with more resolution in racial identity formation (Tatum, 2004). Therefore, it appears that having more same-race friends is associated with changes in racial/ethnic identity status over time. Taken as a whole, the current empirical literature suggests that both intergroup and intragroup contact are related to changes in racial/ethnic identity. The current chapter explores this possibility.

Elementary School

Although the socialization influences of peer interactions begin before elementary school, most of the research literature begins to consider peer influences more systematically beginning in elementary school. Indeed, this tendency reflects a reality for youths; for many, elementary school marks the first consistent contact with peers and a concurrent separation from the homogeneity of family life. Given this change of context, it is important to consider how both direct peer interaction and larger contextual settings may influence this young population in terms of both their friendship choices as well as reflections on their ethnic/racial selves.

Related to findings supporting intergroup contact theory, the racial/ethnic composition of the school in which youths attend elementary school appears to have an important impact on how they view themselves in terms of their race/ethnicity. Among African American and white fourth-grade school children, the racial/ethnic identity of students in a predominantly white, predominantly African American, and two heterogeneous elementary schools was compared (Dutton, Singer, & Devlin, 1998). Using children's spontaneous mention of race or ethnicity as an indication of racial/ethnic identity, researchers found that children in the two integrated schools mentioned race/ethnicity more frequently than children in the predominantly white school; and in general African American children were more likely to mention race/ethnicity than their white counterparts. While this study was not able to offer completely equivalent comparisons of participants in terms of school context (e.g., no African American student was interviewed from the predominantly white school, so this minority perspective could not be offered), it does suggest that intergroup interaction increases the prominence of race for both white and African American elementary school students.

Although not a direct measure of peer relationships, school and classroom racial/ethnic composition also has implications for peer nominations. For example, when asked about their racial/ethnic friendship preferences, students in the heterogeneous and predominantly white schools were more likely to nominate an other-race friend than students attending the predominantly African American school (Dutton et al., 1998). This finding is partially supported by other research confirming the role of both context and individual ethnicity/race on friendship choices. For example, Aboud, Mendelson, and Purdy (2003) found that both African American and white students in a predominantly white school were more likely to report having same-race as compared to other-race friends. In examining reciprocal nominations of "best friends" across grades, older white boys reported having significantly more same-race friends as compared to other-race friends. Interestingly, longitudinal analyses examining the stability of these reciprocal nominations over time found that other-race friendships were less stable than same-race friendships and that students were less likely to form new cross-race friendships over time. Examining racial/ethnic composition at the classroom level, research suggests that Latino, Asian, white, and African American youth all show a preference for same-ethnicity peers; however, this preference was stronger for youths in classrooms that included more same-ethnicity peers (Bellmore, Nishina, Witkow, Graham, & Juvonen, 2007).

Given the relatively limited autonomy that is available to elementary school students in nearly all domains of life, friendship seems to be one area where youths are able to assert their own choices. This research suggests that these choices may be motivated by racial/ethnic stratifications and that this tendency may increase over time. Yet, this picture is not an entirely bleak statement on racial stratification; instead, it seems that increased intergroup contact can increase liking for the outgroup. Given that racial stratification of friendship appears to be a reality for elementary school social settings, it is interesting to consider how the quality of these relationships may vary. In a study of African American and white elementary school students attending a predominantly white school (50% white, 30% African American, 20% other) in Canada, researchers examined various indices of friendship quality (Aboud, Mendelson, & Purdy, 2003). All students reported a difference in quality of same- and cross-race friendships, with same-race friendships rated as more intimate. In addition, white students' prejudice against their African American peers was associated with fewer cross-race friendships and reports of lower-quality cross-race friendships; yet, no associations between prejudice and friendship dimensions were observed for the African American students. That prejudice is not a salient consideration for African American students in their friendship choices seems sensible, as these prejudices are often targeted at their own ingroup (e.g., African Americans). Yet, the larger social context may still have its effects for this group; in a recent study of African American third, fourth, and fifth graders, Rowley and colleagues found that children who reported having more African American friends (same-race interactions) also reported expecting more discrimination in cross-race interactions. This finding applied regardless of larger contextual considerations such as classroom racial composition (Rowley et al., 2008). In addition to preference for same-race friends, there are clearly qualitative differences in both the stability and soundness of these relationships. For white youth, some of these differences can be attributed to prejudiced attitudes toward the out-

group; for African American youths, some of these differences have implications for their expectations of judgment and bias. It appears that awareness of and sensitivity to differential treatment of peers based on racial/
ethnic characteristics is a reality for youths, even at this young age.

The quality of interracial interactions and specifically expectations of
discrimination can also interact with racial/ethnic evaluations of the self.
Research has found that African American youths who hold their racial/
ethnic identity close to themselves also anticipate that others will judge them
based on this identity; in contrast, African American youths who believe
that others hold their racial/ethnic group in high esteem did not worry about
such judgments (Rowley et al., 2008). Specifically, third-, fourth-, and fifth-
grade African Americans were administered the Multidimensional Inventory of Black Identity (MIBI; Sellers et al., 1997) and questioned about
perceptions of racial discrimination; students high on racial centrality (i.e.,
racial identity is an integral component of one's self-construal) reported
more expectations of discrimination, while students high in public regard
(i.e., feeling that others view one's racial/ethnic group positively) reported
fewer expectations of discrimination, and these findings were consistent
across grades. Further, no relationship was found between private regard
(i.e., feeling good about being a member of one's racial/ethnic group) and
expectations of discrimination. These findings suggest that integral components of racial identity may have different implications for expectations
in peer relationships, and they offer a more nuanced perspective on racial
identity as a multidimensional construct.

Taken as a whole, the literature on elementary school-age youths finds
that same-race friendships appear to dominate social scenes at an early age,
despite contextual opportunities for cross-race friendships to occur. However, increased heterogeneity and contact with other-race peers does appear
to affect this phenomenon in terms of both friendship construction by race/
ethnicity and self-reflection on one's own racial/ethnic identity. Even when
cross-race friendships are formed among this age group, they tend to be
rated as less intimate as compared to friendships with same-race peers.
Further, the role of perceptions of discrimination in these domains reveals
the importance of discrimination for this young population and suggests
the need for additional research to investigate such relationships in more
diverse populations and contexts.

Middle School

Middle school students represent an emerging adolescent population, and
the literature regarding peer influences on racial identity issues reflects both
the growing centrality of identity processes in personal development and

the increasing role of peers at this age. Further, the systematic study of these constructs becomes more broadly conceived and diversely arranged with this age group, generating a more complex understanding of the relationship between peers and racial/ethnic identity development. This section reviews literature on the effects of school racial/ethnic composition, close friendships, and peer discrimination.

As in the literature on elementary school-age youths, the synthesis of both self-selected relationships and contextual dynamics with regard to racial/ethnic identity has been shown to be a worthwhile endeavor among middle school students. When examining the associations among interracial contact, close friendships with African American and white peers, and changes in racial identity status over 1- and 2-year intervals in a combined sample of African American middle and high school students, Yip and colleagues (Yip, Seaton, & Sellers, 2010) found that reporting more contact with African American peers in classes and clubs at school was associated with an increased probability of change in identity over time. That is, youths who reported more interaction with same-race peers also reported that their racial/ethnic identity was more variable within a 1-year period. In addition, reporting having many close African American friends was also associated with an increased probability of identity change. Interestingly, having many close white friends was also observed to be associated with the increased likelihood of change in one's racial/ethnic identity. Thus, this study suggests that not only does mere contact with same-race peers have an influence on identity development but also youths' choice of same- or different-race friends also influences their racial/ethnic identity development. Moreover, this study found that the effects of contact and close friendships depended upon whether the student attended a predominantly white or racially heterogeneous school. Specifically, youths attending heterogeneous schools who had little contact with African American peers in school and who reported having very few close African American friends were more likely to report a change in racial/ethnic identity status. However, youths attending predominantly white schools and having little contact with African American peers in school were less likely to report a change in their identity status as their number of close white friends increased. Finally, among African American youth attending predominantly white schools who reporting having a lot of contact with African American peers in schools, reporting having few close white friends was associated with having a more stable racial/ethnic identity. Thus, it appears that both effortful relationships (as found in friendships) and more passive contexts (as represented by school demographics) are influential for middle school students, and in markedly distinct ways.

However, not all peer interactions are positive. Given that peers are a primary source of interaction for adolescents, other students are a likely source of perceived prejudice and discrimination (Greene, Way, & Pahl, 2006). Previous research has also established the risk for negative effects of perceived prejudice and discrimination on emotional well-being (Essed, 1990; Phelan, Yu, & Davidson, 1994). Taken in concert, peer influences may be conceived as negative sources of self-information for students. Yet, there is also evidence to suggest that ethnic identity can help to buffer the effects of peer discrimination experiences on academic, social, and mental health outcomes (Wong, Eccles, & Sameroff, 2003). Over a period of 2 years, African American middle school students demonstrated that a strong ethnic identity acted as a protective factor such that it mitigated the plethora of effects of perceived discrimination, including decreases in self-concept of ability, decreases in school achievement, decreases in positive perception of peers, and increases in problem behavior. These findings are bolstered by other research, where high private regard (but not public regard) minimized the effects of depressive symptoms for African American sixth graders (Rivas-Drake, Hughes, & Way, 2008). Overall, for African Americans, a strong sense of ethnic identity seems to help guard against the potential negative contributions of one's peers. Further research has shown, however, that ethnic identity may not serve the same function for other racial/ethnic groups.

One such population group where these relationships differ is Chinese Americans. In a sample of this population, Rivas-Drake et al. (2008) found that racial/ethnic identity did not always buffer the negative effects of discrimination. Instead, this buffering effect was found only for public regard on measures of depression; private regard had no apparent interaction with depression and well-being measures. For Chinese Americans, believing that others generally hold their racial/ethnic group in high regard is apparently useful in helping to deplete the effects of negative regard that they directly experience during instances of discrimination. These isolated negative contributions from one's environment seem to be overcome by the more persistent positive belief system about that environment and one's racial/ethnic identity. However, their own positive feelings about their racial/ethnic group does not seem to translate into a buffer for such experiences, perhaps because there is not such a match between input and belief system. Thus, African Americans and Chinese Americans appear to experience the negative input from peers in very different ways, and these experiences are affected by aspects of their own racial/ethnic self-concept.

Research has also conceptualized racial/ethnic identity as a construct that can be influenced by peer context without regard to the direction or specific nature of such interactions. By utilizing a naturally occurring transition from middle school to high school French, Seidman, Allen, and Aber (2000) investigated the possibility that the salience of racial/ethnic identity might be a fluid factor affected by proximal changes in context. This transition may be marked by a change in the racial/ethnic composition of their school context (e.g., movement to more integrated, equivalent, or less integrated schools), as it was for the samples of African American, Latino, and European American students in this study. Self-report questionnaires on group esteem, exploration, and perceived social transactions were used to measure racial identity and peer interactions. Additionally, the racial/ethnic composition of the school context was operationalized as a change variable of student body and faculty members to account for both middle and high school contexts. Results revealed that the pattern of effects varied greatly between the African American, Latino, and European American students; for African American students, exploration of their racial identity was related to change in perceived daily hassles and perceived social support, while these same factors did not relate to their sense of group esteem. For Latino students, no relationship between changing the school of context and racial identity was found. For European Americans, however, this changing context appeared to have effects in a number of ways: change in racial/ethnic congruence of peers and change in perceived social support were negatively related to exploration of their own racial/ethnic identity, while change in perceived daily hassles was positively related to group esteem. With regard to the contact hypothesis, this research highlights the need to recognize how and with whom inter- and intraracial contact may change over time. This research is also supported by the notion that friendships within and between different racial/ethnic groups may be markedly different (Kao & Joyner, 2006) and can, in fact, expand the formal definition of friends to less central relationships such as classmates and peers. This broader conceptualization deemphasizes the self-selected nature of relationships and demonstrates the importance of incorporating more holistic approaches to context in research designs in order to most accurately reflect the lived experiences of adolescents.

To date, research on middle school students has revealed the complex and dynamic roles that both racial/ethnic identity and peer relationships play. When considering racial/ethnic identity as a self-protective buffer from negative peer feedback, we see both the complexities within identity—the complicated relationships that components of identity have to other areas of mental health—as well as the variation that occurs across racial/ethnic designations. Despite this complicated amalgamation, the importance of inter- and intragroup contact is consistently supported. When we consider the possible changes in these relationships that occur across major transition points in the life of the student, we see support for instability and fluctuation within these relationships such that inter- and intragroup contact is not a static experience. The focus on transitions from middle to high school settings (French et al., 2006) and combined samples of middle and high school students (Yip et al., 2010) present an ample introduction of the research to which we now turn.

High School

As we move to the literature regarding high school students, we begin with an already complex understanding of the social processes involved in racial/ethnic identity development. As demonstrated by the research conducted in elementary and middle school samples, most students enter high school with some notion or acknowledgment of who they are as racial/ethnic individuals. Though these experiences are not qualitatively uniform, they are typically present. The crisis of identity formation has been referred to as "the process of adolescing" (Erikson, 1968, p. 91), and a great deal of research conducted in high school populations acknowledges this sensitive period for both identity development and peer influences. Herein we look to this maturing population at a time when peer influences (e.g., peer pressure) is at an all-time high to further understand the dynamic processes within and potential consequences of racial/ethnic identity development during this critical time period. The relative distribution of ingroups and outgroups, individual identity development, voluntary peer selection, and quality of peer relationships are all important considerations for this age group.

There remains a lack of consensus over the role of context in ethnic identity. While racial/ethnic ingroups and outgroups seem to be meaningful, realistic distinctions for high school students in how these groups function to reflect on the self varies both within and across racial/ethnic target groups. For Mexican-origin students, increased intragroup contact (as measured by statistical representation of racial/ethnic groups within their school) has been associated with a stronger racial identity; it appears that contact with an outgroup member may be a particularly central experience to racial identity for Latino students in that it increases the salience of this identity to their self-concept (Umana-Taylor, 2004). However, there also exists support for an alternative process at play for Mexican-origin and Vietnamese-origin students; that is, increased intergroup contact (as measured by self-reported interactions with peers) has also been found to be associated with stronger racial identity, so that contact with people of other similar ethnic/racial backgrounds may increase the salience of their racial/ethnic identity to their self-concept (Phinney et al., 2000). Further, this finding was stronger for the Vietnamese-origin sample than the Mexican-origin sample. Clearly, research supports not only the intragroup contact theory but also the contact hypothesis. These divergent findings can potentially be explained by the varying ways that peer interaction was measured; that is, support for intragroup contact was found when researchers considered the more peripheral context of schools that students attended, a setting that is largely uncontrolled by the individual. However, support for the contact hypothesis was found when researchers tapped into the more proximal measure of peer choice, an interaction in which students are able to make choices and assert their own autonomy. Together these findings offer evidence that peer relationships and interactions are part of a larger socialization schema that exerts meaningful effects on the identity of the adolescent; in some instances, we see the active contributions of the individual to this schema, and at other times we see their passive belongingness. It is clear that there are diverse experiences of different populations within such a schema.

Inquiry into the role of context in the lives of high school students is not restricted to minority populations; in a mixed-methods approach to European American identity, Grossman and Charmaraman (2009) hypothesized that school context was an influential factor in European Americans' racial identity as well, based on the interplay between their social majority status and a varying statistical presence. Rather than using a scale measurement for racial identity, centrality was measured as the construct of interest in schools where European Americans were embedded as part of the statistical majority, statistical minority, or largely diverse population. While preliminary results showed various themes of centrality emerging from different contexts such that diversity promoted exploration and pride and majority students were marked by homophily or disengagement/unexamined statuses, quantitative results showed that these differences did not emerge, above and beyond socioeconomic status. Thus, it appears that for European Americans contextual influences may have less of an effect than for minority-status students. Perhaps as the historical majority entrenched in a position of power in the United States, European Americans may be less susceptible to the fluctuations of their context in terms of their own self-reflections.

Given the prevalence of ingroup and outgroup distinctions in high school, it is important to recognize the disparities that may exist between how individuals view themselves and how they are viewed by their peers. Often, distinctions on race/ethnicity are extant judgments made by the researchers based on self-reported labels and are considered as absolutes (this tendency is clearly seen in the statistical breakdown of school settings, for example). Accessing crowd affiliation presents a different orientation to what constitutes ingroups and outgroups for African American, Asian American, and Latino students (Brown et al., 2008). "Crowd" is used to represent the racial/ethnic affiliations made between people that are less intimate than friendships but more personal than contextual demographics. Thus, we are given a different perspective on in- and outgroup construction. Further, Brown and colleagues (2008) use both self-report and peer nomination measures to reveal the asymmetrical relationship between self- and other-perceptions in terms of ethnic centrality, friendships, and experiences of discrimination. Indeed, there was asymmetry detected between self-report and peer nominations, and these asymmetries further differed by self-reported racial/ethnic labels of the individual. For African American students, ethnic exclusivity of friends and ethnic centrality were both correlated with peer-nominated affiliation, while self-reported affiliation was only correlated with ethnic exclusivity of friends. For Asian Americans, ethnic exclusivity of friends and perceived ethnic discrimination were correlated with peer-nominated affiliation, while ethnic exclusivity of friends and feelings about ethnicity were correlated with self-reported affiliations. For Latino students, self-reported affiliation was correlated with both perceived discrimination and ethnic exclusivity of friends; other-nominated affiliation was correlated with these measures as well as emphasis on ethnicity. These results demonstrate the disconnect that exists for adolescents with the social implications they assign to their own race/ethnicity versus the social implications that others assign to it; it appears that others overestimate the meaning and importance of one's racial/ethnic identity. From this research it becomes clear that the very interactions that make up the contact hypothesis are both bidirectional and asymmetrical. Though we often conceptualize a single person within a relationship as the "target," perceptions and beliefs regarding ethnicity/race are being generated from both sides. Indeed, this disconnect between how one sees him or herself versus how others see him or her is a vital component of social stratification in American society.

Noting the influences of both the context and the person on peer preferences, research has also observed that racial identity both leads action and is responsive to social settings. Given choices for peer selection in diverse school settings, the peers with whom African American males choose to surround themselves vary systematically by the racial identity status of the individual (Wade & Okesola, 2002). Namely, pre-encounter-status students (i.e., ones who are not actively thinking about race) were likely to select a white or mixed-race peer group or to demonstrate ambivalence over which peer group to select; encounter-status students (i.e., ones who are just beginning to think about the role of race in their lives) were likely to not show a preference for any peer group, and immersion/emersion-status students (i.e., ones who have spent time thinking about race and have an understanding of its role in their lives) were likely to select an all-African

American peer group. These findings reflect themes measured by the Black Racial Identity Attitude Scale, which emphasizes the encounter and exploration processes common to most racial/ethnic identity models, and specifically models its subscales from Cross's (1971) five stages of African American racial identity (RIAS-B; Parham & Helms, 1981). While this research was not able to establish causality, the hypothesized mechanism underlying these relationships derives from the notion that the internal representation of one's racial/ethnic self relates to youths' choice of racial/ethnic peers.

As previously noted, the terms "race" and "ethnicity" are often confounded in the literature, and their respective use often depends on the population at hand. Yet, research suggests that the nuanced nature of race/ethnicity is not simply a methodological consideration or linguistic issue; for Hispanic students, the distinction between race and ethnicity may in fact have very real consequences for their peer relationships (Kao & Vaquera, 2006). Kao and Vaquera (2006) found that, when asked to choose a best friend, there was a high degree of matching between the self-identified ethnicity of Hispanic adolescents and the self-identified ethnicity of this individual (as well as a concurrent yet independent high degree of matching between their self-identified races). While Hispanic adolescents appear to stratify their peer relationships along both racial and ethnic lines, this research does suggest that ethnicity supersedes race in friendship selection (Kao & Vaquera, 2006). For Hispanic adolescents, both racial and ethnic identification appear to have very real implications for friendship selection; this relationship is not random and reflects a more refined understanding of racial and ethnic identities among these youths than research typically reflects. Here we see evidence that intergroup and intragroup contact may reflect more complicated stratifications than has been previously acknowledged.

Yet, we also see that these internal representations do not act in isolation, and in fact there may be peer-influenced processes concurrently at play. Indeed, peer pressure has been found to influence peer selection preferences in high school students, based on racial divisions (Wade & Okesola, 2002). For African Americans, this peer pressure may compel individuals to seek out ingroup interactions rather than outgroup interactions. Specifically, research has found that increased perceptions of discrimination led to African American students not selecting white peer groups as well as showing confusion over which peer group to select (Wade & Okesola, 2002). Taken in concert with the previous results on racial identity development, it is possible that as individuals become more aware of their racial/ethnic selves, they also become more aware of the manners in which they may be judged as such by other people. When considering high school students, it is important not only to contextualize their experiences within peer settings but also to take into account the information they are receiving from such settings. This feedback—for example, peer pressure—may be subtle or explicit and can have real implications for social behavior.

Peer pressure and the feedback offered by peers raise the issue of the quality of relationships. Research shows that experiences of discrimination resulting from peer interaction are a frequent occurrence for many different racial/ethnic minority groups in high school (Greene, Way, & Pahl, 2006). However, these experiences are not uniform in frequency; over a period of 4 years, Asian American and non-Puerto Rican Latino students reported more experiences of discrimination than Puerto Rican and African American peers (Greene et al., 2006). Thus, peers may be negative sources of information about the self, and such negative feedback may be differentially experienced. What remains uniform, however, is the impact of discrimination on self-esteem; these effects can be seen across racial/ethnic groups and are moderated by ethnic identity. Subscales from the Multigroup Ethnic Identity Measure (MEIM; Phinney, 1992) were used to differentiate between Ethnic Identity Achievement (made up of exploration and commitment) and Ethnic Affirmation (made up of pride, belonging, and attachment to one's ethnic group). Indeed, different effects were found in regard to each subscale: while high affirmation had protective effects on self-esteem in the face of peer discrimination, high achievement served to heighten the negative effects on self-esteem. In parallel with processes found in middle school students, we seem to see the more personal side of the contact hypothesis here; despite uncommon interactions with their peers, common experiences with their ethnic identity were found. Further, a more secure sense of self does not always appear to be beneficial when experiencing negative feedback from peers. Once again, evidence supports a nuanced construct of racial/ethnic identity that cannot be considered a single readily definable entity.

Research with high school students demonstrates that contact with peers and racial/ethnic identity development are distinctly related. Taken in sum, evidence suggests that salience of the racial/ethnic self appears to be facilitated by the presence of others, regardless of the ingroup or outgroup distinction of that "other." This observation is not to suggest that this relationship is random or uniform; rather, the experiences of both minority- and majority-status students are dependent on their larger social stratification, their distinct situational context, and the proximity of the relationships they are engaged in. Further, the dimensions that are added when consideration of who that "other" is—from peers to crowds to friends—demonstrate the role of intimacy and agency in these relationships as they correlate with racial/ethnic identity. Within such relationships we see interactions that are bidirectional, asymmetrical, and entirely subjective; it is the ideal goal of research to capture these experiences, as they lead to a more dynamic and sophisticated understanding of racial/ethnic identity as a construct.

Conclusions and Future Directions

Tracing the association between peers and ethnic identity development from elementary through high school, we develop an increasingly complex picture of the relationships among these developmental constructs. The literature among elementary school-age youths focuses primarily on school racial/ethnic composition, peer nominations, friendship quality, and expectations of discrimination. Taken all together, these studies suggest that interactions with same- and different-race peers may significantly affect the youths' feelings about their racial/ethnic identity. The dearth of longitudinal studies on this age group precludes our being able to make definitive causal connections; however, given the relative lack of autonomy in one's choice of school context at this early age, it appears likely that school-level factors are significantly affecting peer choices and racial/ethnic identity development. At the same time, however, even among this younger age group, we observe that youths' racial/ethnic identity also shapes their perception of how others may treat them unfairly (Rowley et al., 2008).

Moving into the middle school literature, where students are likely to be exposed to increasing racial/ethnic diversity and may have more autonomy in their selection of peer affiliations, we find similar forces at play (i.e., peer affiliation, discrimination, school racial/ethnic composition); however, the operationalization and the interaction of these forces become more complex. Moreover, in this age range, we start to see more longitudinal studies that track the associations between context, peers, and racial/ethnic identity over time (French et al., 2006; Yip et al., in press). As such, this body of research allows for conclusions about the dynamic relationship between context, peers, and racial/ethnic identity. In addition, research among middle school-age youths extends beyond African American and white youths to include studies of Asian and Latino youths (Kao & Joyner, 2006; Rivas-Drake et al., 2008), allowing for a more complete picture of some of the differences and similarities among these various racial/ethnic groups. Finally, this literature also begins to address some of the academic and behavioral implications of why it is important to examine these relationships in the first place (Rivas-Drake et al., 2008).

Turning to the oldest age group in this review, again we see the importance of contact, context, peers, discrimination, and friendship choices. As in the middle school literature, we also see an increase in the racial/ethnic groups of interest. Namely, the high school literature includes research on specific ethnic groups (e.g., Vietnamese and Mexican youths) as well as a study of racial/ethnic identity of only European American youths (Grossman & Charmaraman, 2009). In addition to the increasing diversity of samples, there is also an inclusion of methods that extend beyond survey research (Grossman & Charmaraman, 2009). As such, the inferences we draw from this body of research are more nuanced than both the middle and elementary school literature. For the first time, we also see samples stratified by gender (Wade & Okesola, 2002), which adds yet another dimension of social identity to the larger picture. As well, the scope of outcome variables included in the high school literature extends beyond that observed in the elementary and middle school reviews to include second-order effects between racial/ethnic identity and psychological adjustment measures such as self-esteem (Greene et al., 2006). As the interplay between developmental constructs becomes more involved, the directional relationship between these constructs is also more complicated. In this older age cohort, increased autonomy (and, with that, increasingly diverse contexts and intergroup contact) likely means that the relationships among peers, identity, context, and contact interact more synergistically. However, definite conclusions about causal directions would require additional longitudinal research.

Despite the differences across elementary, middle, and high schools, there were also many similarities. The relationships between peer influences and racial/ethnic identity are both widespread in effects and diverse in implications. As we see throughout this review of the literature, children and adolescents are influenced by the people surrounding them—those who are similar to them and those who are different from them alike. Indeed, both intergroup and intragroup contacts play a formative role in racial/ethnic identity development. Yet, these influences are neither absolute nor refined; the influence of peers depends upon the nature of relationships, the context in which those relationships take place, the race/ethnicity of the population at hand, and the race/ethnicity of those populations with which they interact. This perception is most apparent in studies with multiple racial/ethnic populations who do not find consistent results across demographics (e.g., Brown et al., 2008; French et al., 2006a, 2006b; Phinney et al., 2001; Rivas-Drake et al., 2008).

The research reviewed in this chapter presents a wide range of operationalizations of "peer" influences based largely on the age of the participants at hand. Research in elementary schools focuses exclusively on friendships and peer nominations, while research in high schools focuses more exclusively on classmates or student bodies as a whole. Most broadly conceived, peers represent any age demographic that matches the subject of interest; yet, the research tends to attach varying degrees of selectivity and intimacy when defining these relationships. This tendency creates a divide between proximal and distal peer influences, presenting a largely ignored confounding variable with which theory needs to contend.

Furthermore, this research is conducted exclusively in the context of the school (for obvious reasons of convenience). This limitation neglects the potential population of peers an individual may spend extensive time with outside of school, particularly if that individual does not attend school in his or her own community (see Cook, Herman, Phillips, Settersten, 2002, for an exception).

In addition to the types of relationships considered in research, issues of direction and nature also run throughout operationalization. While the literature in discrimination presents an obvious example of negative interactions, the types and quality of interactions are often lost in the methodologies of frequency count or categorical relationships. While friendships are often considered positive relationships, research has shown that children and adolescents treat friends worse than nonfriend peers (Kowalski, 1997, 2001, 2003). This dimension deserves further attention as the literature continues to refine findings and relationships.

From an empirical perspective, the developmental aspect of racial/ethnic identity theory has been virtually ignored by researchers. This oversight is paradoxical, given the central nature of this theme to all proposed models (Cross, 1971; Phinney, 1989; Helms, 1984, 1990). Although longitudinal research covering 2–4 years is becoming more commonplace, the self-report questionnaire measures of racial/ethnic identity most often employed are static operationalizations of a truly fluid concept (Sellers, Shelton, et al., 1998; Yip, 2005; Yip & Fuligni, 2002); they are not used to describe movement from stage to stage but to rather assign a single stage to an individual at an isolated point in time (or multiple isolated points in time). Indeed, they seem to reflect the "personality types" approach that Marcia's (1966) ego identity operationalizations presupposed; yet, racial identity theory rejects this notion and strongly supports developmental trends. Further research is needed to allow the trajectories of racial/ethnic identity, its peer-influenced correlates, and its mental health outcomes to be traced over time. This chapter has focused on a very narrow portion of the social influences children and adolescents encounter on a daily basis, and this shortcoming limits the scope of our conclusions. Even within the school context, peers are not the only interactions experienced—teachers, staff, and administrators all contribute to the context and culture of any school, and their roles in racial/ethnic identity were not addressed. Further, many experiences and much development take place outside of school boundaries, and these undoubtedly play a formative role in children's lives. School settings make up just one component within ecological systems theory (Bronfenbrenner, 1977), and it is necessary to take into account many other settings—from the family to the neighborhood, from the community to the locality's overall socioeconomic status—in order to gain a comprehensive understanding of these intricate processes.

References

Aboud, F. E., Mendelson, M. J., & Purdy, K. T. (2003). Cross-race peer relations and friendship quality. *International Journal of Behavioral Development, 27*(2), 165–173.

Alba, R., & Nee, V. (2003). *Rethinking the American mainstream: Assimilation and comtemporary immigration.* Cambridge, MA: Harvard University Press.

Bellmore, A. D., Nishina, A., Witkow, M. R., Graham, S., & Juvonen, J. (2007). The influence of classroom ethnic composition on same- and other-ethnicity peer nominations in middle school. *Social Development, 16*(4), 720–740.

Bronfenbrenner, U. (1977). Toward an experimental ecology of human development. *American Psychologist, 32,* 513–531.

Brown, B. B., Herman, M., Hamm, J. V., & Heck, D. J. (2008). Ethnicity and image: Correlates of crowd affiliation among ethnic minority youth. *Child Development, 79*(3), 529–546.

Clark, K. B., & Clark, M. P. (1939). The development of consciousness of self and the emergence of racial identification in Negro pre-school children. *Journal of Social Psychology, 10,* 591–599.

Cook, T. D., Herman, M. R., Phillips, M., & Settersten, R. A. (2002). Some ways in which neighborhoods, nuclear families, friendship groups, and schools jointly affect changes in early adolescent development. *Child Development, 73*(4), 1283–1309.

Cross, W. E., Jr., & Fhagen-Smith, P. (1996). Nigrescence and ego-identity development. In P. Pedersen, J. Draguns, W. Lonner, & J. Trimble (Eds.), *Counseling across Cultures.* Thousand Oaks, CA: Sage.

Cross, W. E. (1971). Negro-to-black conversion experiences: Toward a psychology of Black liberation. *Black World, 20*(9), 13–27.

Cross, W. E., Jr., & Fhagen-Smith, P. (2001). Patterns of African American identity development: A lifespan perspective. In B. Jackson & C. Wijeyesinghe (Eds.), *New perspectives on racial identity development: A theoretical and practical anthology* (pp. 243–270). New York: New York University Press.

Crystal, D. S., Killen, M., & Ruck, M. (2008). It is who you know that counts: Intergroup contact and judgments about race-based exclusion. *British Journal of Developmental Psychology, 26*(1), 51–70.

Dutton, S. E., Singer, J. A., & Devlin, A. S. (1998). Racial identity of children in integrated, predominantly White, and Black schools. *Journal of Social Psychology, 138*(1), 41–53.

Erikson, E. H. (1968). *Identity: Youth and crisis.* New York: Norton.

Essed, P. E. (1990). *Everyday racism: Reports from women of two cultures.* Claremont, CA: Hunter House.

Frankenberg, E., & Orfield, G. (Eds.). (2007). *Lessons in integration: Realizing the promise of racial diversity in America's schools.* Charlottesville: University of Virginia Press.

French, S. E., Seidman, E., Allen, L., & Aber, J. L. (2006a). The development of ethnic identity during adolescence. *Developmental Psychology, 42*(1), 1–10.

French, S. E., Seidman, E., Allen, L., & Aber, J. L. (2006b). Racial/ethnic identity, congruence with the social context, and the transition to high school. *Journal of Adolescent Research, 15*(5), 587–602.

Graham, S. (2006). Peer victimization in school: Exploring the ethnic context. *Current Directions in Psychological Science, 15*(6), 317–321.

Greene, M. L., Way, N., & Pahl, K. (2006). Trajectories of perceived adult and peer discrimination among Black, Latino and Asian American adolescents: Patterns and psychological correlates. *Developmental Psychology, 42*(2), 218–238.

Grossman, J. M., & Charmaraman, L. (2009). Race, context, and privilege: White adolescents' explanations of racial-ethnic centrality. *Journal of Youth and Adolescence, 38*(2), 139–152.

Hamm, J. V. (2000). Do birds of a feather flock together?: The variable bases for African American, Asian American, and European American adolescents' selection of similar friends. *Developmental Psychology, 36*(2), 209–219.

Hamm, J. V., Brown, B. B., & Heck, D. J. (2005). Bridging the ethnic divide: Student and school characteristics in African American, Asian-descent, Latino, and White adolescents' cross-ethnic friend nominations. *Journal of Research on Adolescence, 15*(1), 21–46.

Hartup, W. W. (1999). Peer experience and its developmental significance. In M. Bennett (Ed.), *Developmental psychology: Achievements and prospects* (pp. 106–125). New York, NY: Psychology Press.

Hartup, W. W., Campbell, A., & Muncer, S. (1998). The company they keep: Friendships and their developmental significance. *The social child* (pp. 143–163). Hove, UK: Psychology Press.

Helms, J. E. (1984). Towards a theoretical explanation of the effect of race on counseling: A black and white model. *The Counseling Psychologist, 12*(4), 153–165.

Helms, J. E. (1990). *Black and White racial identity: Theory, research, and practice.* New York: Greenwood Press.

Helms, J. E. (1994). The conceptualization of racial identity and other "racial" constructs. In E. J. Trickett & R. J. Watts (Eds.), *Human diversity: Perspectives on people in context (pp. 285–311).* San Francisco: Jossey-Bass.

Hill, N. E., Bromell, L., Tyson, D. F., & Flint, R. (2007). Developmental commentary: Ecological perspectives on parental influences during adolescence. *Journal of Clinical Child and Adolescent Psychology, 36*(3), 367–377.

Hughes, D., Rodriquez, J., Smith, E. P., Johnson, D. J., Stevenson, H. C., & Spicer, P. (2006). Parents' ethnic-racial socialization practices: A review of research and directions for future study. *Developmental Psychology, 42*(5), 747–770.

Kao, G., & Joyner, K. (2006). Do Hispanic and Asian adolescents practice panethnicity in friendship choices? *Social Science Quarterly, 87*(1), 972–992.

Kao, G., & Vaquera, E. (2006). The salience of racial and ethnic identification in friendship choices among Hispanic adolescents. *Hispanic Journal of Behavioral Sciences, 28*(1), 23–47.

Kowalski, R. M. (Ed.). (1997). *Aversive interpersonal behaviors.* New York: Plenum Press.

Kowalski, R. M. (Ed). (2001). *Permitted disrespect: Teasing in interpersonal interactions.* Washington, D.C.: American Psychological Association.

Kowalski, R. M. (Ed). (2003). *Complaining, teasing, and other annoying behaviors.* New Haven: Yale University Press.

Lee, R. M., Noh, C.-Y., Yoo, H. C., & Doh, H.-S. (2007). The psychology of diaspora experiences: Intergroup contact, perceived discrimination, and the ethnic identity of Koreans in China. *Cultural Diversity and Ethnic Minority Psychology, 13*(2), 115–124.

Marcia, J. E. (1966). Development and validation of ego-identity status. *Journal of Personality and Social Psychology, 3*(5), 551–558.

Molina, L. E., & Wittig, M. A. (2006). Relative importance of contact conditions in explaining prejudice reduction in a classroom context: Separate and equal? *Journal of Social Issues, 62*(3), 489–509.

Nier, J. A., Gaertner, S. L., Dovidio, J. F., Banker, B. S., Ward, C. M., & Rust, M. C. (2001). Changing interracial evaluations and behavior: The effects of a common group identity. *Group Processes and Intergroup Relations, 4*(4), 299–316.

Orfield, G. (Ed.). (2001). *Diversity challenged: Evidence on the impact of affirmative action.* Cambridge, MA: Harvard Education Publishing Group.

Parham, T. A., & Helms, J. E. (1981). The influence of black students' racial identity attitudes on preferences for counselor's race. *Journal of Counseling Psychology, 28*(3), 250–257.

Pettigrew, T. F. (1998). Intergroup contact theory. *Annual Review of Psychology, 49,* 65–85.

Pettigrew, T. F., & Tropp, L. R. (2008). How does intergroup contact reduce prejudice? Meta analytic tests of three mediators. *European Journal of Social Psychology, 38*(6), 992–934.

Phelan, P., Yu, H. C., & Davidson, A. L. (1994). Navigating the psychosocial pressures of adolescence: The voices and experiences of high school youth. *American Educational Research Journal, 31*(2), 415–447.

Phinney, J. S. (1989). Stages of ethnic identity development in minority group adolescents. *The Journal of Early Adolescence, 9*(1), 34–39.

Phinney, J. S. (1992). The Multigroup Ethnic Identity Measure: A new scale for use with diverse groups. *Journal of Adolescent Research, 7*(2), 156–176.

Phinney, J. S., & Kohatsu, E. L. (1997). Ethnic and racial identity development and mental health. In K. Hurrelman (Ed.), *Health risks and developmental transitions in adolescence* (pp. 420–443). New York: Cambridge University Press.

Phinney, J. S., Romero, I., Nava, M., & Huang, D. (2001). The role of language, parents, and peers in ethnic identity among adolescents in immigrant families. *Journal of Youth and Adolescence, 30*(2), 135–153.

Portes, A., & Rumbaut, R. G. (2001). *Legacies: The story of the immigrant second generation.* Berkeley: University of California Press.

Quillian, L., & Campbell, M. E. (2003). Beyond black and white: The present and future of multiracial friendship segregation. *American Sociological Review, 68*(4), 540–566.

Rivas-Drake, D., Hughes, D., & Way, N. (2008). A closer look at peer discrimination, ethnic identity, and psychological well-being among urban Chinese American sixth graders. *Journal of Youth and Adolescence, 37*(1), 12–21.

Rotheram, M. J., & Phinney, J. S. (1987). Ethnic behavior patterns as an aspect of identity. In M. J. Rotheram & J. S. Phinney (Eds.), *Children's ethnic socialization: Pluralism and development* (pp. 201–218). Newbury Park, CA: Sage.

Rowley, S. J., Burchinal, M. R., Roberts, J. E., & Zeisel, S. A. (2008). Racial identity, social context, and race-related social cognition in African Americans during middle childhood. *Developmental Psychology, 44*(6), 1537–1546.

Rubin, K. H., Bukowski, W. M., Parker, J. G., Eisenberg, N., Damon, W., & Lerner, R. M. (2006). Peer interactions, relationships, and groups. In N. Eisenberg (Ed.), *Handbook of child psychology: Vol. 3. Social, emotional, and personality development* (6th ed., pp. 571–645). Hoboken, NJ: Wiley.

Seaton, E. K., Yip, T., & Sellers, R. M. (2009). Racial identity and perceptions of discrimination: A longitudinal analysis. *Child Development, 80*(2), 406–417.

Sellers, R. M., Rowley, S. A. J., Chavous, T. M., Shelton, J. N., & Smith, M. A. (1997). Multidimensional Inventory of Black Identity: A preliminary investigation of reliability and construct validity. *Journal of Personality and Social Psychology, 73,* 805–815.

Sellers, R. M., Shelton, J. N., Cooke, D. Y., Chavous, T. M., Rowley, S. A. J., & Smith, M. A. (Eds.). (1998). *A Multidimentional Model of Racial Identity: Assumptions, Findings, and Future Directions.* Hampton, VA: Cobb & Henry.

Sellers, R. M., Smith, M. A., Shelton, J. N., Rowley, S. A. J., & Chavous, T. M. (1998). Multidimensional Model of Racial Identity: A reconceptualization of African American racial identity. *Personality and Social Psychology Review, 2*(1), 18–39.

Tatum, B. D. (2004). Family life and school experience: Factors in the racial identity development of Black youth in White communities. *Journal of Social Issues, 60*(1), 117–135.

Tropp, L. R. (2007). Perceived discrimination and interracial contact: Predicting interracial closeness among Black and White Americans. *Social Psychology Quarterly, 70*(1), 70–81.

Umana-Taylor, A. J. (2004). Ethnic identity and self-esteem: Examining the role of social context. *Journal of Adolescence, 27*(2), 139–146.

Umana-Taylor, A. J., Bhanot, R., & Shin, N. (2006). Ethnic identity formation during adolescence: The critical role of families. *Journal of Family Issues, 27*(3), 390–414.

Wade, J. C., & Okesola, O. (2002). Racial peer group selection in African American high school students. *Journal of Multicultural Counseling and Development, 30*(2), 96–109.

Wong, C. A., Eccles, J. S., & Sameroff, A. (2003). The influence of ethnic discrimination and ethnic identification on African American adolescents' school and socioemotional adjustment. *Journal of Personality, 71*(6), 1197–1232.

Yip, T. (2005). Sources of situational variation in ethnic identity and psychological well-being: A Palm Pilot study of Chinese American students. *Personality and Social Psychology Bulletin, 31*(12), 1603–1616.

Yip, T., & Fuligni, A. J. (2002). Daily variation in ethnic identity, ethnic behaviors, and psychological well-being among American adolescents of Chinese descent. *Child Development, 73*(5), 1557–1572.

Yip, T., Seaton, E. K., & Sellers, R. M. (2010). Interracial and intraracial contact, school level diversity, and change in racial identity status among African American adolescents. *Child Development, 81*(5), 1431–1444.

CHAPTER 9

Dyadic Relationships
from a Cross-Cultural Perspective

Parent–Child Relationships and Friendship

KENNETH H. RUBIN, WONJUNG OH,
MELISSA MENZER, *and* KATIE ELLISON

The development of relationships with significant others is one of the most important tasks that an individual encounters in his or her lifetime. According to Hinde (1987, 1997), relationships are ongoing patterns of interaction between two individuals who acknowledge some connection with each other. In the case of children and adolescents, the social partners with whom interaction is most frequently experienced include parents, siblings, and peers. From Hinde's (1987, 1997) and Stevenson-Hinde's perspective (see Chapter 1, this volume, Figure 1.1), *individuals* bring to social exchanges reasonably stable social orientations (temperament, personality) that dispose them to be more or less sociable, agreeable, and able to regulate their emotions. These social orientations are, in part, biologically based, but they are also the product of interactions with others. It is through their individual dispositions and social interactions that children come to develop a repertoire of social cognitions that aid in understanding the thoughts, emotions, and intentions of others, and together these factors create opportunities for the development of social skills and competencies.

Significantly, the interactions that children have with others are not scattershot. Most early interactions occur with parents and siblings (and, in some cultures, with grandparents and extended family members—aunts, uncles, cousins); subsequently, children's *extra*familial interactions most often occur with peers, particularly friends. Thus, most social interactions are embedded in longer-term *relationships*; moreover, these interactions are influenced by past and anticipated future interactions with their relationship partners. The quality of these relationships is actually defined, in large part, by the characteristics of the partners and the interactions that occur between them. Based on the tenets of attachment theory (Bowlby, 1969), the kinds of relationships individuals form depend on their history of interactions and on the relationships they form with significant others. For example, it has been suggested that the quality of children's friendships depends, in part, on the interactions that the children have had with one another as well as the quality of each child's relationships with primary caregivers.

It is also the case that dyadic relationships are embedded within *groups* or networks of relationships with more or less clearly defined boundaries (families, cliques). Groups are more than mere aggregates of relationships; through emergent properties, such as norms or *shared cultural conventions*, groups help define the types and range of relationships, interactions, and, indeed, individual social inclinations that are likely or permissible (Rubin, Bukowski, & Parker, 2006).

Despite accelerated growth in psychological studies pertaining to culture and cross-cultural comparisons, it is nevertheless the case that the vast majority of studies pertaining to children's relationships have focused primarily on western European and North American samples. However, as is evidenced by the contents of this book, researchers are increasingly examining relationships from a cultural perspective; emerging evidence suggests that there is considerable cultural variability in children's relationship experiences (see Chen, French, & Schneider, 2006, for a review). Given our belief that dyadic relationships are highly significant forces in individual development, in this chapter we review the extant cultural and cross-cultural psychological literature on *parent-child* relationships and children's *dyadic* relationships with *peers* (i.e., friendship).

Relationships from a Cultural Perspective

Does a given relationship construct (e.g., supportiveness) function in the same way in different contexts and cultures? Are there different meanings ascribed to given relationship features when they occur in different cultures? Although it may be the case that parents in all cultures nurture their children to be healthy and to feel secure, there appear to be culture-specific norms with regard to how a child's health and security may best be developed and achieved (Hinde, 1987, 1997). Relatedly, McCall (1988) has argued that there are likely cultural blueprints for interpersonal relationships. We begin this chapter with the assumption that the most developmentally adaptive relationships that children (and young adolescents) experience are those that bring with them positive affect and intrapersonal satisfaction. From this assumption, it is argued that positive affect and satisfaction in close relationships may be a function of very different relationship constructs in specific cultures.

Relationship Constructs and Provisions

Given that social relationships are defined and regulated by the norms, rules, and value systems of culture, there is clearly a need to consider how such close relationships as parent–child relationships and friendships are manifested in various cultures and how the underlying constructs or provisions of these relationships are perceived and evaluated by individuals within different cultures. By the term "provisions," we are referring to such constructs as support, protection, guidance, reassurance of worth, and nurturance (e.g., Weiss, 1974). Other relationship constructs or provisions include intimacy, reliable alliance, instrumental help, companionship, and, importantly, power distribution and distance (e.g., Cutrona & Russell, 1987; Furman, 1996; Laursen, Furman, & Mooney, 2006).

Ultimately, the question being asked is whether some relationship constructs/provisions are viewed as more or less valuable and acceptable in certain cultures (e.g., Rubin & Chung, 2006). From our perspective, the expression of individual *satisfaction* with a relationship informs us about those constructs (e.g., felt support, security, trust, intimacy) that define the quality, value, and acceptability of given relationships. An important conceptual feature of relationship satisfaction is its emphasis on individual variability in the perception and interpretation of close relationships in a given culture (e.g., Harkness, Super, & van Tijen, 2000; Killen & Wainryb, 2000; Schwarz, Trommsdorff, Kim, & Park, 2006; Triandis, 1995).

Many researchers have examined the extent to which relationship constructs are associated with adjustment or maladjustment (see Rubin & Chung, 2006, for reviews). Perceived (and, occasionally, observed) support and warmth in parent–child relationships and friendships have been linked to positive adjustment (e.g., social competence, self-worth), while perceived (and, occasionally, observed) lack of supportiveness and warmth have been associated with internalizing and externalizing problems (e.g., Collins & Laursen, 2004; Laursen & Mooney, 2008; McCartney, Owen, Booth, Vandell, & Clarke-Stewart, 2003). Significantly, most of this body of research has been carried out in Western cultures; relatively few studies of relationship perceptions and their associations with positive and negative developmental correlates and consequences are available in non-Western cultures. Furthermore, little attention has been given to individual differences in perceptions and evaluations about the very meaning of satisfactory relationships in various cultures. Below we review two dimensions that reflect cultural values that may be associated with the types of relationships that children and adolescents may have with parents and peers (friends). These dimensions are characterized by vertical or horizontal relationships and individualist or collectivist values (Hofstede, 1980).

Vertical versus Horizontal Relationships: Power Asymmetry versus Symmetry

One of the central features of dyadic relationships is the extent to which each partner wields power and assumes the dominant status. For example, the parent–child relationship typically involves asymmetrical distributions of power, while putatively *horizontal* relationships such as friendships may be depicted as, to some extent, symmetrical and egalitarian (Hartup & Laursen, 1991; Hinde, 1997; Piaget, 1932; Youniss, 1980). Importantly, Hinde (1997) has argued that power distance and power distribution are properties of the relationship and not of individuals. For example, power distance involves the question "Who takes charge and decides what should be done?" in close relationships. Thus, in some relationships Child A may wield relatively little power, while in others he or she may be the dominant force. Significantly, the distribution of power in close relationships may be influenced by context and culture (for example, in some cultures, males have more power—or expect to have more power—in their relationships with females; Hofstede, 1980).

Owing to differences in maturity, experience, wisdom, and authority, parents are generally viewed as wielding greater relative power than their children (Youniss, 1980). Yet, *in Western cultures*, with the emergence of adolescence, changes often occur in the balance of power and autonomy between the parent and child; with increasing age, the peer group becomes increasingly influential. Thus, as the child develops over time, changes and shifts in closeness and interdependence are evidenced within parent–child relationships and friendships (Laursen et al., 2006; Rubin, Bukowski, et al., 2006).

While it has been surmised that there are distinctive differences in the power distributions of parent–child relationships and friendships, Hinde (1997) has argued that *every* relationship is unique in at least some aspects. Although the peer relations of children and young adolescents are thought to be relatively symmetrical and equal on dimensions of power and control, there may be considerable variations in power and autonomy. For example, when one participant in a friendship exercises more power, it results in the other's relative decrease in autonomy. According to Hinde, what matters is the latter's *perception* of this power asymmetry. Agreement versus disagreement or acceptance versus rejection of the power distance between friends may affect their perceptions and evaluations of their relationship. Disagreement about where power lies may lead to conflict within the relationship and dissatisfaction (Hinde, 1997). But it is also possible that there are cultural variations in the relative acceptance of power distance (i.e., disparities) within particular relationships; in some cultures, power distance in particular relationships may be expected and accepted; in others, it may reflect dysfunctional social affiliations.

Individualism and Collectivism

Relative power, or power distance, is but one dimension that distinguishes interactions and relationships in various cultures (Hofstede, 1980). The constructs of *individualism* and *collectivism* are well known among those who study cultural values and orientations (Hofstede, 1980; Triandis, 1995). Although researchers have typically employed a dichotomous approach in their studies of individualism and collectivism, it has become increasingly commonplace to question the existence of a distinct, clear-cut cultural dualism (Killen & Wainryb, 2000; Wainryb, 2004). Rather, researchers who study cultural values and dimensions are likely to consider them as more or less collectivist and more or less individualist in their orientation.

Western cultures are considered to have a cultural bias toward relatively more emphasis on the socialization of independence by encouraging autonomy, assertiveness, and self-reliance. Eastern (e.g., Asian and Arab) and southern (e.g., African, Central and South American) societies are characterized as relatively more collectivist and are likely to place relatively greater emphasis on conformity, compliance, respect for authority figures, and interdependence in social relationships (Hofstede, 1980; Hui & Triandis, 1986).

Families of European background in Western cultures tend to value warmth and nonpunitive methods of discipline in parent–child relationships; such *authoritative* parenting styles have been associated with children's positive social, emotional, and academic outcomes (Baumrind, 1978; Eisenberg et al., 2008). In addition, the frequent parental use of *psychological* controls (e.g., guilt and love withdrawal) among European parents in Western cultures is related to such undesirable children's developmental outcomes as emotional distress and negative self-esteem (for a review, see Barber, Stolz, & Olsen, 2006). It is argued that psychological control intrudes on the development of children's sense of a positive self. On the other hand, parents' *behavioral* control (e.g., monitoring) seems to be associated with such desirable developmental outcomes as academic achievement and lack of delinquency, because it provides children with guidance without risking individuation processes. Such findings are typically attributed to the mainstream European American values of autonomy, individuation, and independence in the United States (Barber et al., 2006). Conceptually these values also reflect a lesser degree of power distance (hierarchy) in parent–child interactions within Western cultures.

In contrast, psychological and behavioral controls in parent–child relationships have not been found to be associated with children's negative outcomes in East Asian cultures (Chao & Tseng, 2002; Greenfield, Keller, Fuligni, & Maynard, 2003). Rohner and Pettengill (1985) found that among South Korean children and adolescents—but not among their North American counterparts—strict parental control was associated with adolescents' perceptions of parental warmth and high levels of involvement in parent–child relationships; among North American youths, however, adolescents' appraisals of high parental control were associated with parental hostility or rejection. The authors indicated that Korean adolescents do not consider their parent–child relationships as negative when parents exercise strict control. In another relevant study, Chao (1994) found that many East Asian children considered their parents' strictness, firm control, and demand for obedience as reflecting parental care, warmth, love, and involvement. Taken together, certain characteristics of parenting traditionally considered as negative in many Western cultures may not be considered so in contexts where strict obligations and deference to others' advice (e.g., elders in the family) are emphasized. The latter characterizes many Asian countries with a Confucian cultural heritage, such as China, Japan, and Korea (Chao & Tseng, 2002).

Thus far, the examples already noted refer to the cultural acceptability and interpretation of particular forms of *parenting*. Similar arguments have been made about the cultural acceptance of, and satisfaction with, particular aspects of *relationships*. For example, some researchers have argued that maintaining intimate relationships with parents is a more important developmental task for Asian children and adolescents than for their Western counterparts (Korea Survey, 1991; Lee & Lee, 1990). According to French (2004), in cultures within which the family system is prioritized (e.g., China, Japan, Korea), the significance of extrafamilial relationships (e.g., friendships) is somewhat diminished. In such cultures, individuals are more likely to turn to family members than to nonfamily members for social aid and support. Relatedly, Takahashi, Ohara, Antonucci, and Akiyama (2002) examined the relative significance of parent–child relationships versus friendship among Americans and Japanese individuals ranging in age from 20 to 64. The findings indicated that affection toward friends was higher within the American than the Japanese sample.

The East Asian findings noted above have been supported by recent studies in Middle Eastern and North and East African countries. Cultural values within these countries tend to be more collectivist and parenting practices more authoritarian, relative to societies in the West (Dwairy & Achoui, 2006). Traditionally in these countries the family is viewed as more important than the individual, emphasizing loyalty, interdependence, and respectfulness toward parents (Kăgitcibaşi, 1996, 2005). Recent research indicates that Arab youths in Lebanon report higher levels of interdependence and asymmetric power distribution (hierarchy) in their parent–child relationships; these youths also report higher levels of satisfaction with their parent–child relationships (e.g., Dwairy & Achoui, 2006; Dwairy, Achoui, Abouserie, & Farah, 2006). Similarly, the *Arab Woman Development Report* (2003) showed that approximately 87% of Arab female youths in Lebanon and Bahrain evaluated their parent–child relationships as good to excellent. In an extensive cross-regional study (Algeria, Saudi, Lebanon, Palestine, Egypt, Jordan), results revealed that, despite the increase in modernization in Arab societies, high levels of interdependence and connectedness were evidenced in parent–child relationships; autonomy and individuation were not positively viewed, regardless of the degree of modernization, country, and parents' education (Dwairy et al., 2006). Thus, Arab children and youths report high levels of satisfaction with the parent–child relationship when the parent exhibits relatively high levels of control and harsh punishment and low levels of expressed warmth (e.g., Dwairy, 2004).

Last, in a study of American, Korean, and Middle Eastern (Omani) young adolescents, determinants of satisfaction with the mother–child and father–child relationship were compared and contrasted (Rubin et al., 2006). The results revealed complex distinctions between the very meanings of mother– and father–child relationships in the three cultures. For example, in the United States, when young adolescents viewed their mothers and fathers as clearly dominant in the parent–child relationship (that is, the relationship was perceived as hierarchical or vertical in nature), they also perceived the relationship to be characterized by negativity (e.g., conflict, punitiveness) and by a relative lack of positivity (e.g., affection, intimacy). This pattern of relations between constructs was identical for mother– and father–child relationships. In South Korea and Oman, the more the mother– and father–child relationships were perceived to be hierarchical/ vertical by young adolescents, the more the relationships were viewed as *positive*. Moreover, in Oman the more the father–child relationships were perceived to be hierarchical/vertical, the less the relationships were characterized by negative interactions (e.g., conflict and punishment). This pattern was not the case in either the United States or Korea. Further analyses revealed that young adolescents' relationship satisfaction with their mothers and fathers was predicted (1) in the United States by high amounts of affection and intimacy and by low negativity and verticality; (2) in South Korea, by high amounts of affection and intimacy and low negativity; (3) in Oman, by high amounts of paternal affection and intimacy and low paternal negativity. And finally, the more the father–child relationship was viewed as hierarchical/vertical, the *more* satisfied Korean and Omani young adolescents were with the relationship. Indeed, in Oman, satisfaction with the mother–child relationship was also predicted by verticality in the relationship (not by positivity, nor by negative interactions). This study reveals clearly that in a culture (the United States) within which autonomy and individuality are promoted young adolescents are dissatisfied when their parents are viewed as adhering to a hierarchical, top-down relationship perspective. In accordance with cultural notions pertaining to filial piety (or "hyo"; Kim, 2006), although verticality in mother–child relationships was positively associated with negative interactions, Korean young adolescents viewed their relationships with their fathers as positive if the fathers were viewed as adhering to a hierarchical, top-down relationship perspective. And finally, in Oman, where hierarchical relationships reflect respect and the acceptance of power, young adolescents viewed their relationships with their fathers and mothers as positive if their parents were viewed as adhering to a hierarchical, top-down relationship perspective.

Taken together, the aforementioned conceptual frameworks and empirical findings suggest that cultural norms, values, and orientations may influence the salience, interpretations, and perceptions of acceptable and desirable qualities in close relationships. In the remainder of this chapter, we review relevant research pertaining to two specific types of relationships, namely, the parent–child attachment relationship and friendship.

Attachment Relationships and Culture

It has been proposed that the attachment relationship between the child and his or her primary caregiver (most often, the mother) derives from a biologically rooted behavioral system that is marked by the infant's natural proximity-seeking to caregivers for safety, security, and support (Ainsworth, Blehar, Waters, & Wall, 1978; Bowlby, 1969). The attachment system regulates both physical and psychological safety in the context of close relationships. Perceived danger, stress, and threats to the accessibility of attachment figures activate attachment responses. When children with *secure attachments* are threatened, they tend to seek out those with whom they feel secure and protected; in this way, these figures serve as "safe havens." In novel environments, attachment figures also serve as "secure bases" from which children (Ainsworth et al., 1978) and adolescents (Allen et al., 2003) can explore unfamiliar people, objects, and activities.

Insecure attachments fall into several subcategories. In unfamiliar contexts, the *insecure–avoidant* child does not seek proximity to and comfort from the primary caregiver; rather, the child often avoids him or her. The *insecure–ambivalent* child is hesitant to explore novelty in the presence of the primary caregiver and is extremely distressed upon separation from him or her. A third category of insecure attachment, *disorganized*, describes children who do not engage in any clear attachment activities, often displaying bizarre behaviors instead.

Generally, attachment theorists and researchers have argued that a child who has experienced warmth, sensitivity, and responsiveness from a parent or caregiver will develop a secure pattern of attachment (e.g., Ainsworth et al., 1978). Significantly and consistently, a secure attachment relationship has been found to predict such positive outcomes as self-esteem and social competence later in childhood and adolescence (e.g., Ainsworth, 1991; Allen, Moore, Kuperminc, & Bell, 1998; Rose-Krasnor, Rubin, Booth, & Coplan, 1996). On the other hand, insecure attachments are associated with subsequent social maladjustment, including internalizing and externalizing difficulties (e.g., Burgess, Marshall, Rubin, & Fox, 2003; Chango, McElhaney, & Allen, 2009; Fearon, Bakermans-Kranenburg, van IJzendoorn, Lapsley, & Roisman, 2010).

Culture and Attachment

One of the primary tenets of attachment theory is that the formation of a secure, caring, and protective relationship with a primary caregiver is the outcome of evolution and a culturally universal value (van IJzendoorn & Sagi-Schwartz, 2008). This assumption implies that such notions as the secure base for exploration are reinforced by the attachment figure regardless of culture. Unsurprisingly, the relationship between culture and attachment has proved to be a somewhat controversial topic; for example, the cross-cultural universality of attachment *theory* has been questioned. Critics of the universality position often argue that attachment theory emphasizes autonomy, independence, and individuation as defining competence; as noted above, these values are rooted in Western ideals. Critics also emphasize that caregiver sensitivity may be culturally defined and thus differ among societies (e.g., Rothbaum, Weisz, Port, Miyake, & Coplan, 2000). Consequently, traditional measures of attachment, such as the Strange Situation (Ainsworth et al., 1978), may not be relevant in all cultures. Central to this latter debate is that most studies have been conducted in the West and that most measures assessing the attachment relationship were developed in Western laboratories. This situation has led to reasonable questions of conceptual and methodological ethnocentrism (Rothbaum et al., 2000). While the earliest work on parent–child attachment was conducted in Uganda (Ainsworth, 1967), most subsequent research has taken place in the United States and western Europe. Furthermore, many non-Western attachment studies have yielded mixed results. This circumstance has led several researchers to question whether attachment theory (and/or the methods used to assess it) is equally relevant across cultures.

During the 1980s, several studies questioned the applicability of the Strange Situation procedure in particular, and attachment theory in general, to certain cultures. Grossmann, Grossmann, Franz, and Wartner (1981) used the Strange Situation to evaluate attachment behaviors in German infants and toddlers. Results suggested an overrepresentation of insecure–avoidant (A) babies relative to the numbers found in North American laboratories. In addition, contrary to North American findings (in which approximately two-thirds of infants were classified as securely attached), only one-third of the German babies were securely attached to their mothers.

Research conducted within Israeli kibbutzim discovered disproportionate numbers of insecure–ambivalent (C) infants (Oppenheim, Sagi, & Lamb, 1988). Follow-up studies several years later found that children who were classified as securely attached as infants were more likely to demonstrate independence, achievement orientation, and empathy than those children who were found to have an insecure–ambivalent attachment as infants. These results suggested that the higher prevalence of insecure attachment was not necessarily endemic to, or "normal" within, the culture, since some of the negative outcomes associated with insecure attachments elsewhere in the world were still experienced.

Again, during the 1980s, several attachment studies were conducted in Japan; just as was the case with the German and Israeli samples, the results varied from those reported for North American infants. Thus, for example, Miyake, Chen, and Campos (1985) found that the insecure–ambivalent (C) classification was overrepresented in a sample of Japanese infants. Significantly, however, more than two-thirds of infants were securely attached, an even higher proportion than that found in most Western studies; also, there were no reported instances of insecure–avoidant attachments. Similarly, Takahashi (1986) reported high rates of insecure–ambivalent, relatively normal (similar to worldwide norms) rates of secure, and no cases of insecure–avoidant attachments. These results have led to assertions that the dominant assumptions of attachment theory, in particular the secure base hypothesis, are not relevant in Japan, especially given that Asian culture is relatively more accepting of interdependence (collectivism) than independence (individualism) (e.g., Rothbaum et al., 2000). In support of this assertion, the Japanese results have been replicated in other Asian cultures (e.g., Zevalkink, Riksen-Walraven, & Van Lieshout, 1999). It has been argued further that research protocols such as the Strange Situation and the Attachment Q Sort, designed by Western scientists, may be less valid in Japanese and other Asian cultures than in the cultures where the measures were developed. Yet, other research in Japan and elsewhere in Asia, however, has not supported these claims (e.g., Behrens, Hesse, & Main, 2007; Li, Jing, & Yang, 2004).

Several studies have taken place in Africa and are worth noting. Kermoian and Leiderman (1986) studied the Gusii of southwestern Kenya. Both mothers and other caretakers commonly rear Gusii infants, with the care provided by mothers mostly limited to meeting physical (particularly nutritional) needs. A Strange Situation procedure, slightly modified, found about two-thirds of Gusii infants to be securely attached to their mothers, despite the fact that the mothers rarely play with their infants. Interestingly, the nonmaternal caretakers of the infants, who mostly interact in play and social settings, showed lower rates of secure attachment to the babies. This finding suggests that, at least for infants, the strongest attachment was generally formed with the caregiver who provides for the babies' physical needs.

Tomlinson, Cooper, and Murray (2005) found that South African toddlers living in extreme poverty had secure attachment rates similar to those worldwide. They noted that the majority of parents were able to provide a secure home environment, which was reflected by the high proportion of secure attachments. Of those who were insecurely attached, the largest subcategory was insecure–disorganized, found in one-fourth of the children. The researchers hypothesized that this finding could be unique to the high-poverty sample, living in an area where exposure to violence and abuse are common for children. This particular finding, however, is most likely not unique to South Africa—in a meta-analysis of disorganized attachment in North American samples, for example, children living in low-socioeconomic environments were overrepresented (van IJzendoorn, Schuengel, & Bakermans-Kranenburg, 1999). Certainly, more research of this kind is needed in diverse areas (relative to socioeconomic status).

Overall, the results from cross-cultural studies on the parent–child attachment relationship reveal that in most of the world a majority of children are securely attached to a parent but that the proportion of children falling within any one of the insecure subcategories may vary widely. The rates of secure attachment do appear to be relatively steady worldwide, in both Western and non-Western cultures as well as those with nontraditional family and caregiving arrangements.

The major debate that has occupied the cross-cultural research on parent–child attachment has much to do with the psychological meanings of behavior across culture. The *form* that behaviors take (the ways things look) may appear identical from culture to culture (Whiting & Child, 1953);

yet, given that cultures vary in their customs and belief systems (Harkness & Super, 2002), any particular form (e.g., a behavior or an interaction) may be viewed as having a different *function* across cultures. Expressed another way, the psychological "meaning" attributed to any given social behavior is, in large part, a function of the ecological niche in which it is produced and exhibited (Bornstein & Cheah, 2006). An excellent example, in this regard, is the discussion between researchers and theorists about the conceptual distinction between attachment security/insecurity and the Japanese construct of *amae* (Behrens, 2004; Rothbaum et al., 2000). Some have argued that the early research findings indicating an overrepresentation of insecure–ambivalent (C) babies in Japan reflected the Eastern view that during infancy and early childhood parents reinforce child behaviors that to Westerners would appear to reflect dependency and clinginess. In an alternative interpretation, these same behaviors have been viewed by some as reflecting a desirable sense of interdependency, or *amae*, rather than signs of an insecure attachment relationship (Rothbaum et al., 2000).

Importantly, this Western view of Eastern meanings (Rothbaum et al., 2000) has been challenged by several researchers. For example, Behrens (2004) has argued that dependency does not constitute *amae*, although remaining in close proximity to the mother in unfamiliar situations may be responded to with warmth and indulgence. Indeed, Vereijken, Riksen-Walraven, and Van Lieshout (1997) asked Japanese experts to describe the construct of *amae* using the Attachment Q Sort. The authors found that measures of *amae* and dependency in 14- and 24-month-old children were not significantly correlated with an index of secure attachment. Also, Japanese mothers viewed secure attachment behavior as desirable, whereas *amae* and dependency-related behaviors were not viewed in the same light by the same Japanese mothers.

Taken together, cross-cultural attachment research reveals how careful one must be in interpreting *forms* of social behavior. Clearly, the *form* may be identical, but yet the *function* may differ; as such, it is probably the case that Western researchers would do well to study the cultural meanings of this, that, or the other behavior in concert with those researchers who have a personal history within the cultures of interest. In short, this is a call for collaboration between researchers in different cultures for whom given *forms* of behavior or relationships are viewed as demonstrating different *functions*. And while one entertains thoughts about this latter proposal, it also bears noting that much remains unknown in the cross-cultural and cultural parent–child attachment literature. For one thing, we know little about the implications of various attachment classifications for infants and children in the long run. While Western researchers have found that attachment security predicts positive social and emotional outcomes (e.g., Ainsworth, 1991; Allen et al., 1998; Rose-Krasnor et al., 1996; van Ijzendoorn

& Bakermans-Kranenburg, 1996) and insecure attachments predict internalizing and externalizing difficulties (e.g., Burgess et al., 2003; Moss, Bureau, Beliveau, Zdebik, & Lepine, 2009; Chango et al., 2009), there is a lack of cross-cultural research regarding the outcomes surrounding infant and childhood attachment. In addition, few researchers have approached the cross-cultural study of attachment from a developmental perspective—how do attachments change over time, from childhood into adolescence and beyond? Finally, there remain many areas of the world within which attachment research appears to be almost nonexistent (e.g., Latin America, South Asia, eastern Europe). Again, this is a relative vacuum that requires much greater attention.

Friendship and Culture

In some cultures, parents and adult figures remain the most important judges of acceptable behaviors throughout childhood; in other cultures, the peer group becomes an increasingly important adjudicator of acceptable behavior and relationships with increasing age. These observations being the case, a central issue is the degree to which peer interactions and relationships are encouraged or even allowed. In Western cultures, for example, children are generally encouraged to interact with peers and form relationships with them. It is believed that the development of close extrafamilial relationships augurs well for the child's future well-being. However, in kin-based societies, peer interactions may be discouraged because parents fear the potential for competition and conflict (Edwards, 1992). In addition, interactions and relationships with siblings may take the place of peers in many kin-based societies (e.g., Gaskins, 2006).

Hinde (1987) has argued that culture is a driving force in how peer interactions and relationships play out (Rubin, Cheah, & Menzer, 2010). For example, cultural beliefs and norms shape how people respond to and evaluate individual characteristics, behaviors, and interactions in the peer group. In the following sections, we review cross-cultural research related to peer relationships, with a specific focus on friendships.

Friendship

Friendships typically comprise the first significant nonfamilial relationships that children develop with others. Friendships may be defined as reciprocal egalitarian relationships in which both partners acknowledge the relationship and treat each other as equals. Friendships are typically characterized, in Western research, by companionship, a shared history, and mutual affection.

The Functions and Meanings of Friendship

Friendships serve to provide (1) support, self-esteem enhancement, and positive self-evaluation; (2) emotional security; (3) affection and opportunities for intimate disclosure; (4) intimacy and affection; (5) consensual validation of interests, hopes, and fears; (6) instrumental and informational assistance; and (7) prototypes for later romantic, marital, and parental relationships. Friendships also offer children an extrafamilial base of security from which they may explore the effects of their behaviors on themselves, their peers, and their environments (Rubin, Bukowski, & Parker, 2006).

From a Western perspective, Parker and Gottman (1989) have argued that young children's friendships are based on the maximization of excitement and amusement levels in play. During middle childhood, friendships allow children to learn behavioral norms and develop necessary social skills. Finally, in adolescence, friends assist in identity development and self-exploration. These assumptions are grounded in the existing research on what friendship means to children of different ages. For example, Bigelow (1977) identified a developmental sequence of children's friendship expectations, that progressed from an emphasis on friends as those providing rewards to a view of friends as those who have similar interests, understand one another, and engage in self-disclosure. Selman (1980) viewed children as miniphilosophers for whom beliefs about friendship shaped both their friendship expectations and behaviors, identifying six friendship issues: formation, closeness and intimacy, trust and reciprocity, jealousy, conflict resolution, and termination. Five developmental stages of friendship understanding were described within each issue, ranging from a view of friendship as a momentary physical interaction based on proximity to an understanding that friendship develops through the integration of psychological dependency and independence. With development, children gain a better understanding of the psychological nature of friendship, acknowledge interdependency among friends, recognize the need to balance autonomy and intimacy, coordinate social perspectives, and show mutual respect for each other's viewpoint. The developmental stage sequence proposed by Selman has been supported in a number of studies (e.g., Gurucharri, Phelps, & Selman, 1984; Keller & Wood, 1989; Selman, 1980) conducted in North America and western Europe.

Of the limited extant cross-cultural research, it has been suggested that children come to understand the meanings of friendship in different ways and at different development rates across cultures. For example, Gummerum and Keller (2008) studied friendship reasoning among 7-, 9-, 12-, and 15-year-olds from China, Germany, Iceland, and Russia. Among the 7-year-olds, the Russian children were found to have the highest level of friendship understanding, while Chinese and German youths were found to have the least sophisticated understanding. Among the 9-, 12-, and 15-year-olds, the Russian *and* Chinese children were significantly higher in their level of friendship understanding than Icelandic and German children. These latter findings suggest that Chinese children appear to have a more dramatic change in friendship reasoning from age 7 to 9. One might argue that the results reflect a stronger collectivist, interdependency orientation in China and Russia—countries in which such group-oriented collectivist phenomena as the "Young Pioneers" were once important institutions.

Although cultural differences are apparent in the levels of sophistication that children demonstrate in their understanding of friendship as a relationship, this field of study is only in its infancy. Perhaps, then, researchers would do well to continue this line of research, within and across cultures, by interviewing children and young adolescents about the very meaning of friendship (Bigelow, 1977; Keller, Schuster, & Edelstein, 1993; Selman, 1980). And perhaps youths should be asked some very basic questions that may produce different answers across cultures: What *is* a friend and a friendship? What is it that defines a *good* friendship? How does one *become* a friend with another person? How does one *end* a friendship? How does one recapture closeness in a friendship after one has had a disagreement? Given that relationships within various cultural communities are differentiated along such continua as individualism/autonomy, collectivism/connectedness, power distance, and uncertainty avoidance (Hofstede, 1980, Markus & Kitayama, 1991; Triandis, 1995), strong, well-thought-out, conceptually based cross-cultural research programs on developing better understanding of the meaning of friendship are merited.

Friendship Provisions and Culture

In cultures within which friendships are considered one of very few relationships guaranteeing societal success, both intimacy and exclusivity should be regarded as the most important aspects of a friendship (Triandis, Bontempo, Villareal, & Asai, 1988). In support of this conjecture, researchers have found that intimacy is more important in the friendships of children in Korea (French, Lee, & Pidada, 2006) and Cuba (Gonzalez, Moreno, Schneider, 2004) than in those of North American children. At the same time, not all putatively collectivist cultures evidence differences from relatively individualistically oriented cultures. For example, children in collectivist Indonesia do not differ from North American children with respect to friendship intimacy (French, Pidada, & Victor, 2005); and Indonesian children also appear to be more inclusive rather than exclusive in their friendships. Sharabany (2006) highlighted variability within collectivist cultures as well, but between Arab and Israeli children. Arab culture values kin-based over non-kin-based friendships and beliefs in a patriarchal organization of the community. The Israeli children in Sharabany's study resided in kibbutzim (small collective communities in which property and responsibilities are shared). Israeli children were found to engage in more intimate disclosure and reported lower conflict with their best friends than did their Arab counterparts.

An emphasis on trust within friendships has also been found to differ among cultures. For instance, young Russian children are found to use trust to define friendships more often than Icelandic children of the same age (Gummerum & Keller, 2008). Furthermore, whereas the prevalence of conflict is generally similar across cultures, the means by which conflict is resolved differs (French, Pidada, Denoma, McDonald, & Lawton, 2005). For example, Indonesian children disengage when confronted with conflict in an effort to decrease tension, whereas North American children are more likely to confront one another to resolve conflict. Disengagement in the face of potential conflict and peer animosity is the preferred choice among Chinese children and adolescents (Xu, Farver, Chang, Yu, & Zhang, 2006). This form of behavior is referred to as the *ren* strategy and is indicated by refraining from argument or confrontation with friends and peers. Significantly, this strategy is unlike problem-focused avoidance because Chinese children who utilize *ren* are not avoiding or running away from the situation. When Chinese children choose *ren* as a coping strategy, they do not participate in confrontation but, rather, directly attempt to elicit *ren* from the peers with whom they are interacting. This method of coping is used to encourage social harmony and group orientation—outcomes that are likely to strengthen ongoing friendships and to be attractive to those with whom one may wish to initiate a friendship.

Friendship Prevalence and Stability

Approximately 75–80% of Western children have a mutual best friendship (Rubin, Bukowski, & Parker, 2006), and these friendships are remarkably stable. Triandis et al. (1988) have argued that friendships are more stable in non-Western, more collectivistic cultures than in individualistic cultures where friendships are supposedly more fluid. However, some researchers have found evidence that contradicts this contention; for example, the friendships of children from South Korea, a collectivist nation, are both more stable and exclusive than those of Indonesian children, also a collectivist nation (French et al., 2006). Within individualist cultures, Schneider, Woodburn, Soteras-de Toro, & Udvari, (1997) found that Italian children, particularly girls, report more stable friendships than Canadian children. With regard to prevalence, French, Jansen, Riansari, and Setiono (2003) found that Indonesian and North American children have roughly the same number of friendships. Otherwise, the literature on culture and friendship prevalence and stability is practically nonexistent.

Friendship Homophily

Most children engage in friendships with peers who are similar to themselves in observable characteristics, such as age, sex, race, ethnicity, and social behaviors. For example, with regard to multicultural and ethnically diverse nations, children in the United States are more likely to choose same-race or -ethnicity peers as friends than other peers (Howes & Wu, 1990; Kao & Joyner, 2004). This tendency to form same-race friendships has been documented from the preschool through high school years, with a peak in intensity during the developmental periods of middle and late childhood (Aboud & Mendelson, 1998). In other diverse nations, such as Germany, researchers have found that immigrants tend to develop friendships with others of the same ethnicity (Titzmann, Silbereisen, & Schmitt-Rodermund, 2007). Furthermore, new immigrants are more likely to develop intraethnic friendships than immigrants who have lived in Germany for longer periods of time, suggesting the significance of acculturation and shared values in friendship formation (Titzmann & Silbereisen, 2009).

Ethnicity, Race, and Friendship

Beyond the rather limited cross-cultural developmental work on friendships, there have been studies of race, ethnicity, and friendships within culturally diverse nations. In general, there is considerable evidence suggesting that children and adolescents form friendships with same-race/-ethnicity peers (see Graham, Taylor, & Ho, 2009, for a recent review). From preschool through high school, with a peak of intensity during middle and late childhood, there is a tendency for students to interact more often with same-race/-ethnicity peers more often than with cross-race/-ethnicity classmates (e.g., Way & Chen, 2000). Given these differences in the quantity of social interactions with same-race/-ethnicity peers, it is unsurprising that race/ethnicity homophily exists in friendship partners (Kao & Joyner, 2004). But there is some evidence to suggest that acculturation may influence the prevalence of cross-racial/-ethnicity friendships. For example, although Kawabata and Crick (2008) have reported that Latino(a) Americans are highly likely to engage in same-ethnicity friendships, Updegraff, McHale, Whiteman, Thayer, & Crouter (2006) have found that when Mexican American parents were acculturated into European American culture, their children were more likely to have diverse social networks.

In terms of friendship *quality*, Aboud, Mendelson, and Purdy (2003) reported that the same-race and cross-race friendships of European Canadian and African Canadian children were similar in quality, although same-race friendships appeared to be more intimate. Schneider, Dixon, and Udvari (2007) reported that East Asian Canadians had higher-quality friendships with same-ethnic peers than with cross-ethnic peers, whereas Indian Canadians and European Canadians did not differ qualitatively in their same-ethnic and cross-ethnic friendships. Finally, whereas European American children generally rate their friendships as high in positive friendship qualities, other racial/ethnic groups within North America are less inclined to do so (e.g., Aboud, et al., 2003; Way, 2006). For example, Way and colleagues (Way, Cowal, Gingold, Pahl, & Bissessar, 2001) found that Chinese American young adolescents, particularly boys, reported that their friendships were relatively low in quality. In contrast, Latina American girls had relatively high-quality and intimate friendships relative to African American and Chinese American youths.

In sum, the extant literature on same- and cross-race friendship, albeit limited in the number of studies and their scope, suggests that some same-ethnic and cross-ethnic friendships are more similar than they are different. Yet, given the sparse database, clearly much more work is required before a conclusion may be drawn about qualitative differences or similarities in the friendship prevalence, stability and quality of same-race/-ethnicity and interracial/-ethnicity friendships (see Graham et al., 2009, for a recent and relevant review).

In summary, the majority of psychological research on children's friendships has involved middle-class European-American and western European children and young adolescents. Within North America and western Europe, little attention has been paid to culture and the meanings, provisions, occurrence, and stability of friendship, and the extent to which similarity (i.e., homophily) influences friendship (for exceptions, see Azmitia, Ittel, & Brenk, 2006; Graham & Cohen, 1997; Way, 2006). Beyond North America and western Europe, surprisingly little research on peer relationships has focused on friendship.

This relative lack of cultural and cross-cultural research is rather surprising, given that relationships within various cultural communities are differentiated along such continua as individualism versus autonomy, collectivism versus connectedness, power distance, and uncertainty avoidance (Hofstede, 1980; Markus & Kitayama, 1991; Triandis, 1995), each of which has a relationship connotation. For example, in cultures that are relatively more collectivist, connectedness and conformity within long-term relationships as well as within the community at large are highly valued. This attribution being the case, the choice of one's friends may be constrained by adult (parental) influence. Moreover, extrafamilial friendships may remain less influential than one's relationships with parents and family members throughout the childhood and adolescent years.

In contrast, in relatively more individualist cultures, children and young adolescents may be freer to make their own choices of friendship, may value independence, and may more readily relinquish their extrafamilial relationships when individual needs are not being met. And in such cultures autonomy and extrafamilial friendships may assume more and earlier significance than is the case in more collectivist cultures. These "thoughts" about childhood and early adolescent friendships are just that, as comparatively little evidence currently exists to support these conjectures.

As noted earlier, *power distance* is a relevant construct that distinguishes among cultures. Some cultures value relationships that are relatively more egalitarian, whereas others primarily value a hierarchical relationship structure (Hofstede, 1980). In this context friendship, when explored through the lens of culture, may reflect greater or lesser propensities in the directions of either dominance versus submissiveness or egalitarianism versus collectivism.

Lastly, *uncertainty avoidance* involves the extent to which cultures feel comfortable in unstructured situations (Hofstede, 1980). According to Hofstede, uncertainty-avoiding cultures try to minimize the possibility of such situations by adhering to strict laws and rules, and on the philosophical and religious level by a belief in *absolute truth*. Consequently, one may expect that rules and regulations pertaining to relationships are clearly demarcated through socialization practices. In such cultures, friendships may be selected by parents, not children. And the choice of friendships may be marked by perceived similarities in familial or cultural beliefs and traditions. These notions may be particularly valid for immigrant families (and especially parents) that aspire to cultural (and ethnic or religious) connectedness to their children. In cultures that are more accepting of uncertainty, there may be greater tolerance for philosophical and religious diversity. In this regard, there may be greater degrees of freedom accorded to the nature of the friendship, who might be considered an allowable friend (by parents and family), and how autonomous/independent the friendships (and the individuals) can be. Again, many of these notions have yet to be examined.

Concluding Remarks: Parent–Child Relationships, Friendship, and Development in a Cultural Context

In this chapter, we have reviewed the cross-cultural literature that relates to children's dyadic relationships—specifically, parent–child relationships and friendships. From our perspective, most cross-cultural research on relationships has been dominated by an *etic* framework; Western (mostly North American and western European) researchers have, by and large, assumed that such relationship constructs as attachment and friendship are of equivalent relevance and can be assessed in the same ways across all cultures. However, as we have observed throughout this chapter, this perspective may cause researchers to overlook or miss social conventions that are related to a specific construct in one culture but are completely unrelated in another culture.

Among the many future directions the literature on children's dyadic relation should take are the study of relations between relationships systems and the long-term outcomes of different types of relationships. In the first case, attachment theorists propose that the child who receives responsive and sensitive parenting from the primary caregiver forms an internal working model of that caregiver as trustworthy and dependable when needed, as well as develops a model of the self as someone who is worthy of such care (Bowlby, 1969). Through experience with a responsive and sensitive caregiver, the child learns reciprocity in social interactions (Elicker, Englund, & Sroufe, 1992) and a set of specific social skills that can be used in relationships that extend beyond the child–caregiver relationship. Also, the securely attached child is able to use the caregiver as a secure base for exploration (Ainsworth et al., 1978), including the exploration of relationships with peers. Thus, there is a compelling rationale for proposing that the quality of the parent–child relationship engenders a set of internalized relationship expectations that affect the quality of friendships with peers.

Indeed, researchers have found that children with secure attachments to parents have more friends and their friendships are of better quality than those of insecurely attached children (e.g., Kerns, Klepec, & Cole, 1996; Rubin et al., 2004; Youngblade & Belsky, 1992). Interactions between friendship dyads comprising two securely attached members are more positive, fair, intimate, and responsive than interactions within dyads comprising only one securely attached member. Moreover, securely attached adolescents are viewed by their best friends as being more altruistic and more conciliatory after conflict; also, they are more satisfied with their friendships than the friends of anxious–avoidant or anxious–ambivalent adolescents. While there generally are associations between parent–child attachments and later peer and friend relationships, a child's attachment relationship to parents is not absolutely deterministic of their later relationships with friends. There are children who are insecurely attached to parents and yet form high-quality friendships. In this way, a good friendship may compensate for the child's insecure attachment to parents (Rubin et al., 2004).

There are virtually no studies of the relations between the quality of the attachment relationships and the quality of extrafamilial relationships beyond North America and western Europe. This failing represents a vacuum of significant proportions not only empirically but also theoretically. A central tenet of attachment theory is that secure attachments predict competent, supportive, and satisfactory friendships and romantic relationships (Furman, Simon, Shaffer, & Bouchey, 2002). It would certainly behoove researchers to investigate cross-culturally these relations among relationship systems.

As for the long-term outcomes of supportive, secure, and satisfactory dyadic relationships, several North American and western European researchers have examined relations between relationship systems and the manner in which experiences in both familial and extrafamilial relationships may interact to influence psychosocial functioning (e.g., Booth-LaForce et al., 2006; Rubin et al. 2004). A central focus has been on whether and how friendships may serve to moderate the association between parent–adolescent relationship quality and psychosocial functioning.

To begin with, children who feel secure and supported by their primary caregivers have been shown to have higher levels of perceived competence in multiple domains (Kerns et al., 1996) as well as higher self-esteem (Simons, Paternite, & Shore, 2001), and fewer feelings of loneliness (Kerns et al., 1996). Furthermore, relatively lower security has been associated with both internalizing and externalizing problems (Granot & Mayseless, 2001; McCartney, Owens, Booth, Vandell, & Clarke-Stewart, 2003). The quality of the child–parent attachment relationship has been linked with social competence and adjustment and maladjustment from early childhood through adolescence. As children mature, however, relationships outside of the home, specifically their friendships, may influence adjustment directly. For example, the long-term influence of friendship quality in early adolescence has been demonstrated in a 12-year longitudinal study by Bagwell, Newcomb, and Bukowski (1998). These researchers found that adolescents without friends, compared with those with friends, had lower self-esteem and more psychopathological symptoms in adulthood. Whether or not friendship predicts psychological outcomes in non-Western countries is, as yet, unknown.

Given the significance of both parent–child relationships and friendships in early adolescence, one may speculate that these relationships interact in meaningful ways to predict adjustment. Thus, the parent–adolescent relationship and friendship processes may be associated with psychosocial functioning in at least three ways. First, as we have already noted, each may make an independent, unique contribution to predicting adjustment outcomes. Second, the parent–adolescent relationship may provide the basis for the formation of friendships, which in turn are related to psychosocial adjustment. Third, the relation between the parent–adolescent relationship and functioning may be moderated by friendship quality. According to Bowlby (1969), adjustment at any particular stage is the result of the interaction of the individual's past experiences with current relationships in the larger social environment. Therefore, the early parent–adolescent relationship and friendship experiences may interact with each other to influence psychosocial functioning (e.g., Laible, Carlo, & Raffaelli, 2000). Specifically, a high-quality friendship may buffer the impact of a qualitatively poor parent–adolescent relationship (Booth, Rubin, & Rose-Krasnor, 1998). We do not suggest that only one of these models is the "correct" model. Rather, it is more likely that all three processes take place in varying degrees and, most important, may diverge significantly across cultures.

All in all, there appears to be much to do in the study of culture and dyadic relationships. We have proposed several new lines of research, and we welcome other such theoretically based research programs, some of which may well be under way already.

References

Aboud, F., & Mendelson, M. (1998). Determinants of friendship selection and quality: Developmental perspectives. In W. Bukowski & A. Newcomb (Eds.), *The company they keep: Friendship in childhood and adolescence* (pp. 87–112). New York: Cambridge University Press.

Aboud, F., Mendelson, M., & Purdy, K. (2003). Cross-race peer relations and friendship quality. *International Journal of Behavioral Development, 27,* 165–173.

Ainsworth, M. (1967). *Infancy in Uganda.* Baltimore, MD: Johns Hopkins University Press.

Ainsworth, M. (1991). Attachments and other affectional bonds across the life cycle. In C. M. Parkes, J. Stevenson-Hinde, & P. Marris (Eds.), *Attachment across the life cycle.* London: Routledge.

Ainsworth, M., Blehar, M., Waters, E., & Wall, S. (1978). *Patterns of attachment.* Hillsdale, NJ: Erlbaum.

Allen, J. P., McElhaney, K. B., Land, D. J., Kuperminc, G. P., Moore, C. W., O'Beirne-Kelly, H., et al. (2003). A secure base in adolescence: Markers of attachment security in the mother adolescent relationship. *Child Development, 74,* 292–307.

Allen, J. P., Moore, C., Kuperminc, G., & Bell, K. (1998). Attachment and adolescent psychosocial functioning. *Child Development, 69,* 1406–1419.

Arab Woman Developmental Report. (2003). Alfatat al Arabeyah al Moraheqah [The Arab adolescent girls]. Beirut, Lebanon: Kawtar.

Azmitia, M., Ittel, A., & Brenk, C. (2006). Latino-heritage adolescents' friendships. *Peer relationships in cultural context* (pp. 426–451). New York: Cambridge University Press.

Bagwell, C., Newcomb, A., & Bukowski, W. (1998). Preadolescent friendship and peer rejection as predictors of adult adjustment. *Child Development, 69*(1), 140–153.

Barber, B. K., Stolz, H. E., & Olsen, J. A. (2006). Parental support, psychological control, and behavioral control: Assessing relevance across time, culture, and method. *Monographs of the Society for Research in Child Development, 70,* Serial No. 282, 1–137.

Baumrind, D. (1978). Parental disciplinary patterns and social competence in youth. *Youth and Society, 9,* 239–276.

Behrens, K. (2004). A multifaceted view of the concept of amae: Reconsidering the indigenous Japanese concept of relatedness. *Human Development, 47,* 1–27.

Behrens, K. Y., Hesse, E., & Main, M. (2007). Mothers' attachment status as determined by the Adult Attachment Interview predicts their 6-year-olds' reunion responses: A study conducted in Japan. *Developmental Psychology, 43, 1553–1567.*

Bigelow, B. (1977). Children's friendship expectations: A cognitive-developmental study. *Child Development, 48*(1), 246–253.

Booth, C., Rubin, K., & Rose-Krasnor, L. (1998). Perceptions of emotional support from mother and friend in middle childhood: Links with social–emotional adaptation and preschool attachment security. *Child Development, 69,* 427–442.

Booth-LaForce, C. L., Oh, W., Kim, A., Rubin, K. H., Rose-Krasnor, L., et al. (2006). Attachment, self-worth, and peer-group Functioning in middle childhood. *Attachment and Human Development, 8,* 309–325.

Bornstein, M. H., & Cheah, C. S. L. (2006). The place of "culture and parenting" in the ecological contextual perspective on developmental science. In K. H. Rubin and O. Boon Chung (Eds.), *Parental beliefs, parenting, and child development in cross-cultural perspective* (pp. 3–33). London: Psychology Press.

Bowlby, J. (1969). *Attachment and loss: Vol. 1. Attachment.* New York: Basic Books.

Burgess, K. B., Marshall, P. J., Rubin, K. H., & Fox, N. A. (2003). Infant attachment and temperament as predictors of subsequent externalizing problems and cardiac physiology. *Journal of Child Psychology and Psychiatry, 44,* 819–831.

Chango, J. M., McElhaney, K. B., & Allen, J. P. (2009). Attachment organization and patterns of conflict resolution in friendships predicting adolescents' depressive symptoms over time. *Attachment and Human Development, 11,* 331–346.

Chao, R. K. (1994). Beyond parental control and authoritarian parenting style: Understanding Chinese parenting through the cultural notion of training. *Child Development, 65*(4), 1111–1119.

Chao, R., & Tseng, V. (2002). Parenting of Asians. In M. H. Bornstein (Ed.), *Handbook of parenting: Social conditions and applied parenting* (2nd ed., Vol. 4, pp. 59–93). Mahwah, NJ: Erlbaum.

Chen, X., French, D., & Schneider, B. (2006). Culture and peer relationships. In X. Chen, D. French, & B. H. Schneider (Eds.), *Peer relationships in cultural context* (pp. 3–20). New York: Cambridge University Press.

Collins, W. A., & Laursen, B. (2004). Parent–adolescent relationships and influences. In R. Lerner & L. Steinberg (Eds.), *The handbook of adolescent psychology* (pp. 331–362). New York: Wiley.

Cutrona, C. E., & Russell, D. (1987). The provisions of social relationships and adaptation to stress. In W. H. Jones & D. Perlman (Eds.), *Advances in personal relationships* (Vol. 1).

Dwairy, M. (2004). Parenting styles and psychological adjustment of Arab adolescents. *Transcultural Psychiatry, 41*(2), 233–252.

Dwairy, M. & Achoui, M. (2006). Introduction to three cross-regional research studies on parenting styles, individuation, and mental health in the Arab societies. *Journal of Cross-Cultural Psychology 37,*(3), 221–229.

Dwairy, M., Achoui, M., Abouserie, R., & Farah A., (2006). Parenting styles, individuation, and mental health of Arab adolescents: A third cross-regional research study. *Journal of Cross-Cultural Psychology, 37*(3), 262–272.

Edwards, C. P. (1992). Cross-cultural perspective on family-peer relations. In R. D. Parke and G. W. Ladd (Eds.), *Family-peer relationships: Modes of linkage* (pp. 285–316). Hillsdale, NJ: Erlbaum.

Eisenberg, N., Valiente, C., Losoya, S., Zhou, Q., Cumberland, A., Liew, J., et al. (2008). Understanding mother–adolescent conflict discussions: Concurrent and across-time prediction from youths' dispositions and parenting. *Monographs of the Society for Research on Child Development* (Vol. 72).

Elicker, J., Englund, M., & Sroufe, L. (1992). Predicting peer competence and peer relationships in childhood from early parent–child relationships. *Family–peer relationships: Modes of linkage* (pp. 77–106). Hillsdale, NJ England: Lawrence Erlbaum Associates, Inc.

Fearon, R. P., Bakermans-Kranenburg, M. J., van IJzendoorn, M. H., Lapsley, A.-M., & Roisman, G. I. (2010), The significance of insecure attachment and disorganization in the development of children's externalizing behavior: A meta-analytic study. *Child Development, 81,* 435–456.

French, D. C. (2004). The cultural context of friendhips. *ISSBD Newsletter, 28,* 19–20.

French, D., Jansen, E., Riansari, M., & Setiono, K. (2003). Friendships of Indonesian children: Adjustment of children who differ in friendship presence and similarity between mutual friends. *Social Development, 12,* 606–621.

French, D., Lee, O., & Pidada, S. (2006). Friendships of Indonesian, South Korean, and U.S. youth: Exclusivity, intimacy, enhancement of worth, and conflict. In X. Chen, D. French, & B. H. Schneider (Eds.), *Peer relationships in cultural context* (pp. 379–402). New York: Cambridge University Press.

French, D., Pidada, S., Denoma, J., McDonald, K., & Lawton, A. (2005). Reported peer conflicts of children in the United States and Indonesia. *Social Development, 14,* 458–472.

French, D., Pidada, S., & Victor, A. (2005). Friendships of Indonesian and United States youth. *International Journal of Behavioral Development, 29,* 304–313.

Furman, W. (1996). The measurement of friendship perceptions: Conceptual and methodological issues. In W. M. Bukowski, A. F. Newcomb, & W. W. Hartup (Eds.), *The company they keep: Friendship in childhood and adolescence* (pp. 41–65). New York: Cambridge University Press.

Furman, W., Simon, V. A., Shaffer, L., & Bouchey, H. A. (2002). Adolescents' working models and styles for relationships with parents, friends, and romantic partners. *Child Development, 73,* 241–255.

Gaskins, S. (2006). The cultural organization of Yucatec Mayan children's social interactions. *Peer relationships in cultural context* (pp. 283–309). New York: Cambridge University Press.

Gonzalez, Y., Moreno, D., & Schneider, B. (2004). Friendship expectations of early adolescents in Cuba and Canada. *Journal of Cross-Cultural Psychology, 35,* 436–445.

Graham, J., & Cohen, R. (1997). Race and sex as factors in children's sociometric ratings and friendship choices. *Social Development, 6,* 355–372.

Graham, S., Taylor, A. Z., & Ho, A. Y. (2009). Race and ethnicity in peer relations research. In K. H. Rubin, W. Bukowski, & B. Laursen (Eds.), *Handbook of peer interactions, relationships, and groups* (pp. 394–413). New York: Guilford Press.

Granot, D., & Mayseless, O. (2001). Attachment security and adjustment to school in middle childhood. *International Journal of Behavioral Development, 25,* 530–541.

Greenfield, P., Keller, H., Fuligni, A., & Maynard, A. (2003). Cultural pathways through universal development. *Annual Review of Psychology, 54,* 461–490.

Grossmann, K. E., Grossmann, K., Franz, H., & Wartner, U. (1981). German children's behavior toward their mothers at 12 months and their fathers at 18 months in Ainsworth's strange situation. *International Journal of Behavioral Development, 4,* 157–181.

Gummerum, M., & Keller, M. (2008). Affection, virtue, pleasure, and profit: Developing an understanding of friendship closeness and intimacy in Western and Asian societies. *International Journal of Behavioral Development, 32*(3), 218–231.

Gurucharri, C., Phelps, E., & Selman, R. (1984). Development of interpersonal understanding: A longitudinal and comparative study of normal and disturbed youths. *Journal of Consulting and Clinical Psychology, 52,* 26–36.

Harkness, S., & Super, C. M. (2002). Culture and parenting. In M. H. Bornstein (Ed.), *Handbook of parenting: Vol. 2. Biology and ecology of parenting* (2nd ed., pp. 253–280). Mahwah, NJ: Erlbaum.

Harkness, S., Super, C. M., & van Tijen, N. (2000). Individualism and the "Western mind" reconsidered: American and Dutch parents' ethnotheories of children and family. In S. Harkness, C. Raeff, & C. M. Super (Eds.), *Variability in the social construction of the child* (*New Directions for Child and Adolescent Development*, 87, pp. 23–39). San Francisco: Jossey-Bass.

Hartup, W. W., & Laursen, B. (1991). Relationships as developmental contexts. In R. Cohen & A. W. Siegel (Eds.), *Context and development* (pp. 253–279). Hillsdale, NJ: Erlbaum.

Hinde, R. A. (1987). *Individuals, relationships, and culture.* Cambridge, UK: Cambridge University Press.

Hinde, R. A. (1997). *Relationships: A dialectical perspective.* Hove, UK: Psychology Press.

Hofstede, G. (1980). *Culture's consequences: International differences in work-related values.* Beverly Hills, CA: Sage.

Howes, C., & Wu, F. (1990). Peer interactions and friendships in an ethnically diverse school setting. *Child Development, 61,* 537–541.

Hui, C. H., & Triandis, H. C. (1986). Individualism–collectivism: A study of cross-cultural researchers.

Kăgitcibaşi, C. (1996). *Family and human development across cultures: A view from the other side.* Hilsdale, NJ: Erlbaum.

Kăgitcibaşi, C. (2005). Autonomy and relatedness in cultural context. *Journal of Cross-Cultural Psychology, 36,* 403–422.

Kao, G., & Joyner, K. (2004). Do race and ethnicity matter among friends?: Activities among interracial, interethnic, and intraethnic adolescent friends. *Sociological Quarterly, 45,* 557–573.

Kawabata, Y., & Crick, N. (2008). The role of cross-racial/ethnic friendships in social adjustment. *Developmental Psychology, 44*(4), 1177–1183.

Keller, M., Schuster, P., & Edelstein, W. (1993). Universal and differential aspects of the development of socio-moral reasoning: Results from a study of Icelandic and Chinese children. *Zeitschrift fü Sozialisationforschung und Erzienhungssoziologie, 13,* 149–160.

Keller, M., & Wood, P. (1989). Development of friendship reasoning: A study of interindividual differences in intraindividual change. *Developmental Psychology, 25*(5), 820–826.

Kermoian, R., & Leiderman, P. H. (1986). Infant attachment to mother and child caretaker in an East African community. *International Journal of Behavioral Development, 9,* 455–469.

Kerns, K., Klepac, L., & Cole, A. (1996). Peer relationships and preadolescents' perceptions of security in the child-mother relationship. *Developmental Psychology, 32,* 457–466.

Killen, M., & Wainryb, C. (2000). Independence and interdependence in diverse cultural contexts. In S. Harkness, C. Raeff, & C. M. Super (Eds.), *Variability in the social construction of the child* (pp. 5–21). San Francisco: Jossey-Bass.

Kim, K. W. (2006). "Hyo" and parenting in Korea. In K. H. Rubin & O. B. Chung (Eds.), *Parenting beliefs, parenting, and child development in cross-cultural perspective* (pp. 207–222). New York: Psychology Press.

Korea Survey (1991). *The youth of the world and Korea.* Seoul, Korea: Korea Survey Gallup Polls.

Laible, D., Carlo, G., & Raffaelli, M. (2000). The differential relations of parent and peer attachment to adolescent adjustment. *Journal of Youth and Adolescence, 29,* 45–59.

Laursen, B., Furman. W., & Mooney, K. S. (2006). Predicting interpersonal competence and self-worth from adolescent relationships and relationship networks: Variable-centered and person-centered perspectives. *Merrill-Palmer Quarterly, 52*(3), 572–600.

Laursen, B., & Mooney, K. S. (2008). Relationship network quality: Adolescent adjustment and perceptions of relationships with parents and friends. *American Journal of Orthopsychiatry, 78,* 47–53.

Lee, E. H., & Lee, K. W. (1990). *The Korean mothers' socialization process for children* (in Korean). Seoul: Ehwa Women's University.

Li, X., Jing, J., & Yang, D. (2004). Characters of 75 infants' attachment toward their mothers. *Chinese Mental Health Journal, 18,* 291–293.

Markus, H., & Kitayama, S. (1991). Culture and the self: Implications for cognition, emotion, and motivation. *Psychological Review, 98*(2), 224–253.

McCall, G. J. (1988). The organizational life cycle of relationships. In S. Duck (Ed.), *Handbook of personal relationships: Theory, research, and interventions* (pp. 467–486). New York: Wiley.

McCartney, K., Owen, M. T., Booth, C., Vandell, D. L., & Clarke-Stewart, K. A. (2003). Testing a maternal attachment model of behavior problems in early childhood. *Journal of Child Psychology and Psychiatry, 44,* 1–14.

Miyake, K., Chen, S., & Campos, J. J. (1985). Infant temperament, mother's mode of interaction, and attachment in Japan: An interim report. *Monographs of the Society for Research in Child Development, 50,* 276–297.

Moss, E., Bureau, J., Beliveau, M., Zdebik, M., & Lepine, S. (2009). Links between children's attachment behavior at early school-age, their attachment-related representations, and behavior problems in middle childhood. *International Journal of Behavioral Development, 33,* 155–166.

Oppenheim, D., Sagi, A., & Lamb, M. E. (1988). Infant-adult attachments on the Kibbutz and their relation to socioemotional development 4 years later. *Developmental Psychology, 24,* 427–433.

Parker, J., & Gottman, J. (1989). Social and emotional development in a relational context: Friendship interaction from early childhood to adolescence. In T. J. Berndt & G. W. Ladd (Eds.), *Peer relationships in child development* (pp. 95–131). Oxford, UK: Wiley.

Piaget, J. (1932). *The moral judgment of the child.* Glencoe, IL: Free Press.

Rohner, R. P., & Pettengill, S. M. (1985). Perceived parental acceptance-rejection and parental control among Korean adolescents. *Child Development, 56*(2), 524–528.

Rose-Krasnor, L., Rubin, K. H., Booth, C. L., & Coplan, R. J. (1996). Maternal directiveness and child attachment security as predictors of social competence in preschoolers. *International Journal of Behavioral Development, 19,* 309–325.

Rothbaum, F., Weisz, J., Pott, M., Miyake, K., & Morelli, G. (2000). Attachment and culture: Security in the United States and Japan. *American Psychologist, 55,* 1093–1104.

Rubin, K., Bukowski, W., & Parker, J. (2006). Peer interactions, relationships, and groups. In N. Eisenberg, W. Damon, & R. M. Lerner (Eds.), *Handbook of child psychology: Vol. 3. Social, emotional, and personality development* (6th ed., pp. 571–645). New York: Wiley.

Rubin, K., Cheah, C., & Menzer, M. (2010). Peers. In M. Bornstein (Ed.), *Handbook of cultural developmental science* (pp. 223–237). New York: Psychology Press.

Rubin, K. H. & Chung, O. B. (Eds.). (2006). *Parental beliefs, parenting, and child development in cross-cultural perspective.* London: Psychology Press.

Rubin, K., Dwyer, K., Booth-LaForce, C., Kim, A., Burgess, K., & Rose-Krasnor, L. (2004). Attachment, friendship, and psychosocial functioning in early adolescence. *The Journal of Early Adolescence, 24,* 326–356.

Rubin, K. H., Oh, W., Ashktorab, S., Rhee, U., Jung, S., & Kim, A. H. (2006, July).
Children's perceptions of their parent–child relationships: A cross-cultural study of US, South Korea, and Oman. Paper presented at invited symposium, Social Relationships in Changing Cultural Context (X. Chen & R. Sharabany, Co-Chairs). (Invited Paper Symposium). 19th biennial meeting of the International Society for the Study of Behavioral Development, Melbourne, Australia.

Schneider, B., Dixon, K., & Udvari, S. (2007). Closeness and competition in the inter-ethnic and co-ethnic friendships of early adolescents in Toronto and Montreal. *The Journal of Early Adolescence, 27*, 115–138.

Schneider, B., Woodburn, S., Soteras-de Toro, M., & Udvari, S. (2005). Cultural and gender differences in the implications of competition for early adolescent friendship. *Merrill-Palmer Quarterly, 51*, 163–191.

Schwarz, B., Trommsdorff, G., Kim, U., & Park, Y.-S. (2006). Intergenerational support: Psychological and cultural analyses of Korean and German women. *Current Sociology, 54*(2), 315–340.

Selman, R. (1980). *The growth of interpersonal understanding: Developmental and clinical analyses.* New York: Academic Press.

Sharabany, R. (2006). The cultural context of children and adolescents: Peer relationships and intimate friendships among Arab and Jewish children in Israel. In X. Chen, D. French, & B. H. Schneider (Eds.), *Peer relationships in cultural context* (pp. 452–478). New York: Cambridge University Press.

Simons, K., Paternite, C., & Shore, C. (2001). Quality of parent/adolescent attachment and aggression in young adolescents. *The Journal of Early Adolescence, 21*, 182–203.

Takahashi, K. (1986). Examining the strange-situation procedure with Japanese mothers and 12-month-old infants. *Developmental Psychology, 22*, 265–270.

Takahashi, K., Ohara, N., Antonucci, T. C., & Akiyama, H. (2002). Commonalities and differences in close relationships among the Americans and Japanese: A comparison by the individualism/collectivism concept. *International Journal of Behavioral Development, 26*, 453–465.

Titzmann, P., & Silbereisen, R. (2009). Friendship homophily among ethnic German immigrants: A longitudinal comparison between recent and more experienced immigrant adolescents. *Journal of Family Psychology, 23*, 301–310.

Titzmann, P., Silbereisen, R., & Schmitt-Rodermund, E. (2007). Friendship homophily among diaspora migrant adolescents in Germany and Israel. *European Psychologist, 12*(3), 181–195.

Tomlinson, M., Cooper, P., & Murray, L. (2005). The mother–infant relationship and infant attachment in a South African peri-urban settlement. *Child Development, 76*, 1044–1054.

Triandis, H. C. (1995). *Individualism & collectivism.* Boulder, CO: Westview Press.

Triandis, H., Bontempo, R., Villareal, M., & Asai, M. (1988). Individualism and collectivism: Cross-cultural perspectives on self-ingroup relationships. *Journal of Personality and Social Psychology, 54*, 323–338.

van IJzendoorn, M. H., & Bakermans-Kranenburg, M. J. (1996). Attachment representations in mothers, fathers, adolescents, and clinical groups: A meta-analytic search for normative data. *Journal of Consulting & Clinical Psychology, 64*, 8–21.

van IJzendoorn, M. H., & Sagi-Schwartz, A. (2008). Cross-cultural patterns of attachment: Universal and contextual dimensions. In J. Cassidy & P. R. Shaver (Eds.), *Handbook of attachment* (2nd ed., pp. 880–905). New York: Guilford Press.

van IJzendoorn, M., Schuengel, C., & Bakermans-Kranenburg, M. (1999). Disorganized attachment in early childhood: Meta-analysis of precursors, concomitants, and sequelae. *Development and Psychopathology, 11*, 225–249.

Vereijken, C., Riksen-Walraven, J., & Van Lieshout, C. (1997). Mother-infant relationships in Japan: Attachment, dependency, and amae. *Journal of Cross-Cultural Psychology, 28*, 442–462.

Wainryb, C. (2004). Is and ought: Moral judgments about the world as understood. In B. Sokol & J. Baird (Eds.), *Mind, morals, and action: The interface between children's theories of mind and socio-moral development*. San Francisco: Jossey-Bass.

Way, N. (2006). The cultural practice of close friendships among urban adolescents in the United States. In X. Chen, D. French, & B. H. Schneider (Eds.), *Peer relationships in cultural context* (pp. 403–425). New York: Cambridge University Press.

Way, N., & Chen, L. (2000). Close and general friendships among African American, Latino, and Asian American adolescents from low-income families. *Journal of Adolescent Research, 15*, 274–301.

Weiss, R. S. (1974). The provisions of social relationships. In Z. Rubin (Ed.), *Doing unto others* (pp. 17–26). Englewood Cliffs, NJ: Prentice-Hall.

Whiting, J., & Child, I. (1953). *Child training and personality: A cross-cultural study*. New Haven, CT: Yale University Press.

Xu, Y., Farver, J., Chang, L., Yu, L., & Zhang, Z. (2006). Culture, family contexts, and children's coping strategies in peer interactions. In X. Chen, D. French, & B. H. Schneider (Eds.), *Peer relationships in cultural context* (pp. 264–280). New York: Cambridge University Press.

Youngblade, L., & Belsky, J. (1992). Parent-child antecedents of 5-year-olds' close friendships: A longitudinal analysis. *Developmental Psychology, 28*, 700–713.

Youniss, J. (1980). Parents and peers in social development: A Sullivan–Piaget perspective. Chicago: University of Chicago Press.

Zevalkink, J., Riksen-Walraven, J., & Van Lieshout, C. (1999). Attachment in the Indonesian caregiving context. *Social Development, 8*, 21–40.

PART IV

ADAPTIVE AND MALADAPTIVE
SOCIAL FUNCTIONING

CHAPTER 10

Morality, Exclusion, and Culture

MELANIE KILLEN *and* ALAINA BRENICK

Conceptual Overview

Children's social, emotional, and moral development occurs in a cultural context. Over the past two decades, research in developmental science has demonstrated the vast and myriad ways in which culture plays an important role in how children form concepts, acquire language, develop social competence, and construct morality. How culture plays a role is quite complicated and varies for each phenomenon under investigation. The goal of this chapter is to review current literature on how culture plays a role in children's evaluations of peer exclusion, and particularly exclusion that involves intergroup attitudes. Recently, developmental psychologists have studied children's intergroup attitudes, defined as judgments, beliefs, and biases that exist about members of outgroups, and how these judgments are related to group identity (Bennett & Sani, 2004) and peer exclusion (Killen, Sinno, & Margie, 2007).

Culture is relevant for the topic of intergroup peer exclusion in several ways. First, cultural membership, in the form of social identity, has been shown to contribute to patterns of peer exclusion. Social identity theory proposes that as children develop an identification with their group, then peers from different groups, such as those based on culture, become members of the "outgroup"; rejecting members of the outgroup enhances and reinforces the identity of the ingroup (Nesdale, 2004; Rutland, 2004). This type of rejection has been shown to manifest itself in the context of everyday peer exclusion in school and home settings (Killen, Sinno, et al., 2007). Second, cultural membership is a significant factor affecting why children exclude others based on culture.

Societal and cultural expectations contribute to the formation of ingroup identity. When children hear negative messages about members of other cultures, the distinctions between the ingroup and outgroup are reinforced. Studying how messages from parents reinforce peer exclusion reflects cultural influences on children's exclusion of one another. Third, how children develop group identity and the factors that contribute to peer exclusion need to be understood from diverse cultural perspectives (Rutland, Killen, & Abrams, 2010). What constitutes legitimate reasons for exclusion in one culture may be viewed as negative reasons in another culture. For example, exclusion based on gender in one culture has different connotations in another culture, particularly when gender expectations (stereotypical and nonstereotypical) have unique cultural meanings. In fact, an important question is, To what extent does exclusion based on gender or other group categories generalize across cultures? This question may be usefully posed for any group membership category, such as gender, race, ethnicity, and particularly for "cultural" identity.

To address these issues, in this chapter we review the literature on peer exclusion in a range of cultural contexts. As we discuss in more detail later, we apply a social cognitive domain model to understanding issues of social exclusion (Killen, Sinno, et al., 2007; Hitti, Mulvey, & Killen, in press), which proposes a "culture by context by domain" theory. This interactive theory holds that comparisons of children from different cultural backgrounds requires detailed analyses of the context of interactions as well as the domain of social issues under investigation. Rarely does "culture," alone, account for differences between groups of children from two different parts of the world. This is so because other factors, such as the context of interactions or the domain of social judgments, contribute to how individuals make judgments (Turiel, 2002). This situation is the case "within cultures," and it is also the case "between cultures." Further, other variables such as gender, age, and socioeconomic status (SES) play a role in contributing to cultural comparisons. Thus, when comparing how Koreans and Americans evaluate peer exclusion, for example, it is necessary to analyze how the context of exclusion (for example, rejection, exclusion, victimization) and the domain of exclusion (is it reasoned about in terms of fairness, group identity, or personal choice?) bear on how Koreans and Americans evaluate exclusion (Park & Killen, 2010). For these reasons, which are spelled out in more detail in this chapter, we view culture as a multifaceted construct, requiring extensive analyses that include the context and domain of interactions and judgments.

In general, the cultural context of exclusion is an understudied but much needed focal point for understanding children's social development as well as patterns of peer rejection and exclusion. Because much of the research on cultural exclusion has been conducted from an intergroup perspective, a brief review of developmental intergroup attitudes follows next.

Developmental Intergroup Attitudes

Research on intergroup attitudes stems from social psychology, which has devoted more than 50 years to understanding the outcomes of intergroup attitudes that reflect prejudice, stereotyping, and discrimination (Dovidio, Glick, & Rudman, 2005; Dovidio, Hewstone, Glick, & Estes, 2010). While children's prejudice has been investigated for more than two decades (see Aboud, 1988), the topic of intergroup attitudes has recently awarded a more expansive role in child development research, focusing on the developmental origins of intergroup attitudes and how these attitudes reflect the emergence of prejudice, discrimination, and stereotyping as well as exclusion (Aboud & Amato, 2001; Abrams & Rutland, 2008; Levy & Killen, 2008; Quintana & McKown, 2007).

What makes child developmental intergroup research different from adult intergroup research is the necessity of determining the ways in which children's social cognitive and cognitive abilities constrain their responses, judgments, and intentions toward others, and particularly regarding the relationship between the ingroup and the outgroup. To accomplish these aims, developmental psychology researchers analyze children's interpretations of a number of dimensions, including the social context (where does prejudice or bias occur?), types of relationship (who is involved? peer, adult, or family?), the forms of identification with the ingroup (am I a member of this group, what is the nature of my affiliation, and how much do I value it?), social experiences (what is the nature of my history of intergroup contact and experiences with discrimination?), social categorization (who is a member of the ingroup or the outgroup?) and the social construal (what meaning do I give to the situation?). This type of contextual analysis has been applied to peer exclusion as well as the general area of childhood prejudice (Killen, Richardson, & Kelly, 2010).

For the most part, developmental intergroup research has demonstrated how negative biases about others are often maintained by attitudes from the "majority" group, that is, the dominant social, ethnic, or gender group, in a given social context. As articulated by political and social theorists, hierarchical relationships within and between cultures are often maintained by conventions and stereotypical expectations, which too often perpetuate power and status relationships (Nussbaum, 1999; Turiel, 2002). Using both explicit (judgments, evaluations) as well as implicit (reaction times, ambiguous pictures tasks) methodologies, research has shown how status differences in peer relationships (which contribute to prejudice and exclusion) begin in early childhood and evolve throughout childhood, adolescence, and into adulthood (for reviews, see Abrams & Rutland, 2008; Killen, Sinno, et al., 2007; Levy & Killen, 2008). As we subsequently describe, research on peer exclusion from an intergroup perspective complements research on peer rejection from a peer relations perspective (Chen & French, 2008; Rubin, Bukowski, & Parker, 2006).

Peer Rejection and Exclusion

Over the past decade, research has demonstrated that there are times in which children exclude others for reasons that do not pertain to the behavioral characteristics of the individual children but to their group membership (Abrams & Rutland, 2008; Killen, Sinno, et al., 2007; Nesdale, 2004, 2008). This finding is in contrast to the bulk of research on peer relationships in childhood, which focuses on individual behavioral characteristics that put children at risk for rejecting others or being rejected (Asher & Coie, 1990; Bierman, 2004; Rubin et al., 2006). Typically, research has focused on individual differences in social skills, demonstrating that children who lack social skills (e.g., ones who are fearful, socially anxious, and shy) put themselves at risk for being rejected by others, and treated as "victims." In addition, children lacking social skills, such as being aggressive or insensitive to social cues, put themselves at risk for rejecting others, that is, becoming "bullies." This research makes predictions about the relationships between social deficits and peer rejection and has been important for understanding patterns of aggression, social withdrawal, anxiety, and depression in childhood (Rubin et al., 2006). Social deficits that contribute to negative social outcomes include limitations on interpreting social cues, judging the intentions of others, resolving conflicts constructively, and acquiring the basics of peer group entry rituals (Boivin, Hymel, & Hodges, 2001; Dodge et al., 2003; Parker & Asher, 1987).

Research on social competence from a peer relations perspective has called attention to the cultural meaning of personality traits that contribute to peer rejection (Bierman, 2004; Chen & French, 2008). For example, Chen and his colleagues have conducted extensive research on how cultural norms and values affect how one exhibits sociability (Chen & French, 2008), and they have demonstrated that how peers respond to peer rejection varies by culture, at least in their research studies conducted in China and Canada (Chen, DeSouza, Chen, & Wang, 2006). While children in

Canada and China both displayed reticent behavior in peer situations, for example, Canadian children responded with overt refusal, whereas Chinese children responded more positively. These findings indicate that the bases for peer rejection may vary by culture such that what counts as a reason to reject in one culture (e.g., reticence) would not be viewed as a basis for rejection in another culture. This analysis tells us that even behaviors that have a biological basis, such as temperament, need to be understood in a cultural context. Group membership, the focus of intergroup peer exclusion research, reflects societal expectations and norms as well, that both define an individual and at the same time often serve to justify exclusion.

Peer exclusion based on group membership often reflects prejudice, stereotyping, and bias. This perspective differs from the typical peer rejection approach because implicit intergroup biases are pervasive in society and exist among socially well-functioning individuals; thus, the focus is less on clinical diagnoses of children at the extremes of peer social competence and is more on how cultural expectations of inclusion and exclusion manifest themselves in children's interactions, judgments, and relationships (Abrams, Hogg, & Marques, 2005; Baron & Banaji, 2006; Killen, Sinno, et al., 2007; Rutland, Cameron, Milne, & McGeorge, 2005). Further, the "intervention" focus would not be on social competence training programs for outliers (shy and fearful or aggressive children) but rather on prejudice-reduction programs targeted at the majority groups (i.e., broadly, all children). The theoretical models that guide this research stem from social-cognitive theories as well as social identity theories that are described in the next section.

Social-Cognitive Domain Theory

Social-cognitive domain theory provides a theoretical framework for examining social reasoning about exclusion, prejudice, stereotyping, and intergroup bias in childhood (Killen, Richardson, & Kelly, 2010). This model has identified three categories of social reasoning—the moral (fairness, justice, equality, rights), the socially conventional (traditions, customs, etiquette, rituals), and the psychological (personal individual discretion, autonomy, theory of mind)—that coexist within individual evaluations of social issues (Smetana & Turiel, 2003; Turiel, 1983; Turiel, 2002) and that are reflected in social reasoning about gender and racial exclusion (Killen, Henning, Kelly, Crystal, & Ruck, et al., 2007). For example, exclusion may be viewed as wrong and "unfair" (morally), or as legitimate to make the group work well (conventional), or as legitimate owing to personal prerogatives and choice (psychological). The social-cognitive domain model differs from Kolhberg's global stage theory of moral development (Kohlberg,

1971) in that these types of justifications exist in parallel in development, emerge at a very early age, and change in terms of their breadth, criteria, and nature. This approach is consistent with many domain-specific views in cognitive development (Keil, 2006).

With age and experience, adolescents become more aware of the roles of social conventions in maintaining structure and order in society. In middle adolescence, social conventions are prioritized owing to a strict acceptance of the importance of social structure (Turiel, 1983), reflecting the increased importance of social identity and group functioning. When evaluating intergroup exclusion among youths from different social cliques (Horn, 2003) and ethnic groups (Killen, et al., 2007; Killen, Lee-Kim, McGlothlin, & Stangor, 2002), middle adolescents rate exclusion as more acceptable in peer and group contexts than do younger children, particularly for reasons relating to autonomy and personal choice in friendship, group identity, norms, and functioning. Their previously prosocial and inclusive attitudes toward intergroup interaction are subordinated to group norms.

As an illustration of empirical research from the social-cognitive domain model on children's reasoning about exclusion, Killen and Stangor (2001) investigated the forms of reasoning used by children and adolescents when evaluating exclusion from activity-based peer groups who share interests (e.g., ballet, baseball). The role of group membership (gender and race) was introduced by asking children about exclusion of an individual who did not fit the stereotypical expectations of the group (e.g., gender: excluding a boy from ballet, a girl from baseball; race: excluding a white student from basketball or a black student from a math club) (Killen & Stangor, 2001). For straightforward exclusion decisions (e.g., "Is it all right or not all right to exclude a boy from a ballet club?"), the vast majority of first, fourth and seventh graders evaluated such exclusionary acts as unfair and morally wrong. Shared interests were viewed as more important than stereotypical issues.

When asked to make judgments that were complex, however, such as who the group should pick when only one space was available and two children wanted to join—one who matched the stereotype and one who did not (e.g., "A boy and girl both want to join ballet—who should the group pick?")—with increasing age, participants focused more on group functioning considerations and picked the child who best fit the stereotype. Despite using moral reasoning to evaluate the straightforward exclusion vignette, the older sample used more social conventional reasoning than did their younger counterparts when picking a new group member in the inclusion/exclusion scenario. Thus, with increasing age, adolescents' awareness of group functioning considerations were given priority to their own concerns about fairness or equal opportunity in the more straightforward contexts (Horn, 2003; Horn, 2006).

These findings also indicated that multiple forms of reasoning coexist within individual thinking about an issue. Adolescents did not use only one form of reasoning (as would be characterized in a general stage model) but instead used forms of reasoning from different domains of knowledge (moral and social–conventional). The contextual aspect of social cognition has been validated by many studies. Adolescents will give priority to morality and fairness, even in complex situations. Thus, the task for research is to identify the salient contextual factors that contribute to children's and adolescents' decision making. The salience of reasoning for interpreting children's and adolescents' decision making has been demonstrated in many aspects of children's and adolescents' lives (Smetana, 2006; Turiel, 2006). The research discussed here provides evidence for the importance attached to reasoning about peer exclusion and peer rejection.

What remains to be better understood is what underlies group functioning considerations in exclusion situations. On the one hand, a concern for making groups work well could be a legitimate issue as it relates to social coordination and group cohesiveness. On the other hand, a concern for group functioning could be merely a proxy for stereotypical assumptions and outgroup bias. When all-male executive board rooms of the past century were asked to include women, many members balked at the idea, citing the need to preserve the group and to maintain "group order." The idea of admitting women was viewed as disruptive and unconventional. Most likely, both forms of group functioning were operative—both a concern for a lack of precedents, and an underlying set of stereotypes about women. To some extent, these two dimensions are related in that stereotypical views about women's business knowledge or personality traits, if true, would be disruptive as well as incompatible with a business approach, and the outcome would be that including women would be unlikely to help to make the group "work well." Yet, when challenged and shown that the assumptions are false (as a group category label), then the notion of what makes the group function well changes. As change comes about, individuals are differentiated from norms so that eventually women who espouse the norms of the group (i.e., probusiness and assertive) come to be preferred over men who espouse norms of the outgroup. This example also illustrates what happens when expectations about personality traits are confused with stereotypical expectations about groups and group functioning. Thus, stereotypical expectations about personality traits assigned to women interfere with expectations about group functioning. Exclusion based on personality traits can be argued as legitimate as a basis for exclusion when the personality traits interfere with group functioning. Do individuals evaluate exclusion based on group membership as different from exclusion based on personality traits? Further, as alluded to earlier, to what extent is this distinction culturally unique or generalizable?

In a recent study, Park and Killen (2010) investigated whether children's evaluations of peer rejection based on personality traits differed from rejection based on group membership, and the extent to which these judgments were culturally generalizable. In this study, Korean (N = 397) and U.S. (N = 333) children and adolescents (10 and 13 years of age) evaluated personality (aggression, shyness) and group (gender, nationality) characteristics as a basis for peer rejection in three contexts (friendship rejection, group exclusion, victimization). Children evaluated 12 scenarios in all: three peer rejection scenarios (friendship rejection, peer group exclusion, and peer victimization) in which there were four different types of exclusion: two based on personality traits (shy, aggressive) and two based on group memberships (different nationality, different gender). The friendship rejection context was one in which one child did not want to be friends with another child; the exclusion context was one in which a group did not want a child to join them in their club, and the victimization context was one in which a group repeatedly teased and taunted a child. For each context, the excluded child was alternatively shy, aggressive, of a different nationality, or of a different gender.

Overall, peer rejection based on group membership was viewed by this study's respondents as more unfair (reflecting moral reasons) than peer rejection based on personality traits, supporting both social domain research as well as social identity research on peer exclusion (Killen, Sinno, et al., 2007; Nesdale et al., 2007). Social domain research has proposed that group membership would be viewed as unfair (moral reasons), in contrast to exclusion based on personality characteristics, which could be viewed either in terms of group functioning (socially conventional reasons) or personal choice (psychological reasons) (Killen, 2007). Social identity theory has proposed that rejection in the context of group membership is more similar to prejudice than rejection in the context of personality characteristics; group identity reflects a complex interaction among ingroup and outgroup members (Nesdale, 2008).

Additionally, a closer examination of the responses in the Park and Killen study (2010) indicated that participants viewed it as most legitimate to reject a peer who was aggressive and least legitimate to exclude one based on nationality. Rejecting a peer based on shyness was not considered as legitimate as rejecting one based on aggression (and rated about the same as rejection based on gender). The findings for context indicated that children viewed friendship rejection as more legitimate than group exclusion or victimization and used more personal choice reasoning for friendship rejection than for rejection in any other context, again supporting social domain theory. Social domain theory would predict that friendship rejection would be justified based on personal decisions about friendship choice. In contrast victimization is viewed as wrong based on moral reasons such as harm to the victim.

The findings also provided support for the culturally generalizable nature of social reasoning about peer exclusion; Korean and U.S. children were not significantly different on most measures of peer rejection. In fact, the only significant cultural differences were that Korean children viewed exclusion based on nationality as more legitimate than did U.S. children, and Korean children viewed exclusion based on aggression as more legitimate than did U.S. children. These findings support our "culture by context by domain" theory because culture, taken alone, did not account for the differences in evaluations of exclusion across the board but rather only with respect to two factors. Surprisingly, Korean children did not view shyness as a less legitimate reason to exclude than did U.S. children, contrary to cultural theorizing about shyness as a more "normative" behavior in Korea than in the United States. This finding could be attributable to several factors. First, this study included children who were 10 and 13 years of age; much of the previous data on reticence as a positive behavior in Chinese children reflected research conducted with younger children. Second, shyness was described as "a quiet child who reads by him- or herself and is ignored by other children." This form of shyness describes a different quality, potentially, from "reticence," which is a form of social withdrawal. Thus, further research is required to fully understand the role of culture in defining various forms of shyness as a basis for peer exclusion and rejection. For the most part, the findings confirmed the generalizability of social reasoning about peer rejection, and particularly regarding the distinction between exclusion based on personality traits as more legitimate than exclusion based on group membership.

Developmental Subjective Group Dynamics

Understanding the dynamic role of group identity and group membership in the evaluation of social exclusion requires an examination of how children weigh ingroup and outgroup norms (Abrams & Rutland, 2008). At an early age children develop an understanding of the different groups that constitute their social world and begin to identity with these groups (Bennett & Sani, 2004; Ruble et al., 2004; Ruble, Martin, & Berenbaum, 2006). These groups range from broad social categories, such as culture, ethnicity, or gender, to unique groups such as the family and temporary but significant groups, such as the school class. According to social identity theory (Tajfel & Turner, 1979), by excluding others from their social group, children are able to bolster their sense of social identity (Nesdale, 2004; Verkuyten & Steenhuis, 2005) and present a positive public self to their peer group (Rutland, 2004; Rutland et al., 2005). An emphasis on bolstering one's own identity is what can lead to the justification of exclusion of others.

The developmental subjective group dynamics model (Abrams & Rutland, 2008; Abrams et al., 2003; Abrams, Rutland, Cameron & Ferrell, 2007) holds that children develop a dynamic relationship between their judgments about peers within groups and about groups as a whole (i.e., intergroup attitudes). As children's social-cognitive development changes and they experience belonging to social groups, they are more likely to integrate their preferences for different groups with their evaluations of peers within groups based on particular characteristics or behaviors (Aboud & Amato, 2001; Nesdale, 2004; Tajfel & Turner, 1979). For example, a group of children identifying with a sports team may begin to change their attitudes about a member of the ingroup "team" who acts like, or prefers, members of a rival team (the outgroup). This change in children's social cognition means they can often both exclude a peer because he or she is from a different social group (i.e., intergroup bias) and exclude a peer from within their own group who deviates from the group's socially conventional norms (i.e., intragroup bias), such as increased liking expressed for an outgroup member. What is interesting, then, is that group membership, alone, is not what contributes to exclusion, but rather the dynamic between group identity and group norms.

Research following this developmental intergroup approach (Abrams & Rutland, 2008; Abrams, Rutland, & Cameron, 2003) has investigated intergroup exclusion by constructing an experimental paradigm to examine how children would evaluate ingroup and outgroup peers who either showed "normative" (loyal) behavior or "deviant" (disloyal) behavior. In experiments using nationality as the group membership factor (e.g., English and German groups), children were first asked to rate how they felt toward the ingroup as a whole and the outgroup as a whole (i.e., intergroup exclusion). Then the children heard descriptions of normative and deviant peers who were either in the same or a different group. Normative peers made two positive statements about the group, while deviant peers made one positive statement about the group but also one positive statement about the other group.

Studies in intergroup contexts that used national groups (Abrams et al., 2003), summer school groups (Abrams et al., 2007), and minimal or "arbitrary" groups (Abrams, Rutland, Ferrell, & Pelletier, 2008) have shown that when evaluating potential targets of exclusion children simultaneously prefer those from other social groups and exclude those within their peer group that do not threaten the socially conventional norms central to their group. In addition, studies (e.g., Abrams et al., 2003; Abrams et al., 2008) have shown that these different forms of social exclusion are more strongly linked among older children that are more motivated to support their ingroup (i.e., show high intergroup bias or identify more strongly). This finding indicates that both types of social exclusion are related to the children's sense of social identity and their desire to maintain intergroup differences.

Yet, what about when the deviance that threatens the group arises not in the social-conventional domain but in the moral domain? This distinction has been shown to emerge early in development (by age 3 or 4 years) and guides how children interpret rules, transgressions, and responses to peers and adults regarding social interactions and encounters. How do children weigh their concerns about group identity (preserving the group norms) with moral beliefs about fairness and justice? This intergroup and intragroup conflict is central to social life for children and adults, and understanding this developmental trajectory sheds light on exclusion and prejudice in adulthood.

To undertake an examination of the interplay of cultural identity, social norms, and social reasoning, it is first necessary to describe studies that have been conducted on each one of these constructs and to consider specifically how culture plays a role in group identity and social norms.

Culture and Exclusion

As discussed earlier, much of the current developmental research on intergroup inclusion and exclusion has focused solely on gender and race, and relatively little has examined cultural attitudes that invoke stereotypes and negative intergroup opinions. By examining cultural groups rather than gender and race, we move beyond groups that are often defined primarily by stable lifelong categories. Cultural groups and cultural identity include stable, unchanging components as well as those beliefs, conventions, and traditions that group members self-select and choose to identify with. Below we review several recent studies that have systematically examined the intersection between culture and morality in interpersonal and intergroup relations.

Killen, Crystal, and Watanabe (2002) and Park, Killen, Crystal, and Watanabe (2003) examined the influence of the participant's culture and context of exclusion on the exclusion judgments of first, Japanese and American and, second, Korean, Japanese, and American children, respectively. Both of the studies utilized samples of 4th, 7th, and 10th graders and followed the same methodology. In the two studies the children were asked to evaluate scenarios of exclusion based on one of six factors: (1) aggressive behavior; (2) unconventionality in dress (wearing strange clothes to a fancy restaurant); (3) unconventionality in public behavior (acting like a clown in the movie theater); (4) cross-gender behavior; (5) ineptness in sports; and (6) personality (acting sad or lonely at a picnic). Their evaluations were assessed in terms of an evaluative judgment (is it all right or not all right to exclude?), conformity (should the excluded child change his or her behavior to fit in?), and self-perceived differences (is the participant similar to or different from the excluded child?). The results of both of the studies yielded no overall differences between the exclusion evaluations of the Japanese and American participants. Both groups place priority on group functioning in some scenarios and individual choice in others.

Further, Park et al. (2003) found that Japanese, Korean, and American participants generally found exclusion to be wrong overall, with the Korean participants perceived to be the most tolerant of the three groups. While the Korean children offered similar evaluations of exclusion when it was predicated on the aggressive behavior of the excluded child, amid all of the scenarios, they were most willing to exclude when the exclusion was based on the unconventionality of the public behavior of the excluded child, again supporting our interactional theory about culture and context.

A recent set of studies was designed to examine how Israeli-Jewish and Arab children (in Israel, Jordan, and the Palestinian Territories) evaluate conflict resolution, intergroup peer encounters, and exclusion situations (Brenick et al., 2007; Brenick et al., 2010; Cole et al., 2003). These studies have been framed by the social-cognitive domain model, identifying moral, social–conventional, and psychological reasoning as basic aspects of children's social judgments (see Smetana, 2006; Turiel, 2006). Specifically, these studies have examined the stereotypes and moral judgments related to intergroup relations among Jewish-Israeli, Palestinian-Israeli, and Palestinian-Arab preschoolers (Cole et al., 2003) as well as Jewish-Israeli, Palestinian-Israeli, Palestinian-Arab, and Jordanian preschoolers (Brenick et al., 2010; and see Brenick et al., 2007). This research has found that, while children involved in the Arab-Israeli conflict tend to hold negative stereotypes toward the outgroup, they also make prosocial moral justifications in evaluating potential interpersonal transgressions and certain instances of intergroup exclusion. These studies have also found that children's intergroup judgments vary, depending the context of the intergroup interaction, and are influenced by group membership (Brenick et al., 2007).

Children were assessed in terms of their knowledge of Israeli and Arab cultural symbols, their understanding of the cultural similarities between the two groups (Brenick et al., 2007; Cole et al., 2003), their stereotypes of members of the other group (e.g., Israeli-Jewish children were asked

about Arabs, and Arab children were asked about Jews), their social judgments about vignettes detailing dilemmas involving everyday peer conflict
resolution, and how these changed after viewing specified *Sesame Street*
programming (Brenick et al., 2007; Cole et al., 2003). Cole et al.'s (2003)
assessment included the evaluation of everyday scenarios with Jewish and
Palestinian peers that involved turn-taking on swings, sharing toys (cars or
dolls), and playing a game of hide-and-seek. For example, the swings story
would be explained as follows:

> Shira, who is Jewish, and Aisha, who is Arab, are playing in the
> park. Shira is on the swings. Aisha wants to swing, but there is
> only one swing. What will happen next? Aisha, the Arab girl, will
> push Shira, the Jewish girl, off the swing and then get on it, or,
> Aisha, the Arab girl, will say "Can I have a turn on the swing?"
> and then wait until Shira, the Jewish girl, gets off.

For each vignette, each child selected one of the two possible resolutions
and then justified his or her answer. The findings from this study showed
that all three groups of children (Israeli-Jewish, Israeli-Palestinian, and
Palestinian-Arab) held negative stereotypes about the outgroup and lacked
an understanding of the cultural similarities prior to viewing the *Sesame
Street* program. At the pretest, both Israeli-Jewish and Palestinian children
also lacked knowledge about the cultural symbols of the other group. In
terms of their social reasoning, the pretest responses were highly prosocial, indicating that children find these potential moral transgressions as
opportunities to offer the benefit of the doubt and attribute positive intentions to outgroup members. In other words, even though these children
held negative conceptions of the outgroup, they were not yet applying them
to intergroup interactions.

In an extension of the Cole et al. study (2003), Brenick and colleagues
(2010) assessed the stereotyped knowledge and social reasoning about
intergroup exclusion of Israeli-Jewish, Israeli-Palestinian, Palestinian-Arab,
and Jordanian children. Brenick et al. (2010) analyzed how children evaluated and justified their evaluations of exclusion contexts in which a child
was excluded based on country of origin (being excluded from a play group
because he or she was from a "different country"), cultural stereotypes,
(being excluded from a party because he or she was from a culture that
typically wore a different type of "party hat"), and language (not being
helped and being excluded from getting "ice cream" because he or she
spoke a different language). For instance, the vignette titled "Ice Cream"
featured a group of children who all spoke the same language, posing the
question whether they should first stop and help another child who spoke a
different language and had fallen while they were running to the ice cream

truck or whether they should get their ice cream and then help the child. These scenarios coupled the moral considerations of fairness with socially conventional norms and determined the factors that were most salient to the children.

The results varied across contexts and across cultural groups. Stereo-typed knowledge results for this sample differed slightly from those of Cole et al. (2003). While both the Palestinian and Jordanian children held nega-tive stereotypes about the other, the Israeli-Jewish children provided more neutral traits, and the Israeli-Palestinian children provided more positive traits. Social reasoning about all three scenarios differed by cultural group. Palestinian children, overall, were the most accepting of exclusion and were more likely to use stereotyped reasoning when justifying exclusion of a child who spoke a different language or came from a different country but group-functioning reasoning when justifying exclusion of a child with different cultural customs. Israeli-Jewish and Israeli-Palestinian children tended to be the least accepting of exclusion and utilized more prosocial and inclusive reasoning. Jordanian children, however, showed both inclu-sive and exclusive judgments and reasoning; they exhibited concerns for inclusion as well as group functioning.

These findings confirmed that children who hold negative stereotypes about the outgroup will not necessarily appeal to that stereotyped knowl-edge when weighing the possibilities of intergroup friendships and play. While these children held negative attitudes of members of the outgroup, they did not indiscriminately act on them. This set of findings yielded posi-tive implications for prejudice reduction and coexistence. However, it also warrants further examination of these processes in older children and ado-lescents to determine whether the relationships between stereotyping and evaluations of intergroup interactions remain constant and, if not, how and when any subsequent differences manifest themselves.

While these studies found that the majority of participating children held negative stereotypes about the other group (though the Palestinian-Israeli group held primarily neutral to positive stereotypes), this perception did not directly carry over into the reasoning the children offered in their evaluations of the intergroup conflict scenarios. The types of justifications provided by the children differed by cultural group. Yet, all groups of chil-dren showed prosocial and inclusive reasoning in their responses (Brenick et al., 2007; Brenick et al., 2010; Cole et al., 2003).

In a study with older children in the Netherlands, Gieling, Thijs, and Verkuyten (2010) examined Dutch adolescents' tolerance of the cultural beliefs and practices of the Muslim population in the Netherlands. This study was conducted in the context of an extensive research program by Verkuyten and colleagues to understand Dutch adolescents' views about Muslims, asylum seekers, and recent immigrants from North Africa in the

Netherlands (Verkuyten, 2008). The study by Gieling, Thijs, et al. (2010) took a different approach from research in which participants are asked directly about exclusion of one member of a cultural group, as has been described in most of the studies reviewed in this chapter.

Instead, in this study, analyses were conducted on Dutch-majority adolescents' views of tolerance of, and evaluation of practices of, a minority group (Muslims) that has experienced exclusion by the majority. In addition, the researchers conducted a second study in which they examined whether the view that maintaining one's own minority culture in a majority society was related to evaluations of cultural practices. All participants were asked to evaluate a series of beliefs and practices of the Muslim population in terms of their conventionality, acceptability, wrongfulness, harmful consequences, and personal nature. Four scenarios—a student wearing a headscarf, a teacher refusing to shake hands with a parent of the opposite-sex, an Islamic school for only Muslim children, and an imam making antihomosexual proclamations—were described to participants for their evaluation. The findings for the first study (Study 1) demonstrated that participants evaluated all four practices by using multiple forms of reasonsing—personal, socially conventional, and moral. Thus, the issues were multifaceted, drawing on moral (unfairness), conventional (traditions), and personal (choice) domains to evaluate these acts.

In the second study (Study 2), analyses of tolerance revealed that participants were more tolerant of acts considered to be a personal issue and less tolerant of acts that pertained to moral issues (socially conventional acts were in the middle). Furthermore, participants were more tolerant of the particular practices than of campaigns for public support of these practices. One's level of education, in-group identification, and multiculturalism had much stronger effects in the nonmoral than in the moral domain. Older adolescents were less tolerant than younger ones, which also reflected the fact that, with increased age, respondents viewed the issues as more complicated or multifaceted. These findings demonstrated that exclusion of a minority group by the majority is often condoned through cultural expectations about minority groups. Thus, children's lack of tolerance was attributed more to cultural messages than to individual differences in social competence and interaction.

Owing to sociopolitical changes, in some countries peer exclusion exists among respondents sharing the same—as well as a different–ethnic heritage. In Germany, for example, exclusion may pertain to members of the same ethnic groups—former West Germans and former East Germans (reflecting the fall of the Berlin Wall in the late 1980s)—as well as between Germans and Turks—even though Turkish families migrated to Germany for employment several generations ago. Feddes, Noack, and Rutland (2009) conducted a longitudinal study to examine direct and extended cross-ethnic friendship effects on outgroup evaluations among German and Turkish children (ages 7–11) who were enrolled in ethnically heterogeneous elementary schools. Their results showed that, among ethnic-majority children but not ethnic-minority children, direct cross-ethnic friendship predicted positive outgroup evaluations over time. This longitudinal study demonstrated a causal direction between greater direct cross-ethnic friendship and more positive outgroup attitudes among ethnic-majority children. The effect of increased cross-group friendships on more positive intergroup attitudes and less exclusion was shown in part to result from changes in the children's perceived social ingroup norms about cross-ethnic friendship relations.

The experience of cross-group friendships encouraged children to think that their ingroup viewed these friendships as normal, and therefore they showed more positive intergroup attitudes. These findings were in line with previous research in the United Kingdom that found that both direct and extended contact promoted more positive social ingroup norms regarding cross-ethnic friendship, which then also resulted in improved intergroup attitudes among majority children (Cameron, Rutland, & Hossain, 2007).

The study by Feddes and colleagues (2009) suggested that in ethnically heterogeneous contexts direct friendship is more effective in changing intergroup attitudes than extended friendship and that social status moderates direct friendship effects. The expectation that cross-race friendships provide important experiences for reducing prejudice and increasing inclusion has been demonstrated in a wide range of cultural contexts. Further, the finding that intergroup contact was more effective for majority (German) than for minority (Turkish) children over the course of 1 year provides further support for the "culture by context by domain" theory because it demonstrates how a specific context of interaction can positively affect children's intergroup attitudes regarding outgroup members in quite different cultural contexts (Germany, the United Kingdom, and the Netherlands).

Cross-Group Friendships and Exclusion

While parents' attitudes toward intergroup friendships play a significant role in defining their children's attitudes toward and engagement in cross-group relationships, high-quality contact with peers (e.g., friendships) has been shown to be significantly related to prejudice reduction (Tropp & Prenovost, 2008). In fact, parental messages have been shown to be significantly related to adolescents' experiences with cross-group friendships. For example, adolescents whose parents are less supportive of cross-group relationships are less likely to engage in cross-group relationships, to achieve deeper levels of intimacy through their cross-group relationships, and to bring cross-group friends into their homes (Edmonds & Killen, 2009).

Additionally, outgroup attitudes also play a critical role in children's and adolescents' perspectives on intergroup relations. Individuals are often highly concerned with how the outgroup will perceive their character when considering the prospect of engaging in intergroup contact. Those who feel threatened or anxious about how they might be viewed by the outgroup frequently distance themselves from the situation or avoid intergroup contact altogether (Mendoza-Denton & Page-Gould, 2008; Tropp & Prenovost, 2008). The role of anxiety in cross-group friendships has been examined in adult samples (Mendoza-Denton & Page-Gould, 2008) and more recently with children (Nesdale et al., 2007).

The experience of positive cross-group friendships can provide increased levels of intimacy that yield positive outcomes in terms of intergroup attitudes and decreases in prejudice. This circumstance creates an environment in which increases in intergroup closeness may flourish. Unfortunately, however, while youths become more adept in their abilities to understand the heterogeneity within and homogeneity across groups (Doyle & Aboud, 1995), a trajectory that would seemingly promote cross-group relations, by middle childhood a decrease in cross-group friendships becomes apparent (Aboud, Mendelson, & Purdy, 2003; Dubois & Hirsch, 1990). Thus, more research on intergroup contact among children and adolescents and the factors that determine what it is about intergroup friendships that influences a child or adolescent's likelihood of engaging in intergroup contact as well as actual experience with cross-group friendships needs to be conducted.

Given the potentially positive impact of intergroup friendships, it is essential to fully understand the complex nature of these relationships. While these topics have begun to be addressed with adults, a developmental approach is necessary for exploring these social psychological processes throughout childhood. From early on, how and why do children and adolescents choose to engage or not engage in intergroup contact? What influences their desire to engage in intergroup contact as well as the effectiveness of such contact? What is the role of culture in this process?

It is important to examine the variables that influence children's and adolescents' desire to engage in intergroup contact. While it has been demonstrated that friendship choices (i.e., who to befriend) are typically considered matters of personal choice, when those decisions involve crossing group boundaries such as race, ethnicity, and culture, children's and adolescents' reasoning also appeals to the moral and social–conventional concerns, indicating the complex nature of these relationships. This complexity is also reflected in the varying evaluations across different contexts of intergroup relations. The extent to which a child thinks members of his or her own group, family, peers, and outgroup members would be in favor of or against contact may be related to whether a child would even consider engaging in intergroup contact, spurring such questions as "Is this something that I'm even allowed to do? encouraged to do? told to actively avoid?" Perceived ingroup and outgroup norms for contact are still an understudied topic in the intergroup literature, especially with children and adolescents—yet, one that can fully benefit from the inclusion of developmental perspectives that feature a history of research on peer and parental relationships.

Additional questions of interest include: "How do I think kids from other groups perceive me? Are they interested in getting to know me? Do they want to avoid me? Will they exclude me? How do they perceive my interest in contact or learning about their group? What drives my perceptions about their interest or lack of interest in contact?" Tropp (2006) found that both minority and majority adults report having higher levels of interest in contact than they perceive the outgroup to have. For children and adolescents, this perception can elicit anxiety and avoidance motivation around intergroup contact rather than lessening intergroup bias (as such contact is intended to promote). These questions of perceived interest, motivation, and expectations for engaging in contact require further investigation.

Both the developmental literature on inclusion/exclusion and the social psychological literature on contact effects have found differences regarding perceptions of, engagement in, and effects of intergroup contact (Cameron, Rutland, Brown, & Douch, 2006; Crystal, Killen, & Ruck, 2008; Hewstone et al., 2005; Killen, Crystal, & Ruck, 2007). While intergroup contact is an effective means of reducing prejudice (Pettigrew & Tropp, 2005), optimal conditions prove more effective in reducing the prejudices of majority-group members than of minority-group members (Wright, Aron, McLaughlin-Volpe, & Ross, 1997). The effects of contact, in general, are stronger for majority-status than minority-status groups overall (Tropp & Prenovost, 2008). Additionally, group differences emerge between majority and minority participants' evaluations of intergroup exclusion, with minority participants rating intergroup exclusion as more wrong than majority participants.

Examining the influences of group norms, meta-perceptions, and expectations about intergroup contact in a variety of cultures will help elucidate the varying levels of engagement in intergroup contact and cross-group friendships and of success in achieving positive intergroup attitudes across majority and minority groups as well as help provide guidelines to prevent negative intergroup interactions. Tracing age-related patterns from childhood to adulthood will provide novel insight into how these developmental changes serve as the foundation for both exclusive as well as inclusive social relationships, attitudes, and beliefs.

Conclusions

Understanding the role of culture on exclusion is complex and has been investigated at multiple levels. At the societal level, exclusion based on culture has resulted in civil wars, strife, and conflict (Opotow, 1990). How does exclusion based on cultural membership begin? What are the origins of exclusion based on culture? To address this issue it is necessary to understand how cultural identity emerges, when it becomes a justification for rejecting others, and how it is justified from a conventional perspective. In straightforward contexts, children and adolescents view exclusion based on a range of categories (culture, gender, ethnicity, race) as wrong from a moral standpoint, invoking reasons that primarily stem from a sense of injustice and a lack of fairness. With increasing age, children gradually adopt an identity that can, at times, serve to justify exclusion. Moreover, messages from parents and society often perpetuate these forms of exclusion, owing to traditions and ingroup identification. Further, situations that are complex or ambiguous are the contexts that are most likely to elicit stereotypical responses and to foster exclusionary decision making. Thus, one of the first places to facilitate more inclusive decision making is the complex or multidimensional contexts. By adulthood, stereotypes become deeply entrenched. To make a difference, it is necessary to intervene during early development, and that requires basic knowledge about how children and adolescents are approaching decision making about peer relationships.

The current patterns of migration during the 21st century pose new challenges for addressing issues relating to exclusion and peer relationships (Malti, Killen, & Gasser, in press). Children are attending schools that were previously homogeneous with respect to some categories (such as culture and ethnicity). The new diversity brings opportunities for intergroup dialogue and friendship; at the same time, diversity can create group alliances that result in outgroup threats and ingroup favoritism. To understand these complexities it is necessary to move beyond a unidimensional theory of culture (as a monolithic variable) and to understand how culture interacts with context and the domain of social interactions and judgments. Moreover, developing interventions to take advantage of the diversity through facilitating friendships rather than antagonisms and ingroup bias will go a long way toward fostering a just and fair society.

Acknowledgments

Melanie Killen was supported by an award from the National Science Foundation (No. 0840492) and by a University of Maryland Summer Stipend. We thank Xinyin Chen and Kenneth Rubin for helpful feedback on the manuscript.

References

Aboud, F. E. (1988). *Children and prejudice*. Oxford, England: Blackwell.

Aboud, F. E., & Amato, M. (2001). Developmental and socialization influences on intergroup bias. In R. Brown & S. L. Gaertner (Eds.), *Blackwell handbook of social psychology: Intergroup relations* (pp. 65–85). Oxford, UK: Blackwell.

Aboud, F. E., Mendelson, M. J., & Purdy, K. T. (2003). Cross-race peer relations and friendship quality. *International Journal of Behavioral Development, 27*, 165–173. Doi: 10.1080/01650250244000164.

Abrams, D., Hogg, M. A., & Marques, J. M. (2005). A social psychological framework for understanding social inclusion and exclusion. In D. Abrams, M. A. Hogg, & J. M. Marques (Eds.), *The social psychology of inclusion and exclusion* (pp. 1–24). New York: Psychology Press.

Abrams, D., & Rutland, A. (2008). The development of subjective group dynamics. In S. R. Levy & M. Killen (Eds.), *Intergroup relations and attitudes in childhood through adulthood* (pp. 47–65). Oxford, UK: Oxford University Press.

Abrams, D., Rutland, A., & Cameron, L. (2003). The development of subjective group dynamics: Children's judgments of normative and deviant in-group and out-group individuals. *Child Development, 74*, 1840–1856.

Abrams, D., Rutland, A., Cameron, L., & Ferrell, J. (2007). Older but wilier: In-group accountability and the development of subjective group dynamics. *Developmental Psychology, 43*, 134–148.

Abrams, D., Rutland, A., Ferrell, J. M., & Pelletier, J. (2008). Children's judgments of disloyal and immoral peer behavior: Subjective group dynamics in minimal intergroup contexts. *Child Development, 79*, 444–461.

Asher, S. R., & Coie, J. (1990). *Peer rejection in childhood*. Cambridge: Cambridge University Press.

Baron, A. S., & Banaji, M. R. (2006). The development of implicit attitudes: Evidence of race evaluations from ages 6 and 10 and adulthood. *Psychological Science, 17*, 53–58.

Bennett, M., & Sani, F. (Eds.). (2004). *The development of the social self*. New York: Psychology Press.

Bierman, K. L. (2004). *Peer rejection: Developmental processes and intervention strategies*. New York: Guilford Press.

Boivin, M., Hymel, S., & Hodges, E. V. E. (2001). Toward a process view of peer rejection and harassment. In J. Juvonen & S. Graham (Eds.), *Peer harassment in school: The plight of the vulnerable and victimized* (pp. 265–289). New York: Guilford Press.

Brenick, A., Killen, M., Lee-Kim, J., Fox, N. A., Leavitt, L. A., Raviv, A. et al. (2010). Social understanding in Young Israeli-Jewish, Israeli-Palestinian, Palestinian, and Jordanian children: Moral judgments and stereotypes. *Early Education and Development, 21*, 1–26.

Brenick, A., Lee-Kim, J., Killen, M., Fox, N. A., Leavitt, L. A., & Raviv, A. (2007). Social judgments in Israeli and Arabic children: Findings from media-based intervention projects. In D. Lemish & M. Gotz (Eds.), *Children, media and war* (pp. 287–308). Cresskill, NJ: Hampton Press.

Cameron, L., Rutland, A., Brown, R., & Douch, R. (2006). Changing children's intergroup attitudes toward refugees: Testing different models of extended contact. *Child Development, 77,* 1208–1219.

Cameron, L., Rutland, A., & Hossain, R. (2007). *Prejudice-reduction through story-reading: Indirect contact in the classroom.* Paper presented at the 37th annual meeting of the Jean Piaget Society, Amsterdam, Netherlands.

Chen, X., DeSouza, A. T., Chen, H., & Wang, L. (2006). Reticent behavior and experiences in peer interactions in Chinese and Canadian children. *Developmental Psychology, 42,* 656–665.

Chen, X., & French, D. C. (2008). Children's social competence in cultural context. *Annual Review of Psychology, 59,* 591–616.

Cole, C., Arafat, C., Tidhar, C., Zidan, W. T., Fox, N. A., Killen, M., et al. (2003). The educational impact of Rechov Sumsum/Shara'a Simsim, a television series for Israeli and Palestinian children. *International Journal of Behavioral Development, 27,* 409–422.

Crystal, D., Killen, M., & Ruck, M. (2008). It's who you know that counts: Intergroup contact and judgments about race-based exclusion. *British Journal of Developmental Psychology, 26,* 51–70.

Dodge, K. A., Lansford, J. E., Burks, V. S., Bates, J. E., Pettit, G. S., Fontaine, R., et al. (2003). Peer rejection and social information-processing factors in the development of aggressive behavior problems in children. *Child Development, 74,* 374–393.

Dovidio, J. F., Glick, P., & Rudman, L. (Eds.). (2005). *Reflecting on the nature of prejudice: Fifty years after Allport.* Oxford, UK: Blackwell.

Dovidio, J. F., Hewstone, M., Glick, P., & Estes, V. (2010). *Handbook of prejudice, stereotyping, and discrimination.* Thousand Oaks, CA: Sage.

Doyle, A., B., & Aboud, F. E. (1995). A longitudinal study of White children's racial prejudice as a social-cognitive development. *Merrill-Palmer Quarterly, 41,* 209–228.

DuBois, D. L., & Hirsch, B. J. (1990). School and neighborhood patterns of blacks and whites in early adolescence. *Child Development, 61,* 524–536.

Edmonds, C., & Killen, M. (2009). Do adolescents' perceptions of parental racial attitudes relate to their intergroup contact and cross-race relationships? *Group Processes and Intergroup Relations, 12,* 5–21.

Feddes, A. R., Noack, P., & Rutland, A. (2009). Direct and extended friendship effects on minority and majority children's interethnic attitudes: A longitudinal study. *Child Development, 80,* 377–390. Doi: 10.1111/j.1467-8624.2009.01266.x.

Gieling, M., Thijs, J., & Verkuyten, M. (2010). Tolerance of practices by Muslim actors: An integrative social-developmental perspective. *Child Development, 81,* 1384–1399., doi: 10.1111/j.1467-8624.2010.01480.x.

Hewstone, M., Cairns, E., Voci, A., Paolini, S., McLernon, F., Crisp, R., et al. (2005). Intergroup contact in a divided society: Challenging segregation in Northern Ireland. In D. Abrams, M. A. Hogg, & J. M. Marques (Eds.), *The social psychology of inclusion and exclusion* (pp. 265–292). New York: Psychology Press.

Hitti, A., Mulvey, K. L., & Killen, M. (in press). Evaluation of social exclusion: The role of group norms, group identity, and fairness. *Anales de Psicologia*(Special issue: Social and developmental aspects of prejudice during childhood and adolescence, Eds. I. Eneso & S. Guerrero).

Horn, S. (2003). Adolescents' reasoning about exclusion from social groups. *Developmental Psychology, 39,* 71–84.

Horn, S. (2006). Group status, group bias, and adolescents' reasoning about treatment of others in school contexts. *International Journal of Behavioral Development, 30,* 208–218.

Keil, F. (2006). Cognitive science and cognitive development. In W. Damon (Ed.), *Handbook of child psychology* (pp. 609–635). Hoboken, NJ: Wiley.

Killen, M. (2007). Children's social and moral reasoning about exclusion. *Current Directions in Psychological Science, 16,* 32–36.

Killen, M., Crystal, D., & Ruck, M. (2007). The social developmental benefits of intergroup contact for children and adolescents. In E. Frankenberg & G. Orfield (Eds.), *Lessons in integration: Realizing the promise of racial diversity in America's schools* (pp. 57–73). Charlottesville, VA: University of Virginia Press.

Killen, M., Crystal, D., & Watanabe, H. (2002). Japanese and American children's evaluations of peer exclusion, tolerance of difference, and prescriptions for conformity. *Child Development, 73,* 1788–1802.

Killen, M., Henning, A., Kelly, M. C., Crystal, D., & Ruck, M. (2007). Evaluations of interracial peer encounters by majority and minority U.S. children and adolescents. *International Journal of Behavioral Development, 31,* 491–500.

Killen, M., Lee-Kim, J., McGlothlin, H., & Stangor, C. (2002). How children and adolescents evaluate gender and racial exclusion. *Monographs of the Society for Research in Child Development* (Serial No. 271, Vol. 67, No. 4). Oxford, England: Blackwell Publishers.

Killen, M., Richardson, C., & Kelly, M. C. (2010). Developmental intergroup attitudes: Stereotyping, exclusion, fairness, and justice. In J. F. Dovidio, M. Hewstone, P. Glick, & V. M. Esses (Eds.), *Handbook of prejudice stereotyping and discrimination* (pp. 97–114). Thousand Oaks, CA: Sage.

Killen, M., & Stangor, C. (2001). Children's social reasoning about inclusion and exclusion in gender and race peer group contexts. *Child Development, 72,* 174–186.

Killen, M., Sinno, S., & Margie, N. G. (2007). Children's experiences and judgments about group exclusion and inclusion. In R. V. Kail (Ed.), *Advances in child development and behavior* (pp. 173–218). New York: Elsevier.

Kohlberg, L. (1971). From is to ought: How to commit the naturalistic fallacy and get away with it in the study of moral development. In T. Mischel (Ed.), *Psychology and genetic epistemology* (pp. 151–235). New York: Academic Press.

Levy, S., & Killen, M. (2008). *Intergroup attitudes and relations in childhood through adulthood.* Oxford, UK: Oxford University Press.

Malti, T., Killen, M., & Gasser, L. (in press). Social judgments and emotion attributions about exclusion in Switzerland. *Child Development.*

Mendoza-Denton, R., & Page-Gould, E. (2008). Can cross-group friendships influence minority students' well-being at historically white universities? *Association of Psychological Science, 19,* 933–939.

Nesdale, D. (2004). Social identity processes and children's ethnic prejudice. In M. Bennett & F. Sani (Eds.), *The development of the social self* (pp. 219–245). New York: Psychology Press.

Nesdale, D., Maass, A., Kiesner, J., Durkin, K., Griffiths, J., & Ekberg, A. (2007). Effects of peer group rejection, group membership, and group norms, on children's outgroup prejudice. *International Journal of Behavioral Development, 31,* 526–535.

Nesdale, D. (2008). Peer group rejection and children's intergroup prejudice. In S. Levy & M. Killen (Eds.), *Intergroup attitudes and relations in childhood through adulthood* (pp. 32–46). Oxford, U.K.: Oxford University Press.

Nussbaum, M. C. (1999). *Sex and social justice.* Oxford, UK: Oxford University Press.

Opotow, S. (1990). Moral exclusion and injustice: An introduction. *Journal of Social Issues, 46,* 1–20.

Park, Y., & Killen, M. (2010). When is peer rejection justifiable?: Children's understanding across two cultures. *Cognitive Development, 24,* 290–301.

Park, Y., Killen, M., Crystal, D. S., & Watanabe, H. (2003). Korean, Japanese, and U.S. students' judgments about peer exclusion: Evidence for diversity. *International Journal of Behavioral Development, 27,* 555–565.

Parker, J. G., & Asher, S. R. (1987). Peer relations and later personal adjustment: Are low-accepted children at risk? *Psychological Bulletin, 102,* 352–389.

Pettigrew, T. F., & Tropp, L. R. (2005). Allport's intergroup contact hypothesis: Its history and influence. In J. F. Dovidio, P. Glick, & L. Rudman (Eds.), *Reflecting on the nature of prejudice: Fifty years after Allport* (pp. 262–277). Oxford, UK: Blackwell.

Quintana, S., & McKown, C. (2007). *The handbook of race, racism, and the developing child.* New York: Wiley.

Rubin, K., Bukowski, W., & Parker, J. (2006). Peers, relationships, and interactions. In W. Damon & R. Lerner (Eds.), *Handbook of child psychology* (pp. 571–645). New York: Wiley.

Ruble, D. N., Alvarez, J., Bachman, M., Cameron, J., Fuligni, A., & Coll, C. G. (2004). The development of a sense of "we": The emergence and implications of children's collective identity. In M. Bennett & F. Sani (Eds.), *The development of the social self* (pp. 29–76). New York: Psychology Press.

Rutland, A. (2004). The development and self-regulation of intergroup attitudes in children. In M. Bennett & F. Sani (Eds.), *The development of the social self* (pp. 247–265). New York: Psychology Press.

Rutland, A., Cameron, L., Milne, A., & McGeorge, P. (2005). Social norms and self-presentation: Children's implicit and explicit intergroup attitudes. *Child Development, 76,* 451–466.

Rutland, A., Killen, M., & Abrams, D. (2010). A new social-cognitive developmental perspective on prejudice: The interplay between morality and group identity. *Perspectives in Psychological Science, 5,* 280–291.

Smetana, J. G. (2006). Social-cognitive domain theory: Consistencies and variations in children's moral and social judgments. In M. Killen & J. G. Smetana (Eds.), *Handbook of moral development* (pp. 119–154). Mahwah, NJ: Erlbaum.

Smetana, J. G., & Turiel, E. (2003). Moral development during adolescence. In G. R. Adams & M. D. Berzonsky (Eds.), *Blackwell handbook of adolescence.* (pp. 247–268). Oxford, UK: Blackwell Publishing.

Tajfel, H., & Turner, J. C. (1979). An integrative theory of intergroup conflict. In W. G. Austin & S. Worchel (Eds.), *The social psychology of intergroup relations* (pp. 33–47). Monterey, CA: Brooks-Cole.

Tropp, L. R. (2006). Stigma and intergroup contact among members of minority and majority status groups. In S. Levin & C. v. Laar (Eds.), *Stigma and group inequality: Social psychological perspectives* (pp. 171–191). Mahwah, NJ: LEA.

Tropp, L. R., & Prenovost, M. A. (2008). The role of intergroup contact in predicting children's inter-ethnic attitudes: Evidence from meta-analytic and field studies. In S. Levy & M. Killen (Eds.), *Intergroup attitudes and relations in childhood through adulthood* (pp. 236–248). Oxford, UK: Oxford University Press.

Turiel, E. (1983). *The development of social knowledge: Morality and convention.* Cambridge, UK: Cambridge University Press.

Turiel, E. (2002). *The culture of morality.* Cambridge, UK: Cambridge University Press.

Turiel, E. (2006). The development of morality. In N. Eisenberg, W. Damon, & R. M. Lerner (Eds.), *Handbook of child psychology: Social, emotional, and personality development* (pp. 789–857). Hoboken, NJ: Wiley.

Verkuyten, M. (2008). Multiculturalism and group evaluations among minority and majority groups. In S. Levy & M. Killen (Eds.), *Intergroup attitudes and relations in childhood through adulthood* (pp. 157–172). Oxford, U.K.: Oxford University Press.

Verkuyten, M., & Steenhuis, A. (2005). Preadolescents' understanding and reasoning about asylum seeker peers and friendships. *Journal of Applied Developmental Psychology, 26,* 660–679.

Wright, S. C., Aron, A., McLaughlin-Volpe, T., & Ross, S. A. (1997). The extended contact effect: Knowledge of cross-group friendships and prejudice. *Journal of Personality and Social Psychology, 73,* 73–90.

CHAPTER 11

The Cultural Context of Child and Adolescent Conflict Management

DORAN C. FRENCH

A ll societies must develop mechanisms to manage interpersonal conflict (de Waal, 1996), in part because this function must occur if close relationships such as friendships, romances, and marriages are to develop and be maintained over time (Gottman & Parker, 1986). Further, conflict management is essential for community cohesion, since uncontrolled conflict, even among children, can seriously disrupt adult relationships and communities (Lambert, 1971). For these reasons, it is important to teach children how to manage their current conflicts effectively as well as to socialize them to deal successfully with those they will experience as adults.

Although the study of conflict management among children and adolescents in different cultures has been limited, there now appears to be converging evidence from countries as diverse as Indonesia (French, Pidada, Denoma, McDonald, & Lawton, 2005), the Netherlands (Goudena, 2006), China (French et al., in press), and Columbia (Chaux, 2005) that there are significant variations across cultures in the management of conflict. This chapter, which is divided into four sections, reviews the evidence underlying this assertion. The first section examines the ways in which conflict management is associated with the dimensions of culture. The second section gives a brief overview of the general issues relevant to understanding child and adolescent conflict, while the third section features a discussion of child and adolescent conflict in North America, Indonesia, and China.

The chapter concludes with some thoughts about methodology and the implications for future research.

Conflict Management and Dimensions of Culture

Social psychologists have suggested that conflict behavior can be understood in part by considering its broad cultural dimensions, principally individualism versus collectivism, and hierarchical organization. This view is consistent with arguments that conflict must be understood within the context of cultural meaning systems that include worldviews, values, and beliefs (Fry, 2000; Ross & Conant, 1992). These systems can affect the manner in which individuals interpret the behavior of others, the extent to which conflicts are permissible within a culture and allowed to exist, the processes by which conflict is manifested, the methods of resolution, and the goals that individuals bring to the particular conflicts.

Conflicts may be conceptualized as struggles between the desires of individuals versus conformity to the expectations of others (Rothbaum, Pott, Azuma, Miyake, & Weiss, 2000; Shantz & Hobart, 1989). Consistent with this perspective, Markus and Lin (1999) argue that central to the organization of meaning and practices pertaining to conflict are cultural perspectives on the extent to which the self is viewed in an individualistic context, or whether the self is conceptualized as embedded within relationships. They argue that persons with individualistic conceptions of self tend to react to conflicts with direct and assertive expression of their desires or views. They also consider it desirable to separate the issue of conflict from the personalities of the individuals involved and to assume that conflicts have a "correct solution." In contrast, persons with an interdependent view of self tend to view conflicts as issues of "relationships." They may consequently avoid confrontation, use mediators, or disengage, with the goal of preventing the conflict from unfavorably impacting relationships.

A second but less explored feature of cultures relevant to the management of conflict is the relative power distance between persons and the extent to which social relationships are ordered hierarchically (Hofstede, 1991). The existence of hierarchies serves to regulate conflict in a manner similar to that in which dominance hierarchies tend to regulate aggression in both human and nonhuman primates (Savin-Williams, 1979).

Within both Korea and China, relationships are structured hierarchically. Thus, conflicts typically occur between persons of similar status because deference is expected to be given to those of higher status (Song, 1996). The hierarchical structure of Chinese and Korean society may be in part a function of Confucian traditions within which relationships, including friendships, are seen as occurring between individuals who are unequal in status (Bond & Hwang, 1986). In contrast, the United States and Canada are relatively low in power distance (Hofstede, 1991), a factor that might account for the typical conflict resolution strategies of conciliation, turn-taking, and individual assertion, strategies that are consistent with norms of equity and individual rights (Ross & Conant, 1992).

Although broad cultural patterns such as "individualism versus collectivism" can be useful in conceptualizing patterns of conflict behavior across cultures, it is important to keep in mind the severe criticisms and limitations associated with their use (Oyserman, Coon, & Kemmelmeier, 2002). These include the heterogeneity of worldviews within a culture, the likelihood that individuals may behave in both a collectivist and an individualist manner depending on the behavior and context, and the difficulties of measuring individualism and collectivism independently from the behavior that the constructs supposedly explain. Despite these caveats, the constructs of individualism and collectivism as well as relative power distance continue to be useful for conceptualizing the cultural differences underlying the manner in which children and adolescents manage conflict, particularly when comparing the United States, Indonesia, and China—countries positioned at the extreme poles of the individualism–collectivism scale.

Children's Conflict Behavior in a Cultural Context

The limited research on culture and the conflict behavior of children appears to be consistent with the Markus and Lin (1999) framework. In general, children from individualist cultures display assertiveness and actively pursue self-interests during conflict episodes. For example, preschool children in the Netherlands were assertive and imposed their personal views during conflicts more often than children in Andalusia, a more collectivist society (Medina, Lozano, & Goudena, 2001); children in central Italy were more efficient than Canadian children at avoiding and resolving conflicts between friends, mainly by maintaining respect for rules (Schneider, Fonzi, Tomada, & Tani, 2000); and Mexican youths reported using concessions and shared principles to resolve interpersonal conflicts to a greater extent than did U.S. youths (Gabrielidis, Ybarra, & Villareal, 1997). Patterns of conflict management of North American, Indonesian, and Chinese youths that will be reviewed later are also consistent with this premise.

Child and Adolescent Conflict

At its most basic level, conflict is defined as overt behavioral opposition (Shantz, 1987), which in most cases is indicated by verbal disagreement. It is important to distinguish conflict from aggression. Aggression is only one of many consequences of conflict; most conflicts do not involve aggression and are settled quickly without adult intervention (Fabes & Eisenberg, 1992; Perry, Perry, & Kennedy, 1992; Shantz, 1987). The distinction between conflict and aggression is particularly relevant when considering how conflict is managed in different cultures. The probability that conflict will lead to aggression varies widely across cultures, with the likelihood of this happening in part a function of cultural norms regarding the acceptability of using coercive control (Björkqvist, 1997; Bond, 2004; Fry, 1988).

Conflict, in contrast to aggression, is also presumed to be growth-enhancing, a position endorsed by developmental theorists, including Piaget, Freud, and Erickson (Shantz, 1987). Conflicts may provide children with opportunities to exercise conventional and moral reasoning (Smetana, Killen, & Turiel, 1991). Empirical evidence that children gain from experiences with conflict is provided by findings that mothers' use of justification during conflicts with their children at 30 months was associated with children's social emotional development six months later (Laible & Thompson, 2002).

Borrowing from the model developed by Kitayama and Markus (1994), conflict management within cultures can be understood in relation to an assortment of socially shared scripts for dealing with provocations. These include cognitive, physiological, emotional processes that in their totality organize the manner in which individuals interpret and respond to various cues. The characteristics of these scripts, the conditions under which they are employed, and the probability that they will be invoked likely vary across cultures.

Conflict Sequences

Conflicts are structured and unfold over time (Shantz, 1987). The conflict sequence can be thought of as occurring in four stages that include (1) preconflict, (2) mutual opposition, (3) conflict termination, and (4) postconflict periods. Processes occurring during each of these stages vary substantially across cultures.

During the preconflict stage, individuals deal with provocations and possible disagreements. The occurrence of conflict depends upon whether or not the individual initiates the conflict by reacting to the provocation. This aspect of conflict has been insufficiently studied, in part because it is difficult to study conflicts that never occur. Nevertheless, it is essential to understand this aspect of conflict management behavior, given the major differences across cultures regarding the acceptability of overt conflict and the many actions undertaken to avoid it (Fry, 2000). Rothbaum et al. (2000) suggest that North Americans view conflict as inevitable and desirable as a method of solving problems. In contrast, Japanese often view conflict as best avoided, although this approach may mean that the issue of contention remains unresolved. As discussed more fully later, a major feature of conflict management in both Indonesia and China includes efforts to prevent overt conflict from occurring, both by withdrawing from the potential conflict and refraining from behavior that might precipitate it.

There has been little exploration of cultural variations in the actions or events that precipitate conflict. In one of the few discussions of this question, Killen and Sueyoshi (1995) suggested that the conflicts of Japanese preschool children are less frequently focused on issues of object disputes than are those of U.S. children.

There have been findings of considerable variability in the manner in which individuals respond once a conflict has been initiated. Sociolinguists have provided rich descriptions of the ways in which children react to an initial opposition, with a wide range of possible responses (Eisenberg & Garvey, 1981). These conflict strategies vary widely, and in some cultures they are in the form of widely adopted and practiced scripts. Indonesian children, for example, frequently avoid encountering the person until such time as the emotions associated with the conflict dissipate (French, Pidada, Denoma, et al., 2005), whereas Italian children sometimes use verbal chants and rhythmic gestures within dispute sequences (Corsaro & Rizzo, 1990). African American children (particularly boys) were observed to exhibit argumentative and confrontational discourse that focused on maintaining their positions of relative power (Goodwin, 1982) and Italian preschool children were observed to practice a form of elaborated disputes typically exhibited by adults, *discussione*, within which the quality of discourse is more important than the actual resolution of the conflict (Corsaro & Rizzo, 1990). These observations of children's disputes provide evidence of the salience of conflict in the lives of children, the sophistication of the conflict strategies that are used by children, and the extent to which their styles of interaction correspond to those used by adults (Garvey & Shantz, 1992).

There is considerable diversity in the manner in which conflicts are resolved across cultures. Fry (2000) suggests that the five methods of negotiation, self-help/coercion, avoidance, toleration, and third-party intervention (including mediation, or decision by a third party) are typically used to settle disputes. There are variations in the use of these different methods across cultures, with negotiation more prominent in individualist cultures and mediation, toleration, and third-party intervention more typically used in collectivist cultures (Markus & Lin, 1999). The manner in which each of these types of resolution methods is exhibited also varies considerably across cultures. For example, Magnis-Suseno (1997) describes third-party mediation in Indonesia as taking place in a large group that collectively seeks consensus about the best solution, whereas Wall and Blum (1991), in contrast, describe third-party mediation in China being undertaken by an authority who prescribes a solution after listening to the opinions of others.

The final stage, which has received little study, is the postconflict period. For some children, this stage consists of reconciliation processes during which children reestablish a positive relationship, a process studied by de Waal (1996) under the rubric of "peacemaking" (Butovskaya, Verbeek, Ljungberg, & Lundarini, 2000). Methods of postconflict conciliation include both explicit (e.g., apology) and implicit methods (e.g., resumption of play) and in some cultures involve the use of scripts, such as the use of rhymes by Swedish and Russian children (Butovskaya et al., 2000). In other cases, the effects of the conflict may continue over time.

Conflict and Relationships

Conflict management must necessarily be considered within the context of the relationship between protagonists. Even 4-year-old children appear sensitive to relationships when evaluating responses to transgressions (Dunn & Slomkowski, 1992). The intertwining of conflict management and relationship development is well illustrated by Gottman and his colleagues' findings that conflict management is essential for the development and maintenance of close relationships across the lifespan (Gottman & Parker, 1986). Laursen, Hartup, and Koplas (1996) suggest that conflict is particularly risky for close friends because of the possible fragility of these important relationships. Consistent with this view, most but not all studies have found that children experience less conflict with friends than they do with nonfriends. Hartup, Laursen, Stewart, and Eastenson (1988), for example, found that preschoolers more often disengaged from conflicts and arrived at more equitable solutions with friends than with nonfriends. But the behavior of friends is likely sensitive to contextual parameters, such as competition demands; in some contexts, friends may have more intense conflicts with their friends than with nonfriends (Hartup, French, Laursen, Johnston, & Ogawa, 1993). Although conflict is likely to differ as a function of friendship status, the specific nature of these effects might vary across cultures perhaps as a function of cultural differences in friendship expectations as well as different norms regarding appropriate behavior with acquaintances.

Developmental Changes in Conflict Management

Given the paucity of longitudinal studies of conflict behavior, the strongest evidence of developmental changes comes from Laursen, Finkelstein, and Betts's (2001) meta-analysis of the resolution of actual and hypothetical conflict situations. They found that adolescents and young adults were observed to solve actual conflicts with negotiation more often than were children. In contrast, all age groups tend to resolve hypothetical conflicts with negotiation. Thus, it appears that as children develop, their actual behavior increasingly corresponds to views about what they "ought" to do. This developmental pattern likely occurs across cultures, and is undoubtedly connected with developmental changes in self-regulation. As previously noted, however, negotiation may be considered a more optimal conflict resolution strategy in individualistic cultures than in others.

Individual Differences in Conflict Management

Although it is useful to talk about broad cultural patterns of conflict management, it is important to recognize that there are often large individual differences within cultures in the extent to which children use various problem-solving methods and in their effectiveness when using them. These variations have been most extensively studied in North America (Crick & Dodge, 1994; Spivack & Shure, 1974).

Common to both the models of Crick and Dodge (1994) and Spivack and Shure (1974) is the notion that individuals approach conflict situations with numerous possible alternative actions available for their use. These are often in the form of "scripts," some of which are well-practiced methods of addressing conflicts; in the United States, these may include coin flipping, playing "rock–paper–scissors," or taking turns. Children likely have multiple scripts within their repertoire that they can draw on. It has been consistently found that successful management of both hypothetical and actual conflicts is associated with other indices of competence, including sociometric status, aggression, and emotional control (French & Waas, 1987; Murphy & Eisenberg, 2002; Putallaz & Sheppard, 1990; Rose & Asher, 1999).

Because the desirability and effectiveness of alternatives varies by culture, socially competent children are most likely to use problem-solving strategies that are consistent with their cultural norms. First, individuals are likely to have been taught through either formal or informal means to use these strategies. Second, because others in the culture are familiar with these strategies, they may meet with more success than would less familiar strategies. Finally, some approaches to conflict may be more consonant with cultural values than are others. Consistent with the analysis of Ogbu (1981), it is likely that individuals who are viewed as competent by others within the culture are most likely to effectively exhibit behavior that is consistent with cultural norms. By closely studying the behavior of socially competent children, it is possible to gain an insider's perspective on the meaning of conflict behavior in various cultures (French et al., 2008).

Conflict Management
in North America, Indonesia, and China

Conflict management practices in North America, Indonesia, and China appear to be consistent with the individualist and collectivist framework presented by Markus and Lin (1999). Despite sharing common features, the differences between Indonesian and Chinese methods of conflict management illustrate the considerable diversity present within collectivist cultures.

North America

Models of conflict resolution prominent among those of European ancestry in North America tend to be based on the notion of individual rights and the attendant idea that successful conflict management involves one's self-assertion of rights. These ideals are reflected in the two most prominent scripts for conflict resolution—namely, entitlement and negotiation—both of which entail mutual respect for one's rights and the desires and rights of others.

North American children learn the principles of entitlement associated with possessing property or using space at a young age and regularly invoke these principles to resolve conflicts with their peers and siblings (Dunn & Munn, 1987; Ross & Conant, 1992). Children as young as 2½ routinely invoke rules of ownership and possession during conflicts, and such arguments are frequently successful (Ross, 1996). Scripts of sharing and turn-taking are further derived from these general principles of rights and obligations, and the relative success of entitlement claims likely derives from the salience of principles of ownership in North America. These principles are used by children to resolve disputes, and parents who intervene in children's conflicts serve to reinforce these principles, in particular those involving sharing (Ross, 1996). Unfortunately, there are few if any cross-cultural studies assessing the use of entitlement justifications to resolve conflict, but it is likely that these are less commonly used in cultures where personal prerogatives and legal rights of possession are less well established (Ross, 1996).

Negotiation and compromise are presumed to be the optimal methods of resolving conflicts. Consistent with these ideals, Sternberg and Dobson (1987) found that college students identified mutual discussion and bargaining as preferred methods of dealing with conflicts with roommates. Even preschool children in the United States endorse negotiation as a method of dealing with hypothetical disputes (Islakandar, Laursen, Finkelstein, & Fredrickson, 1995), and the meta-analysis of Laursen, Finkelstein, and Betts (2001) provides further evidence that negotiation is a preferred method of

resolving hypothetical conflicts at all ages. Findings that socially competent (i.e., popular) U.S. children tend to endorse the use of negotiation as
a strategy to resolve conflicts provides further evidence of the salience of
this conflict resolution script among European Americans (Bryant, 1992).
Although negotiation may be seen as the ideal way of solving conflicts, this
acknowledgment does not necessarily mean that this method is consistently
used; Laursen et al. (2001), in fact, found that actual conflicts were more
often settled with coercion.

Finally, it should not necessarily be assumed that the methods of conflict management typically employed by European American youths are
equally popular with other U.S. ethnic groups. Markus and Lin (1999)
provide an overview of the distinctive styles of conflict management prevalent among European American, Asian American, Hispanic, and African
American adults. Although the ethnic variations in conflict management
among U.S. children have received little study, it is reasonable to expect
that the degree of variation observable among adults would also be present
in children.

Indonesia

Anthropologists have extensively discussed the conflict maintenance methods used by the Javanese and many other ethnic groups in Indonesia (C.
Geertz, 1976; Mulder, 1996). The Javanese word *rukun* describes an ideal
state in which the appearance of interpersonal harmony is maintained
by avoiding outward manifestations of conflict (Magnis-Suseno, 1997).
Included among the many methods used to minimize displays of conflict
are avoiding topics of contention, refraining from interacting with persons
with whom one has conflictual relationships, relying on polite and ritual-
ized forms of interaction, minimizing external displays of strong emotions,
and avoiding expressing strong opinions.

An additional feature of Indonesian social life has been described by
Geertz (1961) as "respect," which entails understanding that there exists a
hierarchical social order and that one is obligated to show respect to those
higher in the social order and kindness to those below. It is particularly
important to refrain from overtly disagreeing with those higher in the hierarchy, although one can privately disagree and covertly disobey their com-
mands. Leaders are responsible for maintaining social order, and thus open
conflict is presumed to reflect poorly on their power (Mulder, 1996).

There are consistent findings that Indonesian youths report low levels
of conflict. Haar and Krahe (1999) compared German and Indonesian adolescents' preferred strategies for resolving hypothetical conflicts with parents, peers, and teachers and found that Indonesian children selected the
confrontational solution less often and the submissive solution more often

than did German adolescents. In two comparative studies Indonesian children and adolescents, respectively, rated their friendships as less conflictual than did U.S. youths (French, Pidada, & Victor, 2005; French, Riansari, Pidada, Nelwan, & Buhrmester, 2001).

French et al. (2005) interviewed U.S. (90% European American) and Indonesian 9- to 11-year-old children to obtain descriptions of their conflicts with peers. Consistent with other studies of conflict, these reported conflicts were short, amicabably settled, and did not involve aggression. Indonesian children more often reported dealing with conflicts by disengaging than did the U.S. children. Some of them described a pattern of disengagement, *musuhan* (acting enemies), in which they avoided the individual with whom they had a disagreement and reengaged when the emotions from the conflict dissipated. These findings are consistent with anthropological reports (Magnis-Suseno, 1997) that describe the widespread practice of maintaining interpersonal harmony by avoiding both the issue of conflict and the conflicting party, a style of dealing with conflict that is exhibited not only in daily life but also in business and political affairs (Friend, 2003).

Further evidence that disengagement is positively regarded as a method of dealing with conflict comes from findings that teacher ratings of competence (popularity and low aggression) were associated with children's reports of disengagement. These results contrasted with findings reporting that disengagement by U.S. children was associated (although not significantly) with teacher ratings of aggression and low popularity. These results suggest that the meaning of *disengagement* differs in these two cultures. In the United States, disengagement appears to be undesirable, reflecting inappropriate passivity and low assertiveness, while in Indonesia, in contrast, this strategy is regarded as the socially competent approach to maintaining interpersonal harmony.

China

Tracing itself back historically through the ideas of Confucius, Chinese consider it important to maintain interpersonal harmony and to attain it by being tolerant, forgiving, and compromising with others (Wall & Blum, 1991). Similar to what is seen among Indonesians; Chinese tend to minimize overt conflict, relying instead on withdrawal or indirect methods of resolution (Bond, 1991). Chinese children exhibit less conflict than North American children. Navon and Ramsey (1989) observed the object possessions in preschool U.S. and Chinese children and found that Chinese children more often shared materials and reacted less defensively and aggressively to attempts by others to take materials. Orlick, Zhou, and Partington (1990) similarly found that kindergarten Chinese children engaged in lower levels of conflict and exhibited more cooperation than their North American peers. Finally, Benjamin, Schneider, Greenman, and Hum (2001) found that elementary-age children from Taiwan reported less conflict in their friendships than did Canadian children.

Dien (1982) argued that Confucian models of conflict resolution provide a framework for resolving conflicts that, unlike Western conceptions, are not based on models of individual rights. In China, it is assumed that morality and justness are present within the natural order of the universe and that, ideally, the true sage possesses insights into this natural order as well as understanding the nuances of specific situations. These assumptions are reflected in the characteristics of community mediation systems described by Wall and Blum (1991) that operate quite differently from the mediation systems commonly employed in the United States, in which mediators are presumed to help individuals negotiate mutually satisfactory solutions. The Chinese systems are not necessarily voluntary, that is, the mediators have the formal authority to intervene in conflicts that come to their attention. Second, they may know the parties involved, and there is no presumption that they are neutral. Third, the goal of mediation is to settle the dispute, not to ensure that all parties are necessarily satisfied with the outcome. Fourth, mediators often tell the participants how they should think and behave and attempt to persuade them to adopt these views.

The use of an authority to manage conflicts is widely used to deal with conflicts in Chinese society. Bond and Hwang (1986) observe that it is typical for conflicts to be managed by group leaders, who are responsible for regulating conflict among persons in a group, mediating disputes, and keeping order.

Insight into the processes by which Chinese children minimize overt conflict was provided by French et al. (in press), who observed how 9-year-old unacquainted Chinese and Canadian children in quartets dealt with the provocation associated with the presence of a single attractive toy. Chinese children displayed patterns of behavior likely to reduce conflict; they more often spontaneously relinquished control to another child and reacted more positively to the attempts by others to obtain the toy. Perspectives on the meaning of these behaviors were seen in comparisons of individuals' behavior and group members' ratings of the extent to which they liked each of the other group members. Using HLM (hierarchical linear modeling) analyses, the authors showed that, within the Chinese groups, children who displayed a more reticent and cooperative style by making relatively few attempts to play with the toy and allowing others to do so were comparatively well liked by other group members. The opposite pattern emerged for Canadian children in that assertiveness was associated with positive group members' liking and passivity with dislike. Thus, it may be inferred that, among Chinese children, avoiding conflict by exhibiting cooperative behavior is associated with competence, whereas assertiveness and success in attaining the resource appears to be most valued in Canadian children.

Also emerging from the French et al. (in press) study was evidence that the "leadership conflict management script" is used by children as well as adults. In some 78% of the Chinese children's groups it was common for one and occasionally two Chinese children to attempt to structure the group's actions by invoking a general rule, a behavior that was less frequently observed in the Canadian groups (46%). That leadership behavior emerged in these groups is remarkable given that the children were age mates and had less than an hour of prior contact. This pattern of involvement likely reflects the prominence of norms within Chinese society for a leader to take charge, a script reinforced in children's lives by the frequent presence of youth leaders who readily assume informal as well as formal authority roles in Chinese classrooms, schools, and communities.

Conclusions

The patterns of conflict maintenance seen in North America, Indonesia, and China are generally consistent with the framework outlined by Markus and Lin (1999). Consistent with their analysis, the conflict behavior of North American youths is characterized by individual assertiveness and a view that negotiation is the optimal approach for resolving conflict. In contrast, the patterns of conflict maintenance in both Indonesia and China are consistent with the view that conflict is typically minimized in collectivist cultures. Particularly salient are the strategies employed by Chinese and Indonesian youths to prevent the occurrence of conflict.

General Conclusions

This chapter concludes with suggestions for further research. These include the need to understand the development of conflict management from childhood to adulthood, the importance of understanding how conflict behavior is associated with other qualities of successful adaptation, and the importance of expanding research on conflict management to assess children in U.S. ethnic groups and in other cultures.

The Development of Conflict Maintenance Competencies

The discussion of conflict management in the United States, Indonesia, and China reveals the considerable parallels between the ways that both children and adults within a given culture deal with conflict. These parallels are reflected in the use of negotiation by North American children, withdrawal by Indonesian children, and leadership scripts by Chinese children—as well as their adult counterparts. This correspondence is striking and deserves further scrutiny. It appears that children learn cultural patterns of conflict maintenance at an early age, employ these within their peer group, and practice and transform these over time. It is likely that the conflict behavior displayed by diplomats and business executives were originally learned and practiced in their respective playgrounds. Missing from this analysis, however, is an understanding of how these development transitions unfold.

Laursen et al. (2001) highlighted the paucity of research on the development of conflict management. The results from the meta-analysis that aggregated the results from multiple studies illustrated a likely developmental course within which even young children have a sophisticated cognitive understanding of appropriate conflict management; with development, their actual behavior comes closer to the ideal. Further research is required to understand how these processes unfold.

Conflict Management and the Development of Children's Competencies

Much of the research on culture and conflict has been descriptive, focusing on the incidence, process, and resolution of conflict (Butovskaya et al., 2000). It is important to expand this research to understand how conflict management is associated with other aspects of development.

Initial efforts have been made to explore how conflict management is associated with social competence (French, Pidada, Denoma, et al., 2005; French et al., in press; Putallaz & Shepard, 1992). Others have assessed the relationship between conflict management and emotional development (Murphy & Eisenberg, 2002), peer relationships (Shantz, 1986), and social cognitive processes (Selman, 1980). Considerably more work needs to be done, particularly if we are to understand whether developmental processes are similar or different across cultures.

It would be useful to assess the extent to which cultural variations exist in children's social-cognitive understandings of conflict and the extent to which these variations are explained by differences in values and practices related to conflict management. Selman's (1980) model suggests that advanced stages of reasoning incorporate mutual solutions and active problem solving of contentious issues. It is possible that somewhat different stages might emerge among youths who are in cultures such as China within which views of individual rights and responsibilities are less prominent. Furthermore, cultural variations in sociomoral reasoning is relevant for understanding how children in various cultures reconcile competing interests in conflict situations (Keller, Edelstein, & Schmid, 1998).

Important efforts have been made to understand the processes by which parenting contributes to the development of conflict management competencies (Laible & Thompson, 2002). Ross and her colleagues (Ross, 1996; Ross & Conant, 1992), for example, have explored the manner in which young children learn the principles of entitlement and use these to resolve conflicts with peers and siblings. Expansion of such research in other cultural groups could illuminate the manner in which parents and others teach children culturally specific conflict management skills (Ross & Conant, 1992).

Expansion of Research Populations

As illustrated by this review, research on children's conflict management has been confined to relatively few cultural and ethnic groups, with most of populations studied in North America, Europe, and Asia. There is a need to expand this research to include populations in other regions of the world, including Africa and Latin America. Such expansion is essential to properly assess the extent to which dimensions of culture such as individualism, collectivism, and power distance are useful in explaining the patterns of conflict management.

It is also important to explore ethnic variations in conflict management among U.S. populations. Markus and Lin (1999) concluded from their review of the very limited research on conflict management among U.S. ethnic groups that it is more difficult to make generalizations about African American and Latino adults than it is about either European or Asian American populations. For example, they describe the conflict management of African Americans as complex, combining elements of communalism with individual self-expression and assertiveness. Given that there has been only limited study of ethnic variation in conflict management of U.S. children's behavior, considerably more research is needed before firm conclusions can be advanced.

References

Benjamin, W. J., Schneider, B. H., Greenman, P. S. & Hum, M. (2001). Conflict and childhood friendship in Taiwan and Canada. *Canadian Journal of Behavioral Science, 33*, 203–211.

Björkqvist, K. (1997). The inevitability of conflict, but not of violence: Theoretical considerations on conflict and aggression. In D. Fry & K. Björkqvist, (Eds.), *Cultural variation in conflict resolution: Alternatives to violence* (pp. 25–37). Mahwah, NJ: Erlbaum.

Bond, M. H. (1991). *Beyond the Chinese face: Insights from psychology.* Hong Kong: Cambridge University Press.

Bond, M. H. (2004). Culture and aggression: From context to coercion. *Personality and Social Psychology Review, 8*, 62–78.

Bond, M. H., & Hwang, K. (1986). The social psychology of the Chinese people. In M. H. Bond (Ed.), *The psychology of the Chinese people* (pp. 213–266). Hong Kong: Oxford University Press.

Bryant, B. K. (1992). Conflict resolution strategies in relation to children's peer relations. *Journal of Applied Developmental Psychology, 3*, 35–50.

Butovskaya, M., Verbeek, P., Ljungberg, T. & Lundarini, A. (2000). A multicultural view of peacemaking among young children. In A. Filippo & F. B. M. deWaal (Eds.), *Natural conflict resolution* (pp. 243–258). Berkeley: University of California Press.

Chaux, E. (2005). Role of third parties in conflicts among Colombian children and early adolescents. *Aggressive Behavior, 31*, 40–55.

Corsaro, W., & Rizzo, T. A. (1990). Disputes and conflict resolution among nursery school children in the U.S. and Italy. In A. Grimshaw (Ed.), *Conflict talk* (pp. 21–66). Cambridge, UK: Cambridge University Press.

Crick, N. R., & Dodge, K. A. (1994). A review and reformulation of social-information processing mechanisms in children's development. *Psychological Bulletin, 115*, 74–101.

de Waal, F. B. M. (1996). Conflict as negotiation. In W. C. McGrew, L. F. Marchant, & T. Nishida (Eds.), *Great ape societies* (pp. 159–172). New York: Cambridge University Press.

Dien, D. S. F. (1982). A Chinese perspective on Kohlberg's theory of moral development. *Developmental Review, 2*, 331–341.

Dunn, J., & Munn, P. (1987). The development of justification in disputes. *Developmental Psychology, 23*, 791–798.

Dunn, J., & Slomkowski, C. (1992). Social understanding. In C. U. Shantz & W. W. Hartup (Eds.), *Conflict in child and adolescent development* (pp. 70–92). New York: Cambridge University Press.

Eisenberg, A. R., & Garvey, C. (1981). Children's use of verbal strategies in resolving disputes. *Discourse Processes, 4*, 149–170.

Fabes, R. A., & Eisenberg, N. (1992). Young children's coping with interpersonal anger. *Child Development, 63*, 116–128.

French, D. C., Chen, X., Chung, J., Miao, L., Li, D., Chen, H., et al. (in press). *Four Children and One Toy: Chinese and Canadian Children Faced with Potential Conflict over a Limited Resource.*

French, D. C., Pidada, S., Denoma, J., McDonald, K., & Lawton, A. (2005). Reported peer conflicts of children in the United States and Indonesia. *Social Development, 14*, 458–472.

French, D. C., Pidada, S., & Victor, A. (2005). Friendships of Indonesian and United States youth. *International Journal for Behavioral Development, 29*, 1–11.

French, D. C., Riansari, M., Pidada, S., Nelwan, P., & Buhrmester, D. (2001). Social support of Indonesian and U.S. children and adolescents by family members and friends. *Merrill-Palmer Quarterly, 47*, 377–394.

French, D. C., & Waas, G. A. (1987). Social-cognitive and behavioral characteristics of peer-rejected boys. *Professional School Psychology, 2*, 103–112.

Friend, T. (2003). *Indonesian destinies*. Cambridge, MA: Harvard University Press.

Fry, D. (1988). Intercommunity differences in aggression among Zapotec children. *Child Development, 59*, 1008–1019.

Fry, D. P. (2000). Conflict management in cross-cultural perspective. In F. Aureli & F. B. M. deWaal (Eds.), *Natural conflict resolution* (pp. 334–351). Berkeley: University of California Press.

Gabrielidis, C., Ybarra, O., & Villareal, L. (1997). Preferred styles of conflict resolution: Mexico and the United States. *Journal of Cross-Cultural Psychology, 28*, 661–677.

Garvey, C., & Shantz, C. U. (1992). Conflict talk. In C. U. Shantz & W. W. Hartup (Eds.), *Conflict in child and adolescent development* (pp. 93–121). New York: Cambridge University Press.

Geertz, C. (1976). *The religion of Java*. Chicago: University of Chicago Press.

Geertz, H. (1961). *The Javanese family: A study of kinship and socialization*. New York: Free Press.

Goodwin, M. (1982). Process of dispute management among urban Black children. *American Ethnologist, 9*, 76–96.

Gottman, J. M., & Parker, J. G. (1986). *Conversations of friends: Speculations on affective development*. Cambridge, UK: Cambridge University Press.

Goudena, P. P. (2006). Real and symbolic entry of children in the social world of peers and parent–child interactions. In X. Chen, D. C. French, & B. H. Schneider (Eds.), *Peer relationships in cultural context* (pp. 247–263). New York: Cambridge University Press.

Haar, B. F., & Krahe, B. (1999). Strategies for resolving interpersonal conflicts in adolescence: A German–Indonesian comparison. *Journal of Cross-Cultural Psychology, 30*, 667–684.

Hartup, W. W., French, D. C., Laursen, B., Johnston, M. K., & Ogawa, J. R. (1993). Conflict and friendship relations in middle childhood: Behavior in a closed-field situation. *Child Development, 64*, 445–454.

Hartup, W. W., Laursen, B., Stewart, M. I., & Eastenson, A. (1988). Conflict and the friendship relations of young children. *Child Development, 59*, 1590–1600.

Hofstede, G. (1991). *Cultures and organizations: Software of the mind*. London: McGraw-Hill.

Islakandar, N., Laursen, B., Finkelstein, B., & Fredrickson, L. (1995). Conflict resolution among preschool children: The appeal of negotiation in hypothetical disputes. *Early Education and Development, 6*, 359–376.

Killen, M., & Sueyoshi, L. (1995). Conflict resolution in Japanese social interactions. *Early Education and Development, 6*, 317–334.

Kitayama, S., & Markus, H. R. (1994). Introduction to cultural psychology and emotion research. In S. Kitayama & H. R. Markus (Eds.), *Emotion and culture: Empirical studies of mutual influence* (pp 1–22). Washington, DC: American Psychological Association.

Keller, M., Edelstein, W., & Schmid, C. (1998). Reasoning about Responsibilities and obligations in close relationships: A comparison across two cultures. *Developmental Psychology, 34*(4), 731–741.

Laible, D. J., & Thompson, R.A. (2002). Mother–child conflict in the toddler years: Lessons in emotion, mortality, and relationships. *Child Development, 73*, 1187–1203.

Lambert, W. W. (1971). Cross-cultural backgrounds to personality development and the socialization of aggression: Findings from the Six Cultures Study. In W. W. Lambert & R. Weisbrod (Eds.), *Comparative perspectives on social psychology* (pp. 49–61). Boston: Little, Brown.

Laursen, B., Finkelstein, B. D., & Betts, N. T. (2001). A developmental meta-analysis of peer conflict resolution. *Developmental Review, 21*, 423–449.

Laursen, B., Hartup, W. W., & Koplas, A. L. (1996). Towards understanding peer conflict. *Merrill-Palmer Quarterly, 1*, 76–102.

Magnis-Suseno, F. (1997). *Javanese ethics and world-view: The Javanese idea of the good life.* Jakarta, Indonesia: Gramedia Pustaka Utama.

Markus, H. R., & Lin, L. R. (1999). Conflictways: Cultural diversity in the meanings and practices of conflict. In D. A. Prentice & D. T. Miller (Eds.), *Cultural divides: understanding and overcoming group conflict* (pp. 302–333). New York: Russell Sage Foundation.

Medina, J. A. M., Lozano, V. M., & Goudena, P. P. (2001). Conflict management in preschoolers: A cross-cultural perspective. *International Journal of Early Years Education, 9*, 153–160.

Mulder, N. (1996). *Inside Indonesian Society: Cultural change in Indonesia.* Amsterdam, Netherlands: Pepin Press.

Murphy, B. C., & Eisenberg, N. (2002). An integrative examination of peer conflict: Children's reported goals, emotions, and behaviors. *Social Development, 11*, 534–557.

Navon, R., & Ramsey, P. G. (1989). Possession and exchange of materials in Chinese and American preschools. *Journal of Research on Childhood Education, 4*, 18–29.

Ogbu, J. (1981). Origins of human competence: A cultural–ecological perspective. *Child Development, 52*, 413–429.

Orlick, T., Zhou, Q. Y., & Partington, J. (1990). Co-operation and conflict within Chinese and Canadian kindergarten settings. *Canadian Journal of Behavioral Science, 22*, 20–25.

Oyserman, D., Coon, H. M., & Kemmelmeier, M. (2002). Rethinking individualism and collectivism: Evaluation of theoretical assumptions and meta-analyses. *Psychological Bulletin, 128*, 3–72.

Perry, D. G., Perry, L. C., & Kennedy, E. (1992). Conflict and the development of antisocial behavior. In C. U. Shantz & W. W. Hartup (Eds.), *Conflict in child and adolescent development* (pp. 301–329). New York: Cambridge University Press.

Putallaz, M., & Sheppard, B. H. (1990). Children's social status and orientations to limited resources. *Child Development, 61*, 2022–2027.

Putallaz, M., & Sheppard, B. H. (1992). Conflict management and social competence. In C. U. Shantz & W. W. Hartup, (Eds.), *Conflict in child and adolescent development* (pp. 330–355). New York: Cambridge University Press.

Rose, A. J., & Asher, S. R. (1999). Children's goals and strategies in response to conflicts within a friendship. *Developmental Psychology, 35*, 69–79.

Ross, H. S. (1996). Negotiating principles of entitlement in sibling property disputes. *Developmental Psychology, 32,* 90–101.

Ross, H. S., & Conant, C. L. (1992). The social structure of early conflict: Interaction, relationships, and alliances. In C. U. Shantz & W. H. Hartup (Eds.), *Conflict in child and adolescent development* (pp. 153–185). Cambridge, UK: Cambridge University Press.

Rothbaum. F., Pott, M., Azuma, H., Miyake, K., & Weisz, J. (2000). The development of close relationships in Japan and the United States: Paths of symbiotic harmony and generative tension. *Child Development, 71,* 1121–1142.

Savin-Williams, R. C. (1979). Dominance hierarchies in groups of early adolescents. *Child Development, 50,* 923–935.

Schneider, B. H., Fonzi, A., Tomada, G., & Tani, F. (2000). A cross-national comparison of children's behavior with their friends in situations of potential conflict. *Journal of Cross-Cultural Psychology, 31,* 259–266.

Selman, R. (1980). *The growth of interpersonal understanding: Developmental and clinical analyses.* New York: Academic Press.

Shantz, C. U. (1987). Conflicts between children. *Child Development, 58,* 283–285.

Shantz, C. U., & Hobart, C. J. (1989). Social conflict and development: Peers and siblings. In T. J. Berndt & G. W. Ladd (Eds.), *Peer relationships in child development* (pp. 71–94). Oxford, UK: Wiley.

Shantz, D. W. (1986). Conflict, aggression, and peer status: An observational study. *Child Development, 57,* 1322–1332.

Smetana, J. G., Killen, M., & Turiel, E. (1991). Children's reasoning about interpersonal and moral conflicts. *Child Development, 62,* 629–644.

Song, Y. J. (1996). Argumentativeness in contexts: A comparison of motivations to argue between South Koreans and North Americans in the contexts of age and relationship (Doctoral dissertation, Ohio University, 1996). *Dissertation Abstracts International, 57,* 3322.

Spivack, G., & Shure, M. B. (1974). *Social adjustment of young children: A cognitive approach to solving real life problems.* San Francisco: Jossey Bass.

Sternberg, R. J., & Dobson, D. M. (1987). Resolving interpersonal conflicts: An analysis of stylistic consistency. *Journal of Personality and Social Psychology, 52,* 794–812.

Wall, J. A., Jr., & Blum, M., (1991). Community mediation in the People's Republic of China. *Journal of Conflict Resolution, 35,* 3–20.

CHAPTER 12

Culture, Families, and Children's Aggression

Findings from Jamaica, Japan, and Latinos in the United States

NANCY G. GUERRA, AMBER J. HAMMONS, *and* MICHIKO OTSUKI CLUTTER

All children (and nonhuman primates) appear to have the capacity for aggression written on their evolutionary birth certificate (de Waal, 2000; Hawley, 1999; Niehoff, 1999). However, actual aggressive behavior varies significantly across and within social and cultural groups. In order to account for this variation, it is important to consider how a child's propensity for aggression is shaped over time and across contexts from birth onward. Indeed, aggression is a complex and multiply determined behavior—whatever biological or genetic differences children bring to the table, these individual characteristics unfold in nested socioecological contexts. Acknowledging the importance of these nested contexts, ecological frameworks have been a mainstay of research on the etiology and prevention of children's aggression for the past several decades (Dodge, Coie, & Lynam, 2006; Guerra & Huesmann, 2004; Metropolitan Area Child Study Research Group, 2002).

Much of this work, particularly within developmental psychology, has emphasized the importance of proximal contexts that provide regular and ongoing venues for social interaction. A primary focus of this research is to understand how children learn aggressive behaviors (and develop related patterns of social cognition) as they interact over time with significant others, including families, friends, classmates, teachers, and mentors. Research has identified characteristics of these relationships that distinguish aggressive children from their less aggressive peers. For example, aggression has been linked to higher levels of rejection by peers (Bierman, Smoot, & Aumiller, 1993), having more-aggressive friends (Tremblay, Mâsse, Vitaro, & Dobkin, 1995), negative and harsh parenting (Patterson, 2002), and low levels of parental monitoring (Pettit, Laird, Dodge, Bates, & Criss, 2001). These characteristics are useful in understanding variations within communities, cultures, and societies.

On the other hand, a separate strand of research has emphasized the influence of more distal contexts on the rates of aggression and violence. Drawing on sociology, anthropology, and cross-cultural psychology, this research has stressed differences in the prevalence of aggression and violence among youths growing up in different neighborhoods, communities, regions, and countries. A primary focus of this research is to identify cultural or subcultural values and practices that characterize groups of individuals and that can increase or decrease the likelihood of aggressive behavior. From this perspective, culture includes the beliefs, norms, values, and shared meanings of any group, whether its members are bound by ethnicity, religion, community, or other shared identities (Staub, 1996).

For example, higher community levels of violence within disadvantaged urban communities in the United States have been associated with a *subculture of violence* characterized by a willingness to use violence (Wolfgang & Ferracuti, 1967) and a *code of the street* based on the threat of vengeance (Anderson, 1999). At the regional level, higher violence rates in the U.S. South have been discussed in terms of a *culture of honor,* in which violence is seen as an appropriate response to violations of personal honor (Nisbett & Cohen, 1996). At the national level, differences in violence rates across countries have been attributed to values that promote or limit aggression. A popular example is the distinction between *individualist* cultures, such as the United States, with relatively high violence rates versus *collectivist* cultures, such as Japan, with low violence rates (Dussich, 2001; Masataka, 2002; White, 1993).

However, it also is the case that contexts are nested and interconnected. In addition to considering the direct effects from each sphere of influence, research also has highlighted the need to assess mediators and moderators to understand the mechanisms of interrelated influence and the conditions under which they occur. For example, just as culture can have a direct effect on aggression if its norms support aggressive behavior and related risk factors, culture can also influence child development and aggression indirectly via its effects on parenting practices. Looking again at the distinction between the United States and Japan, cross-cultural studies have shown that parents in the United States show greater tolerance for young children's willfulness and attention to their own personal needs (increasing the potential for conflict and aggression at an early age), whereas parents in Japan encourage empathy and meeting others' expectations (Kazui, 1997; Rothbaum & Weisz, 1989).

Cultural practices can also moderate observed relations. As an example, the association between aggression and peer rejection has been shown to vary, depending on the overall "value" of aggression within a specific culture or subculture (Hawley, Little, & Rodkin, 2007; Prinstein & Cillessen, 2003). Whether or not aggression portends peer disapproval and rejection also depends on the young person's ability to appropriately calibrate his or her aggression to the demands of the situation. As Vaughn and Santos (2007) discuss, aggressive children who are otherwise socially competent and can call on their aggressive skills only when needed do well in peer groups of all ages, a finding consistent with the historical and anthropological record on aggression and adaptation (Sapolsky, 2004). Thus, the relation between aggression and peer rejection may hinge on the status of aggressive behavior within a specific cultural context and whether an aggressive child is able to strategically use aggression appropriately within this context.

A main theme of this chapter is that culture provides an important lens for understanding how aggression and violence are learned across and within specific contexts. Although ecological models of children's aggression have been at the forefront of etiological and prevention research, the direct and indirect impact of culture has received less attention. To illustrate how cultural norms can account for variations in aggression and violence across different cultural groups, we begin by comparing cultural orientations and societal norms relevant to aggression and violence across three countries characterized by large differences in the rates of serious violence, namely, Jamaica, Japan, and the United States. Although Japan, with low violence rates, typically has been contrasted with the United States, with significantly higher rates, Jamaica now has one of the highest homicide rates in the world, nearly 10 times as high as the United States and more than 100 times higher than Japan. Further, given the diversity of ethnic and cultural groups within a pluralistic society such as the United States, we focus on Latino children and families as a distinct subgroup.

Next, we examine specific processes by which culture can influence children's socioemotional socialization and development as they relate to the learning of aggression. Given considerable empirical support for the role of the family in the development of children's aggression, we focus on how cultural orientations can impact parental socialization and, in turn, increase children's risk for aggressive behavior. Finally, we consider how a focus on culture in studies of children's socialization for aggression can

enhance future research and practice. In particular, we close with suggestions of new directions for culturally sensitive preventive interventions.

Culture, Aggression, and Violence
across Three Cultures:
Jamaica, Japan, and Latinos in the United States

Cross-Cultural Differences in Aggression and Violence

It is often difficult to compare rates of children's aggression across specific
countries. A precise comparison would require a cross-cultural study with
comparable assessments at similar ages in the countries of interest. Although
there are a number of international epidemiological studies of aggression
and violence, to our knowledge there are no developmental studies comparing rates of aggression and violence among children or adolescents in
Jamaica, Japan, and Latinos in the United States. For the purposes of this
chapter, we base such comparisons on the available violence and crime data
for each country, acknowledging the limitations of these data.

We present homicide rates as a proxy for violence because they are
more easily available by country and by ethnic group within the United
States and do not suffer from potential variations in definition (i.e., what
is considered "aggressive" or "criminal" may vary by culture). Although
we do not isolate the rates for youths, homicide typically peaks between
the ages of 16–24 across ethnic and cultural groups (Centers for Disease
Control and Prevention, 2009), suggesting that rates largely are driven by
this age group. Comparing data across Jamaica, Japan, and Latinos in the
United States, the picture is striking.

Consider Jamaica. Since independence in 1962, homicide (and violence)
on this island nation of approximately 2.5 million people has continued to
rise each decade, from 7 per 100,000 population during the 1950s and
1960s to 23 per 100,000 during the 1980s (Moser & Holland, 1997). This
pattern of escalation increased into the 21st century, with rates now higher
than 60 per 100,000 island-wide and reaching over 140 per 100,000 in
the poor communities of inner-city Kingston (Jamaica Constabulary Force,
2009). Not only is the Caribbean one of the highest violence regions in the
world, but Jamaica has the highest homicide rates in the Caribbean. Violence is not limited to homicide—rates for other types of serious and violent
crimes have risen steadily since the 1960s. The problem is so extreme in
some inner-city communities that residents have named them after war
zones or areas notorious for violence, such as "Gaza" and "Tel Aviv" (Harriott, 2008).

In stark contrast, Japan has one of the lowest violence and homicide
rates among the general population and youths in the world, just as rates

across Asia are among the lowest in the world. After the conclusion of World War II, the homicide rate in Japan decreased consistently from 1955 through 1980, after a brief period of increase from 1950 to 1955. The homicide rate decreased from 3.4 per 100,000 population in 1950 (Fujimoto & Park, 1994) to 0.5 per 100,000 in 2005 (United Nations Office on Drugs and Crime, 2009). A similar decline in homicide rates was observed for Japanese youths, as well. The number of youths (ages 14–19) who committed a felony (i.e., homicide, robbery, arson, or rape) was at its highest during the early 1960s, followed by a sharp decline and then cyclical fluctuations into the 21st century. The number of homicides committed by juveniles during the early 21st century ranged from 57 in 2004 to 105 in 2000 (Nawa, 2006). Despite the relatively low rates of homicides among juvenile delinquents in Japan, since the mid-1970s a few definable trends emerged, including a decrease in the average age of delinquents, the spread of delinquency across the socioeconomic spectrum, and an increase in entry-level offenses, such as shoplifting and bicycle/motorcycle theft (Nawa, 2006).

Although homicide rates in the United States are closer to Japan's than to Jamaica's, they are still relatively high. After nearly doubling during the 1960s and 1970s, stabilizing during the 1980s, and rising again in the early 1990s, overall rates declined sharply and then stayed nearly level after 2000 at approximately 5 per 100,000 population. Considering ethnic and cultural variations within the United States, it is important to note that homicide rates are approximately six times higher for African Americans, at over 30 per 100,000, with rates for Latinos falling roughly in the middle, at about 15 per 100,000. Irrespective of ethnicity, rates are comparatively higher for males and young people (Bureau of Justice Statistics, 2009). Violence among Latinos—like that among Jamaicans and for African Americans in the United States—is concentrated in urban areas. Further, Latino homicides are concentrated in certain neighborhoods within urban areas rather than being evenly distributed across cities. However, the picture for Latinos is complicated by the immigrant experience, a cultural experience not shared by African Americans (Martinez, 2002). Indeed, based on 2000 U.S. Census data, 13 million first-generation immigrants, predominantly from Mexico, make up 40% of the Latino population (U.S. Census Bureau, 2002).

Differences in violence rates between countries and within the United States have been attributed, in part, to the well-documented association between poverty and violence (Moser & Holland, 1997). Until recently, the United States and Japan had the highest gross domestic product (GDP) in the world (ranked first and second, respectively, until 2010, when China surpassed Japan) with Jamaica ranked 105th (World Bank, 2009). There are considerable demographic variations within countries, particularly the United States and Jamaica. In the United States, Latino poverty rates are three times those for non-Hispanic whites and greatest among immigrants (*La Raza*, 2009). In Jamaica, poverty is most pronounced in inner-city garrison communities (Moser & Holland, 1997). In both the United States and Jamaica, the highest rates of poverty are concentrated in urban inner-city areas with a high percentage of minority residents—although poverty rather than ethnicity is the strongest predictor of violence (Sampson, 1993). Although poverty and unemployment exist in Japan, there are relatively few areas of concentrated disadvantage compared to the United States and Jamaica (Yamamiya, 2003).

Whatever the demographic circumstances, poverty does not directly lead to increased violence. Rather, economic circumstances create conditions of scarcity, need, and competition for resources not found in more advantaged communities. These conditions can lead to "self-help" systems that socialize violence as an adaptive coping and survival strategy (Buss & Shackelford, 1997; Harriott, 2008). Similarly, wealth does not guarantee immunity from violence, although its forms and functions may change. Systems also are embedded in a larger cultural context. Several prominent dimensions of culture (or cultural orientations) have been suggested to explain cross-cultural variations in behaviors, including violence.

Cultural Orientations and Their Potential Relation to Aggression and Violence

Perhaps the most widely cited approach to capturing the precise dimensions of cultural variability is based on five dimensions detailed by Hofstede, specifically, (1) individualism–collectivism, (2) masculinity–femininity, (3) power distance, (4) uncertainty avoidance, and (5) the long-term versus short-term orientation (Hofstede, 1980). Among these, individualism–collectivism has received the most attention in psychology as an explanatory mechanism for understanding cross-cultural differences as they relate to a variety of outcomes (Oyserman, Koon, & Kemmelmeier, 2002). Examining cross-cultural variations in violence rates in Jamaica, Japan, the United States, and Mexico (given our focus on immigrant Latinos primarily from Mexico), Hofstede's ratings of these countries on each of the five dimensions (see Table 12.1) provide insights beyond the individualism–collectivism distinction and suggest other dimensions of culture to examine in relation to aggression and violence. Each scale ranks from 0 to 100, with 100 representing the highest readings on individualism, masculinity, power distance, uncertainty avoidance, and long-term orientation.

Before discussing how these dimensions may operate in relation to children's socialization for aggression and violence, we provide a brief description of each one. Bear in mind that Hofstede's original study of

TABLE 12.1. Country Ratings on Hofstede's (1980) Dimensions of Cultural Variability

	Individualism–collectivism	Masculinity–femininity	Power distance	Uncertainty avoidance	Long-term versus short-term orientation
Jamaica	39	68	45	13	Not rated
Japan	46	95	54	92	80
United States	91	62	40	46	29
Mexico	30	65	81	82	Not rated

cultural variability was based on detailed interviews with IBM employees in 53 countries during the late 1970s and was not designed to capture cultural dimensions related to child development, aggression, or violence. The Hofstede's measures also are extremely broad dimensions that may actually play out quite unpredictably across various cultures, requiring a more nuanced understanding to link them to variations in children's aggression and violence.

Individualism–Collectivism

This dimension describes the salience of allegiance to the self or to the group within a culture. The fundamental theme of an individualist orientation is the centrality of the autonomous individual, whereas the organizing theme of a collectivist orientation is the centrality of the group (Triandis, 1995). Industrialized Western societies, particularly ethnic groups with a Protestant heritage, typically score high on individualism, with non-Western societies ranking high on collectivism, although there are considerable ethnic divergences within individual societies as well. For example, Latinos in the United States have been characterized as collectively oriented, with a strong emphasis on obligation to both the nuclear and extended family (Marin & Marin, 1991).

Masculinity–Femininity

This distinction has been made along gender-stereotypical lines. Cultures with a high masculinity index (MAS) value achievement and ambition, whereas low-MAS cultures emphasize the quality of life and helping others. High-MAS cultures also have sharply defined and very distinct expectations of male and female roles in society, with masculinity conceptually tied to power and status.

Power Distance

Cultures that are characterized by relatively unequal distributions of institutional and organizational power and unchallenged obedience to authority are regarded as high power distance cultures. For example, the concept of *respeto*, or respect, within Latino culture in Mexico and the United States places great social value on the decision-making roles of authority figures (Marin & Marin, 1991). Typically, the more unequal the distribution of wealth in a culture, the greater the power distance.

Uncertainty Avoidance

High uncertainty avoidance cultures prefer formal rules and structures, with low tolerance for ambiguity. They prefer to avoid uncertainty and dissent, and they strive for consensus. In contrast, cultures with low uncertainty avoidance tend to tolerate dissent and encourage divergent viewpoints.

Long-Term versus Short-Term Orientation

This dimension has also been called "Confucian dynamism," in reference to the selective promotion of the ethics of restraint and perseverance that is found in Confucian teachings. Also emphasized are thrift, a sense of shame, and allegiance to hierarchical structures. This dimension has been used to explain the recent rapid economic development of many Asian countries.

In attempting to account for differences in societal levels of violence, the most likely potential explanatory factor at the broader societal/cultural level is the individualism-collectivism dimension. There has been a general assumption that children growing up in individualist societies with an emphasis on personal success are likely to be more aggressive than children growing up in collectivist societies that emphasize interdependence, sacrifice for the common good, and maintaining harmonious relations with others (Markus & Kitayama, 1991). However, the picture is more complex and most likely is shaped by the economic and historic conditions of the time, the nature of the "collective" or group, and the cultural status of violence as normative behavior with certain groups and subgroups.

Although collectivism emphasizes the common good, it also calls attention to ingroup–outgroup distinctions. Under conditions of scarcity, the power of the group can be used against other groups to leverage resources, leading to clearly demarcated group divisions and increased aggression in the service of the group's "common good," particularly under conditions where violence is more normative. Collectivism also is evident through group cohesion at different levels of social relations. This aspect includes dedication to the family, as seen in both Japanese and Latino American cultures, tight relationships within a geographic community, and identification based on neighborhood groups, as seen particularly in urban Jamaican and Latino enclaves in the United States, and patriotic collectivism based on allegiance to the state or nation, most evident in Japanese society; indeed, Japan is one of the most homogeneous and unified countries in the world (Kawasaki, 1994; Yamamiya, 2003).

Of course, alliances can emerge along a number of different dimensions and based on a range of commonalities. Extended families frequently provide a basis for group allegiance. In some cases, the "family" is created anew through structures such as organized crime and gangs. Within Latino subcultures in the United States, gangs have emerged as unifying groups based largely on the intersection of ethnic origins (e.g., Mexico, Central America, Puerto Rico) and location (including street, neighborhood, community, and region) (Moore, 1991). In Japan, youths who are marginalized from the larger society may band together in an underworld (*yakuza*) that, ironically, relies on collectivist values such as *jingi* (i.e., a moral code emphasizing benevolence and righteousness) to enforce a code of strict allegiance and absolute loyalty to the gang leader (Yamamiya, 2003). In urban Jamaica, group affiliation is defined by a variety of allegiances, including location (street, subdistrict, district), political party affiliation (People's National Party or Jamaica Labour Party), and an informal collection of community governance units ruled by "dons," or bosses (Gray, 2004). In some cases, allegiances emerge over seemingly arbitrary distinctions, such as the current "Gaza-Gully" divide in urban Jamaica linked to which dancehall reggae musician one supports (Vybz Kartel from Gaza or Movado from Gully) (*Jamaica Gleaner*, September 30, 2009).

The important point is that collectivism can serve to unify people within a social group and simultaneously separate them from other groups. Bringing this insight back to children's socialization and the learning of aggression, in cultures where harmony is stressed and group differences minimized, children learn to emphasize cooperation and social responsibility rather than personal desire and need (Whiting & Edwards, 1988). However, in complex urban societies, particularly those with limited or unequally allocated resources, collectivism may be sidetracked in the service of benefitting a specific subgroup. Under these conditions, children not only adopt specific allegiances but also may be more susceptible to polarization and identification with subgroups (such as gangs) from an early age—an orientation that increases the likelihood of aggression and violence against the outgroup. This reasoning suggests that a more useful distinction relevant to understanding aggression and violence would be to differentiate a collectivist orientation "for the common good" of humanity, as contrasted with a collectivist allegiance to one's particular reference group.

Applying this nuanced understanding to differences in aggression and violence between Japan and Jamaica, it is clear that although both societies are considered "collectivist" according to Hofstede's (1980) broad categories, collectivism in Japan operates at a national level for the common good of Japanese society, a practice that discourages conflict and violence, whereas collectivism in Jamaica appears to operate more at the small-group level, similar to more tribally oriented societies, resulting in rivalry, conflict, and competition.

Further, such dimensions as individualism–collectivism operate in tandem with other dimensions of culture. In terms of cross-cultural differences in rates of violence and children's socialization for aggression and violence, it may be the intersection of these dimensions and specific patterns that is most informative. Although we have suggested some reasons why the individualism–collectivism dimension may have some limited explanatory power in attempting to understand the enormous differences in violent crime between Japan and Jamaica, what may be equally important is how these dimensions act *synergistically*. What is most striking about Japan's rankings are its high scores on the masculinity–femininity, uncertainty avoidance, and long-term versus short-term orientation measures. In other words, it may be that collectivism in a relatively homogeneous and prosperous society, combined with values that support striving for consensus, harmony, thrift, a sense of shame, and allegiance to hierarchical structures, generally fosters cooperation and collaboration rather than aggression and violence toward others.

Further, in relation to aggression and violence, it is important to consider the extent to which the operationalization of broader cultural dimensions in a given setting—that is, how they play out in daily life—includes aggression and violence. As an example, the conceptualization of masculinity as representing achievement, status, and the acquisition of wealth does not account for cultural mandates equating masculinity with aggression and coercive control. In resource-poor societies, threats and the use of violence can provide a viable means to achieve status (as well as material goods), particularly for males.

If we were to rate Jamaicans, Japanese, and Latinos in the United States on the association of masculinity with violence, these rank orderings most likely would parallel homicide rankings. For example, although Japan is a patriarchal society that historically has embraced male dominance and achievement, it is not associated with violence but with the maintenance of harmonious relationships—the Japanese are sensitive to collective norms and avoid inappropriate behaviors (Kozu, 1999). In contrast, Jamaica currently would rank high on the association of achievement, status, and wealth with the use of violence within some economically disadvantaged subcultural groups—consider the glorification of male violence in youth-led contemporary dancehall reggae music (*Jamaica Gleaner,* September 30, 2009). Serious violence in Jamaica is dominated by males and often associated with masculinity—"No gun, no girl" is a common expression (Moser & Holland, 1997). Latinos in the United States must contend with cultural mandates for *machismo*-based male aggression and dominance, which ironically seems to increase for immigrants to the U.S. (Stevens, 1973; Sugihara & Warner, 2002). Thus, "violent masculinity" may be a more useful cultural dimension in understanding cultural and subcultural variations in aggression. The impact of violent masculinity on children's socialization for aggression most likely occurs through a range of direct and indirect channels as children learn gender-appropriate behaviors from an early age.

Beyond the links between masculinity and violence in a given subcultural or cultural group, variations in violence and children's socialization within and across various cultural contexts is influenced more generally by norms about the appropriateness of aggressive and prosocial behaviors (Hill, Soriano, Che, & La Fromboise, 1994; Huesmann & Guerra, 1997). These norms can operate at the more general societal level. For instance, frequent media depictions of extreme violence in the United States suggest a general tolerance for violence. Still, that does not mean that all U.S. citizens embrace violence. Although, from a broad cultural viwpoint, violence may be infused into various cultural practices, there still is considerable individual variation within each society: for example, as already noted, regional variations in violence rates in the United States have been linked to a "culture of honor" in the South (Nisbett & Cohen, 1996) Societal norms also are translated into developmental outcomes as they are processed through a range of socializing agents at different developmental stages—that is, families, teachers, peers, and friends all influence children's emerging belief systems about aggression (Huesmann & Guerra, 1997).

How Culture Impacts Socialization for Aggression: Family Processes

Researchers interested in the role of culture in human development have emphasized the role of proximal social contexts in mediating the linkages between cultural values and individual developmental outcomes. For example, Chen and colleagues (Chen, French, & Schneider, 2006) have proposed a contextual–developmental framework, in which social interactional processes serve to mediate cultural influences on human development. In other words, cultural norms and values set the stage for patterns of social interaction that, in turn, impact individual development and behavior. Chen and colleagues have applied their model to examine broad cultural impacts on peer contexts and how these, in turn, affect individual child outcomes. In this chapter, we focus on cultural influences on family practices and parenting that, in turn, are related to variations in children's aggression patterns.

What emerges from our broad cultural comparison of relevant frameworks in Jamaica, Japan, and Latinos in the United States is that these three cultures share important similarities, including collectivist orientation, adherence to fairly rigid gender-based roles and responsibilities, deference to authority figures, and preference for formal rule structures (which is particularly high in Japan). Still, these broad cultural dimensions per se do not shed light on the vast differences in rates of aggression and violence. What may be more important for child outcomes is how these cultural dimensions translate into specific socialization practices. For example, in general, these orientations are likely to result in more authoritarian parenting styles emphasizing child compliance, control, and obedience that have been implicated in negative child outcomes, including increased rates of aggressive and noncompliant behavior across cultures (Chen, Dong, & Zhou, 1997) and adolescent violence and delinquency (Farrington, 1989).

However, just as broad cultural dimensions may look quite different under different conditions, authoritarian parenting, broadly construed, consists of multiple components, including rigid enforcement of rules without explanation, harsh discipline, low levels of affection, high levels of anger and displeasure, and low levels of positive engagement (Baumrind, 1973). These dimensions of authoritarian parenting may operate very differently across cultures (e.g., frequency, intensity) and also vary in meaning, for instance, when used within a context of positive guidance or training (Chao, 1994). Further, the effects of authoritarian parenting on child outcomes has been shown to be moderated by children's interpretation of this behavior (e.g., in relation to perceived parental acceptance or rejection), and this perspective varies within cultures and cross-culturally (Deater-Deckard, Dodge, Bates, & Pettit, 1996; Rohner, Kean, & Cournoyer, 1991).

Such variation suggests that understanding the influence of culture on parenting practices and child behavior requires a more nuanced and holistic assessment of the various features of childrearing and how they play out in different settings. In other words, focusing on any single aspect or component of parenting alone does not account for the meaning of this practice within a particular cultural, historical, and economic environment. Indeed, parenting styles in Jamaica, Japan, and within Latino culture in the United States have all been characterized as controlling, restrictive, or authoritarian; yet, as we have discussed, the effects on children's aggression and violence rates are remarkably different. We propose that cultural variations across these countries influence two particularly salient aspects of parenting that, taken together, create qualitatively different socialization contexts for children's learning of aggression and violence. These are (1) harsh physical punishment and (2) support and encouragement for prosocial and cooperative behavior.

Harsh Physical Punishment and Socialization for Aggression

The use of harsh physical punishment has been linked to subsequent increased aggression and violence in children. In the extreme case, physical abuse is one of the most robust predictors of childhood aggression and youth violence at the individual level (Luntz & Widom, 1994). When parents regularly use physical means of controlling and punishing their children, they send a message that aggression is a normative and effective way to gain compliance. The use of extreme physical discipline can also lead to avoidance of the disciplinary figure, reducing parental opportunities to influence their child. Corporal punishment also can lead to external rather than internal attributions for compliance (Gershoff, 2002). In other words, children learn not to misbehave in order to avoid future punishment, but they do not learn to behave independently in morally and socially acceptable ways (Hoffman, 1983).

Although support and use of harsh physical punishment clearly varies within cultures, it also varies cross-culturally, reflecting a set of culturally transmitted beliefs about appropriate childrearing strategies, the status of children, and legitimate disciplinary agents (e.g., parents, schools, religious organizations) that are translated into laws and policies (Douglas, 2006; Straus, 2001). Parent's "ethnotheories" about child development and parenting provide a frame of reference for understanding and responding to children's behavior within a specific context (Harkness & Super, 1996). Given specific historical and economic conditions, these beliefs, ethnotheories, and related laws also influence accepted standards for the use of corporal punishment (i.e., for which behaviors, how often, by whom, etc.). Presumably, cultures that endorse corporal punishment as a general strategy for childrearing also could vary greatly on conditions for use, particularly among subcultures defined by regional affiliation, religious orientation, and economic status.

Of relevance to our cross-cultural comparison of children's socialization for aggression and violence, corporal punishment is considered justifiable discipline in Jamaica (Smith & Mosby, 2003), Japan (Kozu, 1999), and within Latino subcultures in the United States (Fontes, 2002). At first glance, cultural support for corporal punishment across these cultures calls into question the utility of this construct as a mechanism to explain cross-cultural differences in socialization for aggression and violence. However, there are important variations in the degree to which corporal punishment is a central tenet of beliefs and practices for childrearing, the extent of its use in families and social institutions, and its embeddedness in broader models of parental responsibilities for child development. We propose that these differences can explain some of the variations in violence rates across these cultures over the past few decades (although attitudes worldwide may be evolving away from endorsement of corporal punishment, this trend is a slow process and our comparative data on homicides are based on the past several decades).

Jamaican culture embraces love and peace; yet, parenting is dominated by regular and harsh discipline. Whether it is a result of the brutal history of slavery or religious beliefs based on a literal interpretation of the Bible, physical punishment often is considered a form of "love," with direct reference to the Book of Proverbs (Steely & Rohner, 2006). Flogging or beating cuts across multiple socioeconomic levels and institutions. Although the Jamaican government has accepted its obligation to abide by the recommendations of the United Nations Convention on the Rights of the Child (2005), socially and legally sanctioned forms of discipline in homes and schools still include striking children with hands, sticks, belts, switches, wood, wire, or other objects as well as making children kneel or stand in uncomfortable positions (Meeks Gardner, Powell, & Grantham-McGregor, 2007). Children are punished in these ways for any number of transgressions, including lying, stealing, impoliteness, poor schoolwork, crying too much, not finishing a meal, and not completing their chores (Barrow, 1996). Although data are cross-sectional, increased aggression within Jamaican samples has been shown to correlate with increased experience of corporal punishment (Meeks Gardner et al., 2007).

Japanese childrearing, although traditionally grounded in a patriarchal family structure where hierarchical roles are prescribed and obedience to authority is paramount, both promotes and inhibits the use of corporal punishment as a disciplinary strategy. Although this statement appears to be paradoxical, the underlying quandary has emerged from the untimely emergence of rigid authoritarian families coincident with the virtual absence of legal intervention in Japanese family life (which can increase the likelihood of corporal punishment) combined with a focus on the importance of achieving obedience through the child's internalization of a desire to conform (which should independently decrease the likelihood of external punishments) (Kozu, 1999). Although Japanese society has undergone significant changes in family life in recent years, the stability of the family, the closeness of the mother–child bond, parents' beliefs that they are responsible for their child's behavior, and a tendency to protect and indulge young children have led to childrearing practices that are not overly reliant on corporal punishment as a day-to-day control strategy (Borovoy, 2008; Conroy, Hess, Axuma, & Kashiwagi, 1980).

Latinos in the United States, particularly recent immigrants from Mexico, tend to endorse authoritarian styles of parenting and demand obedience from their children. Several studies have found greater support for and reporting of physical punishment of children among Latino families in the U.S. when compared to European American parents. However, these effects are reduced when parental socioeconomic status is controlled (see Halgunseth, Ispa, & Rudy, 2006, for a discussion). Still, mild forms of physical punishment are embedded in many cultural practices and even take on a symbolic element. For example, a child who has said or done something "stupid" may be knuckled on the top of the head (a *cocotazo*) or a child who swears may be slapped across the mouth (a *tapaboca*). For recent immigrant parents, this style of parenting is particularly problematic as they struggle to understand the norms and laws regarding physical punishment of children in the United States (Fontes, 2002).

As we have noted, serious and repeated physical punishment predicts children's aggression and delinquency within cultures (Luntz & Widom, 1994). However, we have also discussed differences in the use, frequency, and meaning of corporal punishment across cultures that may account, in part, for variations in levels of aggression and violence. When physical discipline administered in a harsh and rejecting manner is a primary mode of parental socialization, such as is the case in Jamaica, it is likely that children learn rules, roles, standards, and values that incorporate the use of aggression and violence. Harsh physical punishment also interferes with the development of internalized standards for behavior and threatens the development of personal autonomy, which should be most problematic during late childhood and adolescence. Poor inner-city Jamaican youths report that they are either "treated like babies" (Brown & Johnson, 2008) or that the lack of parental respect for youths turns into a power struggle, particularly for adolescent males, who turn to the streets for support (Gayle & Levy, 2007).

In contrast, when parenting practices rely on psychological (rather than physical) control for discipline and guidance, the end goal is still compliance, but the means are different, including guilt-inducing strategies and parental intrusiveness. Although this type of parenting generally has not been associated with peer aggression and serious youth violence, it is not without its dark side and does have links with violence. This type of control has been found to lead to anxiety, depression, and loneliness (Barber & Harmon, 2002). Among Japanese youths, this style of intrusive and overprotective parenting has been implicated in the concept of *tokokyohi* (school refusal) or *hikikomori* (the withdrawn). These phenomena reflect total withdrawal from society, in which children (and even young adults) stop attending school, sleep during the day, play video games at night, and sometimes engage in random acts of public aggression or filial violence primarily against their mothers (Borovoy, 2008; Kozu, 1999; Yamamiya, 2003).

Still, parental control strategies must also be understood in the context of positive supports and beliefs about the role of parents in promoting children's prosocial and cooperative behaviors. Cultural beliefs about desirable and positive behaviors are likely to influence parental socialization practices and children's behavior. A common complaint from inner-city Jamaican youths is that "being good" primarily involves not "being bad." In other words, parental affection and support are identified as the absence of disapproval rather than encouragement and support for positive behaviors (Brown & Johnson, 2008). Differential socialization practices to encourage good behavior can also help us to understand cross-cultural differences in learning negative behaviors such as aggression and violence.

Support and Encouragement for Prosocial and Cooperative Behavior

Much of the research on family socialization in Jamaica has emphasized harsh parenting and its negative effects, with relatively little research on the positive and prosocial aspects of Jamaican family socialization. This emphasis does not mean that Jamaican parenting only focuses on children's misdeeds and bad behavior; clearly, there are many positive and loving aspects of Jamaican childrearing that need more in-depth research. In contrast, there is a substantial body of Japanese research on the concept of *ii-ko* (the good child) as well as a number of core cultural concepts in Latino families that highlight the importance of prosocial behavior. Parental socialization that encourages the development of empathy and compassion in children is likely to discourage aggressive and violent acts toward others from early childhood onward. Interestingly, Bowlby's first empirical study on supportive caregiving environments made a connection between the lack of supportive caregiving that encourages empathy and affection and juvenile delinquency (Bowlby, 1944).

In Japanese culture, an important aspect of "the good child" that has been valued since feudal times is social embeddedness, including maintaining harmonious social relationships and being gentle, empathically responsive to others, and willingly compliant with the wishes of others (Olson, Kashiwagi, & Crystal, 2001). In Ruth Benedict's (1954) anthropological account of Japanese parenting behavior, she discusses how Japanese parents continuously enforce a strong need for acceptance in their children that makes "ostracism more dreaded than violence" (pp. 287–288). Consistent with this cultural belief, Japanese parents encourage characteristics that foster social harmony from an early age. Cross-cultural studies of parental socialization have found that Japanese mothers tend to indulge young children, appeal to feelings rather than use their authority, place a high value on self-control of emotion and cooperation, and designate aggressive behaviors as socially insensitive and uncooperative rather than as negative (Kazui, 1997; Olson et al., 2001). For example, when Japanese children display difficult behaviors during a Strange Situation paradigm, Japanese mothers are likely to attribute these to the child's need for security and interdependence, whereas U.S. mothers are more likely to ascribe these behaviors to anger or aggression (Rothbaum, Kakinuma, Nagaoka, & Azuma, 2007).

Overall, significant attention in Japanese society focuses on raising a "good child" who is sensitive to the needs of others, receptive to adult expectations, and motivated by an internal desire to conform to cultural expectations. In group-oriented cultural contexts such as Japan, parental socialization emphasizes the obligatory nature of cooperation and prosocial behavior. In other words, such behavior is not seen as a matter of individual choice—as is typical in Western cultures—but rather as one's duty to the group. *Sasshi*, meaning "mind reading," is valued by Japanese mothers and is an indicator of the child's connection with the social environment (Rothbaum et al., 2007). In fact, having a mind of one's own is seen as less important than readings others' minds (Masataka, 2002).

Latino culture also embraces several norms regarding desirable children's behavior that emphasize the importance of social relationships. For example, *simpatía* places great value on peaceful social relations and the avoidance of conflict. Similar to the Japanese emphasis on social harmony versus individual agency, it discourages assertiveness and personal will. *Personalismo* emphasizes the importance of interpersonal relationships and social connectedness, as contrasted with material gains or personal needs. Respect for authority is mandated through the core cultural concept of *respeto* (respect). In both Japanese and Latino cultures, these values are embedded in strong family networks. However, in contrast to Japanese culture with its emphasis on promoting children's internalization of standards for acceptable behavior, the Latino concept of *respeto* often translates into unquestioning obedience of authority. Recall the high rating on power distance for Mexico reported in Table 12.1. In the absence of legitimate authority figures, however such obedience can easily translate into strong alliances with negative authority figures and strong attachments to negative social groups (Hill et al., 1994).

Further, the stress caused by cultural conflict (labeled "acculturative stress") presents unique challenges for the U.S. Latino families, who must straddle the norms and mandates of both cultures. Latinos who immigrate to the U.S. often find a different cultural environment that may clash with core Latino values and/or be difficult to maintain in a new environment.

As children acculturate to "middle-class American values," some evidence suggests that their shifting cultural value system toward individualism and the cultural values embedded in the U.S. youth culture actually *increases* a variety of negative behaviors, including aggression (Gonzales, Knight, Morgan-Lopez, Saenz, & Sirolli, 2002) and youth violence (Smokowski, David-Ferdon, & Stroupe, 2009). When children acculturate faster than their parents, conflict between loyalty to Latino and mainstream U.S. values can lead to intergenerational conflict and increased aggression (Smith & Krohn, 1995).

Conclusions and Future Directions

We have highlighted the importance of cultural influences on children's learning of aggression and violence by citing examples from Japan, Jamaica, and Latinos in the United States. As we have noted, at the broadest level cross-cultural differences in the rates of aggression and violence may be understood, in part, by comprehending the natural composition of the country, as well as the specific norms, beliefs, and behavioral mandates embedded within this context. Broad cultural dimensions can provide a starting point for understanding differences in aggression and violence across cultures, but how these dimensions play out under specific conditions in each culture is what is most important. For example, collectivism in a high-resource homogeneous culture bound by social obligation, such as Japan, is likely to foster cooperation and compliance rather than aggression. In contrast, collectivism in a low resource culture divided by ingroup–outgroup rivalries, such as Jamaica, is likely to foster competition between groups and higher levels of violence.

Further, culture dictates specific patterns of social interaction in proximal contexts that more directly influence children's developing behavior patterns. U.S. Latinos' higher rates of homicide may be aggravated by issues of acculturation, while Jamaica's very high rates of homicide may be attributable in part to harsh punishments and more impoverished living areas. An important but understudied aspect of culture of relevance to family socialization is the view of the "good child" within different cultures and subcultures. In some way, parental beliefs about the "good parent" hinge on their beliefs about the desired outcomes of parental socialization. Does the good child look out for the welfare of others? Is the good child one who doesn't cause problems and stays out of the way? Is the good child one who obeys without question? Perhaps an important next step for understanding the effects of parental socialization on child behavioral outcomes across and within cultures is to examine these beliefs across multiple cultures and subcultures and to look at their relation to parenting practices and child outcomes.

Family-based programs to prevent children's aggression may also benefit from encouraging discussion of the good child, using cross-cultural illustrations to highlight the positive outcomes from different orientations. For example, if Jamaican youths are dissatisfied with their parents' lack of explicit encouragement of good behavior, this shortcoming may be a culture-specific issue that is modifiable. Developmental literature across cultures appears to suggest that parental support and encouragement of prosocial and cooperative behaviors helps to increase these positive behaviors among youths. Thus, family-based programs for Jamaican youths may emphasize the connections between parental encouragement of good behaviors and desirable child behavioral outcomes.

Culturally sensitive practices typically involve taking an intervention developed within mainstream (often U.S.) culture and adapting it to the conventions and practices of diverse cultural groups. We suggest that we take a step away from a "one-size-fits-all" mindset and propose a slightly different approach. We propose, in short, that cultural sensitivity be expanded to incorporate best practices from multiple cultures. These best practices may begin with a cross-cultural dialogue about how to develop a consensus on how best to encourage desirable child behaviors that enhance children's well-being while preventing antisocial and aggressive behavior regardless of cultural influences.

References

Anderson, E. (1999). *Code of the street.* New York: Norton.

Barber, B. K., & Harmon, E. L. (2002). Violating the self: Parental psychological control of children and adolescents. In B. K. Barber (Ed.), *Intrusive parenting: How psychological control affects children and adolescents* (pp. 15–52). Washington, DC: American Psychological Association.

Barrow, C. (1996). *Family in the Caribbean: Themes and perspectives.* Kingston, Jamaica: Ian Randle.

Baumrind, D. (1973). The development of instrumental competence through socializtion. In A.

D. Pick (Ed.), *Minnesota Symposia on Child Psychology* (Vol. 7, pp. 3–46). Minneapolis: University of Minnesota Press.

Benedict, R. (1954). *The Chrysanthemum and the Sword.* Rutland, VT: Tuttle.

Bierman, K. L., Smoot, D. L., & Aumiller, K. (1993). Characteristics of aggressive-rejected, aggressive-nonrejected, and rejected-nonaggressive boys. *Child Development, 64,* 139–151.

Borovoy, A. (2008). Japan's hidden youths: Mainstreaming the emotionally distressed in Japan. *Culture, Medicine, and Psychiatry, 32,* 552–576.

Bowlby, J. (1944). Forty-four juvenile thieves: Their characters and home life. *International Journal of Psycho-analysis, 25,* 9–52.

Brown, J., & Johnson, S. (2008). Childrearing and child participation in Jamaican families. *International Journal of Early Years Education, 16,* 31–20.

Bureau of Justice Statistics (2009). Homicide rates in the U.S. by gender, age, and ethnicity. Retrieved September 11, 2009, from *www.bjs.gov.*

Buss, D., & Shackelford, T. (1997). Human aggression in evolutionary psychological perspective. *Clinical Psychology Review, 17,* 605–619.

Centers for Disease Control and Prevention. (2009). Youth violence rates in the U.S. Retrieved September 11, 2009, from *www.cdc.gov.*

Chao, R. (1994). Beyond parental control and authoritarian parenting style: Understanding Chinese parenting through the cultural notion of training. *Child Development, 65,* 1111–1119.

Chen, X., Dong, Q., & Zhou, H. (1997). Authoritative and authoritarian parenting practices and social and school performance in Chinese children. *International Journal of Behavioral Development, 21,* 855–873.

Chen, X., French, D., & Schneider, B. (Eds.). (2006). *Peer relationships in cultural context.* New York: Cambridge University Press.

Conroy, M., Hess, R. D., Azuma, H., & Kashiwagi, K. (1980). Maternal strategies for regulating children's behavior: Japanese and American families. *Journal of Cross-Cultural Psychology, 22,* 153–172.

de Waal, F. B. M. (2000). Primates: A natural heritage of conflict resolution. *Science, 289,* 586–590.

Deater-Deckard, K., Dodge, K., Bates, J. E., & Pettit, G. S. (1996). Physical discipline among African-American and European American mothers: Links to children's externalizing behaviors. *Developmental Psychology, 32,* 1065–1072.

Dodge, K. A., Coie, J., & Lynam, D. R. (2006). Aggression and antisocial behavior in youth. In W. Damon (Ed.), *Handbook of child psychology: Vol. 3. Social, emotional, and personality development* (6th ed., pp. 719–788). New York: Wiley.

Douglas, E. (2006). Familial violence socialization in childhood and later life approval of corporal punishment: A cross-cultural perspective. *American Journal of Orthopsychiatry, 76,* 23–30.

Dussich, J. (2001). *Different responses to violence in Japan and America.* New York: Criminal Justice Press.

Farrington, D. P. (1989). Early predictors of adolescent aggression and adult violence. *Violence and Victims, 4,* 79–100.

Fujimoto, T., & Park, W.-K. (1994). Is Japan exceptional? Reconsidering Japanese crime rates. *Social Justice, 21,* 110–135.

Fontes, L. (2002). Child discipline and physical abuse in immigrant Latino families: Reducing violence and misunderstanding. *Journal of Counseling and Development, 80,* 31–40.

Gayle, H., & Levy, H. (2007) *'Forced ripe: How youth of three selected working-class communities assess their identity, support, and authority systems, including their relationship with the Jamaican police* (unpublished report). University of the West Indies, Mona, Jamaica.

Gershoff, E. T. (2002). Corporal punishment by parents and associated child behaviors experiences: A meta-analytic theoretical review. *Psychological Bulletin, 128,* 539–579.

Gonzales, N. A., Knight, G. P., Morgan-Lopez, A., Saenz, D., & Sirolli, A. (2002). Acculturation and the mental health of Latino youths: An integration and critique of the literature. In J. M. Contreras, K. A. Kerns, & A. M. Neal-Barnett (Eds.), *Latino children and families in the United States.* Westport, CT: Greenwood.

Gray, O. (2004). *Demeaned but empowered: The social power of the urban poor in Jamaica.* Kingston, Jamaica: University of the West Indies Press.

Guerra, N. G., & Huesmann, L. R. (2004). A cognitive–ecological model of aggression. *Revue Internationale de Psychologie Sociale, 17,* 177–203.

Halgunseth, L. C., Ispa, J. M., & Rudy, D. (2006). Parental control in Latino families: An integrated review. *Child Development, 77,* 1282–1297.

Harkness, S., & Super, C. (1996). *Parents' cultural belief systems Their origins, expressions, and consequences.* New York: Guilford Press.

Harriott, A. D. (2008). *Bending the trend line: The challenge of controlling violence in Jamaica and the high violence societies of the Caibbean.* Professorial Inaugural Lecture, University of the West Indies, Mona, Jamaica.

Hawley, P. H. (1999). The ontogenesis of social dominance: A strategy-based evolutionary perspective. *Developmental Review, 19,* 97–132.

Hawley, P. H., Little, T. D., & Rodkin, P. C. (Eds.), *Aggression and adaptation: The bright side to bad behavior.* Mahway, NJ: Erlbaum.

Hill, H. M., Soriano, F. I., Chen, S. A., & La Framboise, T. (1994). Sociocultural factors in the etiology and prevention of violence among ethnic minority youth. In L. D. Eron, J. Gentry, & P. Schlegel (Eds.), *Reason to hope: A psychosocial perspective on violence and youth* (pp. 59–97). Washington, DC: American Psychological Association.

Hoffman, M. L. (1983). Affective and cognitive processes in moral internalization. In E. T. Higgins, D. N. Ruble, & W. W. Hartup (Eds.), *Social cognition and social development* (pp. 236–274). New York: Cambridge University Press.

Hofstede, G. (1980). *Culture's consequences: International differences in work-related values.* Newbury Park, CA: Sage.

Huesmann, L. R., & Guerra, N. G. (1997). Normative beliefs and the development of aggressive behavior. *Journal of Personality and Social Psychology, 72,* 1–12.

Jamaica Constabulary Force. (2009). *Island-wide violence trends.* Ministry of National Security, Kingston, Jamaica.

Jamaica Gleaner (2009, September 30), Usian Bolt controversy over Gaza allegiance.

Kawasaki, K. (1994). *Information and contemporary Japanese culture.* Tokyo: Tokyo University.

Kazui, M. (1997). The influence of cultural expectations on mother–child relationships in Japan. *Journal of Applied Developmental Psychology, 18,* 485–496.

Kozu, J. (1999). Domestic violence in Japan. *American Psychologist, 54,* 50–54.

La Raza (2009). Poverty among Latino immigrant populations. Retrieved September 20, 2009, from *www.Laraza.org.*

Luntz, B. K., & Widom, C. S. (1994). Antisocial personality disorder in abused and neglected children grown up. *American Journal of Psychiatry, 151*, 670–674.

Marin, G., & Marin, B. V. (1991). *Research with Hispanic populations.* Newbury Park, CA: Sage.

Markus, H., & Kitayama, S. (1991). Culture and the self: Implications for cognition, emotion, and motivation. *Psychological Review, 98*, 224–253.

Martinez, R. (2002). *Latino homicides: Immigration, violence, and communities.* New York: Routledge.

Masataka, N. (2002). Low anger-aggression and anxiety-withdrawal characteristic to preschoolers in Japanese society with "hikikomori" is becoming a major social problem. *Early Education and Development, 13*, 187–199.

Meeks Gardner, J. M., Powell, C. A., Grantham-McGregor, S. M. (2007). Determinants of aggressive and prosocial behaviour among Jamaican schoolboys. *West Indian Medical Journal, 56*, 34–41.

Metropolitan Area Child Study Research Group. (2002). A cognitive–ecological approach to preventing aggression in urban settings: Initial outcomes for high-risk children. *Journal of Consulting and Clinical Psychology, 70*, 179–194.

Moore, J. W. (1991). *Going down to the barrio.* Philadelphia: Temple University Press.

Moser, C., & Holland, J. (1997). *Urban poverty and violence in Jamaica*, Washington DC: World Bank.

Nawa (2006). Postwar fourth wave of juvenile delinquency and task of juvenile police. In Police Policy Research Center, National Police Academy of Japan (Ed.), *Current juvenile police policy in Japan* (pp. 1–19). Tokyo, Japan: Research Foundation for Safe Society.

Niehoff, D. (1999). *The biology of violence.* New York: Free Press.

Nisbett, R. E., & Cohen, D. (1996). *The psychology of violence in the south.* Boulder, CO: Westview Press.

Olson, S. L., Kashiwagi, K., & Crystal, D. (2001). Concepts of adaptive and maladaptive child behavior: A comparison of U.S. and Japanese mothers of preschool-age children. *Journal of Cross-Cultural Psychology, 32*, 43–57.

Oyserman, D., Coon, H., & Kemmelmeier, M. (2002). Rethinking individualism and collectivism: Evaluation of theoretical assumptions and meta-analyses. *Psychological Bulletin, 128*, 3–73.

Patterson, G. R. (2002). The early development of coercive family processes. In J. B. Reid, G. R. Patterson, & J. Snyder (Eds.), *Antisocial behavior in children and adolescents* (pp. 25–44). Washington, DC: American Psychological Association.

Pettit, G. S., Laird, R. D., Dodge, K. A., Bates, J. E., & Criss, M. M. (2001). Antecedents and behavior-problem outcomes of parental monitoring and psychological control in early adolescence. *Child Development, 72*, 583–598.

Prinstein, M. J., & Cillessen, A. H. N. (2003). Forms and functions of adolescent peer aggression associated with high levels of peer status. *Merrill-Palmer Quarterly, 49*, 310–342.

Rohner, R. P., Kean, K. J., & Cournoyer, D. E., (1991). Effects of physical punishment, perceived caretaker warmth, and cultural beliefs on the psychological adjustment of children in St. Kitts, West Indies. *Journal of Marriage and the Family, 53,* 681–693.

Rothbaum, F., Kakinuma, M., Nagaoka, R., & Azuma, H. (2007). Attachment and AMAE: Parent–child closeness in the United States and Japan. *Journal of Cross-Cultural Psychology, 38,* 465–486.

Sampson, R. J. (1993). The community context of violent crime. In W. J. Wilson (Ed.), *Sociology and the public agency* (pp. 259–286). Newbury Park: Sage.

Sapolsky, R. M. (2004). Social status and health in human and other animals. *Annual Review of Anthropology, 33,* 393–418.

Smith, C. Y., & Krohn, M. D. (1995). Delinquency and family life among male adolescents: The role of ethnicity. *Journal of Youth and Adolescence, 24,* 69–93.

Smith, D. E., & Mosby, G. (2003). Jamaican child-rearing practices: The role of corporal punishment. *Adolescence, 38,* 369–381.

Smokowski, P. R., David-Ferdon, C., & Stroupe, N. (2009). Acculturation and violence in minority adolescents: A review of the empirical literature. *The Journal of Primary Prevention, 30,* 215–263.

Staub, E. (1996). Cultural–societal roots of violence. *American Psychologist, 51,* 117–132.

Steely, A. G., & Rohner, R. P. (2006). Relations among corporal punishment, perceived parental acceptance, and psychological adjustment in Jamaican youths. *Cross-Cultural Research, 40,* 268–286.

Stevens, E. (1973). Machismo and marianismo. *Society, 10,* 57–63.

Straus, M. (2001). *Beating the devil out of them: Corporal punishment in American families and its effects on children.* New Brunswick, NJ: Transaction Publishers.

Sugihara, Y., & Warner, J. A. (2002). Dominance and domestic abuse among Mexican Americans: Gender differences in the etiology of violence in intimate relationships. *Journal of Family Violence, 17,* 315–345.

Tremblay, R. E., Mâsse, L. C., Vitaro, F., & Dobkin, P. L. (1995). The impact of friend's deviant behavior on early onset of delinquency: Longitudinal data from 6 to 13 years of age. *Development and Psychopathology, 7,* 649–667.

Triandis, H. C. (1995). *Individualism and collectivism.* San Francisco: Westview Press.

United Nations Convention on the Rights of the Child. (2005, March). *Global initiative to end all corporal punishment of children: Ending legalized violence against children—Caribbean special report.* New York: United Nations.

United Nations Office on Drugs and Crime. International Homicide Statistics. (2009). Retrieved October 24, 2009, from *www.unodc.org/documents/data-and-analysis/IHS-rates-05012009.pdf*

U.S. Census Bureau (2002). Census 2000 Summary File 3—United States. Retrieved September 10, 2009, from *www.us.gov.*

Vaughn, B. E., & Santos, A. J. (2007). An evolutionary/ecological account of aggressive behavior and trait aggression in human children and adolescents. In P. H. Hawley, T. D. Little, & P. C. Rodkin (Eds.), *Aggression and adaptation: The bright side to bad behavior* (pp. 31–63). Mahway, NJ: Erlbaum.

White, M. (1993). *The material child: Coming of age in Japan and America.* New York: Free Press.

Whiting, B. B., & Edwards, C. P. (1988). *Children of different worlds: The formation of social behavior.* Cambridge, MA: Harvard University Press.

Wolfgang, M. E., & Ferracuti, F. (1967). *The subculture of violence: Towards an integrated theory in criminology.* London: Tavistock.

World Bank. (2009). Country GDP rankings. Retrieved September 21, 2009, from *www.Worldbank.org.*

Yamamiya, Y. (2003). Juvenile delinquency in Japan. *Journal of Prevention and Intervention in the Community, 25,* 27–46.

CHAPTER 13

Psychosocial Functioning
in the Context of Social, Economic,
and Political Change

RAINER K. SILBEREISEN *and* MARTIN J. TOMASIK

This chapter deals with reactions to a particular type of structural change on the macro level of a society, namely, a radical political reform to democracy and the market economy that, during the transformation process, was overlaid with the consequences of negative changes attributable to the globalization of economic activities. Obvious candidates for this particular case of social change are the "new democracies" that developed after the collapse of the socialist block in central and eastern Europe (CEE), from Germany to Poland, Slovakia, the Czech Republic, to the Baltic States, the Ukraine, Belorussia, and Russia. Other countries experienced political change on a much smaller scale, as for example China, but the move toward a market economy was dramatic. The political and economic transformation in all these countries will lead to a new social reality during the lifetime of this generation, but the ultimate result of these processes—which will affect some one-fourth of the world's population (Matutinovic, 1998)—remains to be seen.

A starting point for the type of social change addressed in this chapter is the fall of the Berlin Wall in 1989. In the aftermath of this historical event, the totalitarian regimes of the CEE countries were replaced by systems more open to the rest of the world, including the ideal of parliamentary representation, independent justice, and a clear distinction between the spheres of the state and private life. However, the extent of these changes and their closeness to the Western model of democracy varied by country. With regard to the economy, the system of state-controlled and centrally managed firms was replaced by various forms of private enterprise. This development generally followed the guidelines of a market economy, but the changes varied in the degree to which the reforms specifically followed the Western model. At any rate, these structural changes were quite dramatic in shaking up responsibilities and creating opportunities for individuals to achieve prosperity and well-being.

Besides changes in the political organization of a society, we also have to think about the challenges that emerged as a result of globalization. This catchword describes the process of creating worldwide networks of interdependent actors, mediated through the flow of people, ideas, capital, goods, and other elements. It disregards national borders and promotes the integration of economies, cultures, technologies, and governance mechanisms. According to the 2009 so-called KOF Index of Globalization, which encapsulates all these elements (Dreher, 2006), there were remarkable differences among the transformation countries we have mentioned. Many of the postsocialist countries were counted among the top one-third worldwide in overall globalization impacts (e.g., Poland, Hungary, the Czech Republic, Slovakia, the Baltic States, and even the Ukraine), whereas Russia and China were in the second tier. Looking at social globalization alone (defined in terms of the spread of ideas, information, images, and people), however, China belonged in the bottom one-third, reflecting the limitations of its relatively unchanged political system. Given the emergence in 2008–2009 of a nearly worldwide Great Recession, however, some former stars of globalization such as the Baltic States became instant victims. Nevertheless, all countries mentioned have been under the powerful influence of globalization, for better or for worse.

Neither social change in the broader sense nor in the more limited context of our particular topic has been a major concern of recent psychological research. Nevertheless, recent studies and books under the rubric of "social change" refer to the political and economic transformations we have just cited and analyze in some detail the consequences for psychological adaptation and development (e.g., Silbereisen & Chen, 2010; Silbereisen & Pinquart, 2008). The evidence to date is reported in this chapter, which is divided into four sections. First we outline a framework for the study of the kind of social changes addressed and give examples of the research strategies employed. In the second section, we deal with research that focuses on context, from values that represent the macro context to parent–child relations that illustrate the micro context of the family. The third section examines the results of recent research focused on various aspects of individual adaptation and functioning. The conclusion in the fourth section identifies gaps in our knowledge and addresses future research needs.

A Framework for the Study of Social Change

Unlike sociologists, who deal with societal transformation on the macro level (Nee & Matthews, 1996), we as psychologists are interested in the impact of such changes on individual adaptation and, in this chapter, particularly on socioemotional adaptation and development among young people. Indeed, research on social change has a special appeal for developmental psychology (Pillemer & White, 2005) because it starts with the presumption that contexts and changes therein matter—exactly as Bronfenbrenner's ecological model of development predicted (Bronfenbrenner, 1985)—and then connects variations on the contextual level with variations in individual functioning. Without too much exaggeration, one could claim that research on the role of political and economic transformation provides real-life examples of the power of contexts in shaping human development.

A point of departure for our own framework is Elder's (1974) model and landmark study on the role of social change for individual adaptation and development. Its core element is the mismatch between new demands rooted in social change and established ways of behavior. In order to deal constructively with this mismatch and bring their lives back into balance, individuals are compelled to look for new ways of adapting. This process of regaining control (including its psychological costs and benefits) determines the ultimate psychosocial outcome. This model is reminiscent of coping approaches in psychology (e.g., Lazarus & Folkman, 1984), but on closer scrutiny an important difference becomes clear. The strains are not the independent variable—as in psychological research on stress—but, rather, represent an intervening process between structural changes on the macro level (reflected in difficulties for family functioning) and individual adaptation. Research establishing this link is rare in both disciplines (Aneshensel, 1992). In Elder's (1974) case, the macro part was reflected in financial hardships stemming from economic crises, such as the Great Depression, and major outcomes referred to as life-course achievements.

Our Model of Social Change and Individual Development

Our own approach is depicted in Figure 13.1. Next, we briefly discuss the various conditions and processes shown.

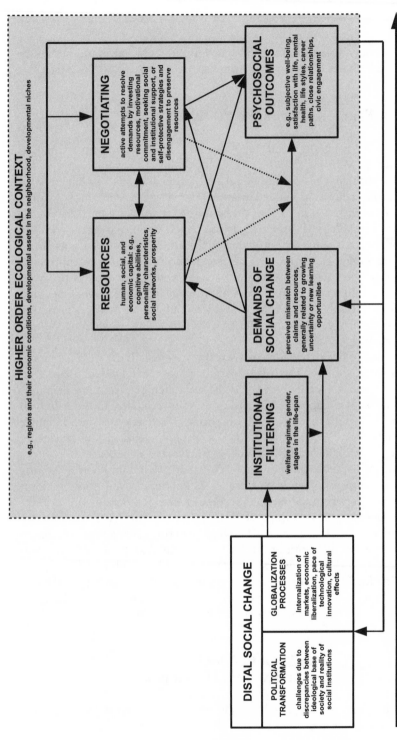

HIGHER ORDER ECOLOGICAL CONTEXT
e.g., regions and their economic conditions, developmental assets in the neighborhood, developmental niches

NEGOTIATING

active attempts to resolve demands by investing resources, motivational commitment, seeking social and institutional support, or self-protective strategies and disengagement to preserve resources

RESOURCES

human, social, and economic capital: e.g., cognitive abilities, personality characteristics, social networks, prosperity

PSYCHOSOCIAL OUTCOMES

e.g., subjective well-being, satisfaction with life, mental health, life styles, career paths, close relationships, civic engagement

DEMANDS OF SOCIAL CHANGE

perceived mismatch between claims and resources, generally related to growing uncertainty or new learning opportunities

INSTITUTIONAL FILTERING

Welfare regimes, gender, stages in the life-span

DISTAL SOCIAL CHANGE

POLITCIAL TRANSFORMATION

challenges due to discrepancies between ideological base of society and reality of social institutions

GLOBALIZATION PROCESSES

Internalization of markets, economic liberalization, pace of technological innovation, cultural effects

INDIVIDUAL LIFE COURSE

FIGURE 13.1. Individual life course.

Challenges

The challenges depicted at the left margin of Figure 13.1 are related to changes of social structures as a consequence of the political transition that began during the early 1990s and that was followed by ongoing economic and social transformations. We distinguish among three interrelated systems, namely, the system of structural challenges on the macro level, the system of contexts varying in level from macro to micro, and the system of individual processes that translate the challenges into outcomes that relate to adaptation and psychosocial development. More specifically, changes on the political and economic levels produce a new equilibrium between uncertainties and opportunities concerning major domains of life. Taking the domain of work after German unification as an example, the formerly state-run firms in East Germany could not effectively compete in worldwide markets without the subsidies supplied in the past, and the required adjustments resulted in surging unemployment or precarious work contracts, particularly in traditional heavy industries.

Societies differ in their understanding of the degree to which groups of individuals need protection from the macro challenges with which they are confronted, and they have developed institutions and regulations aimed at achieving that end. Esping-Andersen (1990) identified certain welfare regimes of this type, which represent "institutional filters" aimed at confronting and coming to terms with the divergent ideologies and practices of the employment, educational, and welfare systems. In societies where the state typically intervenes during times of economic difficulty and where the compatibility of work demands and a happy family life is an important goal of social policies, such as in the Scandinavian model, people are relatively better protected from the exigencies of globalization (Hofäcker, Buchholz, & Blossfeld, 2010).

Contexts

Coming to the system of contexts, the family stands out as the main recipient of the societal challenges, whether filtered by other institutions or not. The role of the family can be characterized by various functions—it secures the economic basis of the household, allocates social positions, provides an arena for recreation, and—last but not least—is an important agent of socialization. All these functions can be affected by social and economic transformations. For instance, the power relations within the family can be changed because the children may adapt more easily to the new circumstances, whereas the parents may be tied to adult commitments (e.g., career paths) that could be irreversibly disrupted by social change without being offered viable alternatives (Elder, Shanahan, & Clipp, 1994; Pinquart, Silbereisen, & Juang, 2004a).

Next to the family are other micro contexts, such as those related to work and leisure, and the meso context, consisting of their intersection. For instance, in many transformation countries the distribution of responsibility between the family and the state as it relates to child care and educational decisions was shifted toward a larger role for the family (Ritter, 2006). These contexts are embedded in what Bronfenbrenner (1985) called the more distant "exo" context (which affects development, although the individual typically is not present). For a child or adolescent, it may be the parent's workplace or the many layers of institutions and physical settings that may powerfully affect an individual, whether or not he or she is a member. Most distant is the macro context of the fabric of a society, including beliefs and worldviews. Prior to transformation in the CEE countries, political control was often based on neighborhood organizations (Schneider, 1994), but these rapidly lost their function under the new democratic rule and as a consequence of economic liberalization (Schmitz, 1995).

Demands

Finally, we turn to the system of individual processes. We call the micro-level manifestations of new societal challenges "demands." They represent the starting point for the individual-level processes that change adaptation and development through repeated cycles of negotiating new demands. In contrast to life events, demands are characterized by persistency and recurrence over prolonged periods of time (Thoits, 1995). Concerning adaptation and development, some instances of demands stemming from social change stand out, such as those resulting from barriers against the achievement of life goals, excessive expectations that overtax capabilities, and inadequate rewards relative to invested effort (Wheaton, 1980). As such demands represent serious risk factors for psychosocial adaptation, they constitute the key subject matter of our analysis.

An example of the challenge–demand linkage that we have in mind is globalization-related constrictions on the market that employers may have to face. In order to stay competitive, they have to pass their own challenges on to the work force (Fenwick & Tausig, 1994). Employees thereafter share a greater risk of layoffs, particularly those who do not enjoy job protection, such as relative novices at the firm. In addition, this particular work sphere demand will spill over to other domains and important life tasks, such as partnership and parenting.

Negotiating Demands

We consider individuals as active producers of their own development and see individual agency as crucial in understanding human development in context (Lerner & Busch-Rossnagel, 1981; Silbereisen, Eyferth, & Rudinger,

1986). In our own research we have relied on a control theoretical approach that differentiates between ways of reacting that actively engage with the issue at hand and attempting to change the balance between demands and behaviors that are no longer adaptive and those that represent a disengagement mode (typically employed when the demands are less central and appear uncontrollable) (Heckhausen, 1999). Referring to this theoretical model allowed us to predict when and why either engagement with or disengagement from the demands of social change is the more adaptive way to deal with such demands. For instance, one criterion for adaptive development was basis congruence between (1) the mode of negotiating demands and (2) the opportunities provided by the social ecology. We hypothesized and found that the social change associated with increasing opportunities required the active negotiation of demands, whereas disengagement was more beneficial when opportunities were decreasing (Tomasik, Silbereisen, & Heckhausen, 2010).

Resources

How people deal with the demands also is a function of available resources, such as social support or personal capabilities. Resources may have a main effect but may also buffer the effect of demands (see Cohen & Wills, 1985). We deem indicators of agency to be a particularly important resource in times of rapid social change. Young people's educational attainment undertaken in the former Soviet Union during the years before the collapse did not necessarily assure oneself—as one might reasonably have expected—more income (Tuma, Titma, & Murakas, 2002), higher social mobility and status (Titma & Tuma, 2005), or a better position in the workforce (Titma & Trapido, 2002) under the new postcommunist system. Rather, higher self-efficacy prior to the political change and, thereby, greater capabilities in dealing flexibly with the new circumstances were more important during the times of transition. Interestingly enough, once the new order had established itself after several years, institutions again became stronger and the markets more regulated, and the traditional measures of social stratification, such as higher educational attainment, regained their relevance (Titma, Tuma, & Roots, 2007). With data gathered both before and during the first years after German unification, Pinquart and colleagues were able to demonstrate the beneficial role of self-efficacy beliefs in determining German adolescents' life satisfaction, future optimism, and educational success (Pinquart et al., 2004a), their psychological distress (Pinquart, Silbereisen, & Juang, 2004b), as well as their general career aspirations and vocational orientation (Pinquart, Juang, & Silbereisen, 2004). High self-efficacy enables one to experience a successful reorientation toward new opportunities through greater expectations of success and a higher motivation to be active in mastering new challenges. Individuals with low self-efficacy, on the other hand, are more prone to worries or anxiety, to self-doubts, and to seeing the new challenges as a threat, which can impede their ability to negotiate social change successfully (Bandura, 1995; Jerusalem & Mittag, 1995).

Outcomes

The possible psychosocial outcomes of social change are manifold, and almost no domain of functioning can be ruled out. Nevertheless, existing research shows a limited number of foci. Given the closeness to sociological thinking, topics related to socialization into important roles concerning work and family—in other words, the resolution of important developmental tasks—play a dominant role. Here we can also include changes in the understanding of what a particular life period, such as one's youth, means for people. Other studies refer to well-being and other forms of positive adjustment, or to delinquency and other forms of maladjustment—both to be seen as generalized indicators of individual adaptation. Finally, there is research referring to particular psychological functions of relevance either to the coping process or to psychosocial outcomes, such as cognitive, motivational, and social capabilities.

Life Cycle

People can be affected by social change at a particular age or stage in the life cycle. For example, the possibilities of dealing with the new conditions in such a way that one at least maintains one's relative position in the social strata may differ remarkably. A case in point is a research study on educational credentials by Zhou and Moen (2001) that compared three cohorts of Chinese workers in urban areas. The workers either entered the labor market during the formative years of the socialist system, later at the time of the Cultural Revolution, or after the 1980s during the more recent era of economic reform. Whereas a college degree was advantageous for all cohorts in achieving a position with government agencies, which endowed one with many premium benefits, this credential aided only the youngest cohort in gaining access to private firms in emerging markets that offered the highest incomes. The relative entrenchment of the oldest cohort in the former system served as an obstacle to others' access to new opportunities.

Pace of Change

A final comment concerns the pace with which social change is expected to affect human adaptation and development. Here a comparison with research on acculturation after migration is helpful. Behaviors rooted in the central beliefs of a culture will show relatively few effects over the short run, while behaviors that are dictated by the requirements of everyday life will change rapidly (Silbereisen & Wiesner, 2000). The almost immediate decline in birthrates in the European transformation countries is a case in point: delaying parenthood when confronted with large-scale uncertainties in one's life is a traditional cultural pattern, and thus the real question is not whether it happens at all but, rather, how long it lasts (Caldwell, 2004).

The Role of Contexts

In this section we want to show how contexts can be affected by the political and economic transformation underlying adaptation and development. We believe that a full understanding of the role of changed contexts in bringing about or influencing demands actually requires addressing the entire pathway from the emergence of the new challenges to consequent changes in individual behavior. The same demand can be rooted in different challenges, and the same challenge can result in different demands, depending on the pathway of contextual change on various levels. However, as we have to draw from diverse research traditions and topics, the evidence is more illustrative than comprehensive.

Macro Context

In the following discussion, we want to exemplify influences on the level of the macro context for adaptation and development. These influences refer to the basic understanding of how people organize their communities in terms of ethnic relationships and value orientations.

Social Cohesion

Characteristic of many transformation societies was a radical shift in the power differential between segments of the population. Especially during the time of transition, in many countries national and cultural identity became an important issue, thereby threatening social cohesion. Depending on the country and the quality of the transformation processes, social cohesion was endangered by actions ranging from ethnic strife, through forced migration, to armed conflict. In some cases, the increase in ethnic consciousness and nationalist pride (Fuller, 2000) potentially threatened chances for the emergence of a democratic society with equal opportunities for psychosocial development, as seen by the work of Kunovich and Deitelbaum (2004). They showed that the growing distrust toward national and ethnic outgroups in the Croatian conflict with Serbia encouraged a return to traditional values, particularly among those living in regions directly affected by the conflict. Interestingly enough, this return to tradition also meant a renaissance of the ideal that bringing up the next generation was properly the traditional role of women.

Depending on the circumstances, the risks for social cohesion may be very circumscribed, however. Data on intermarriage in Latvia (Monden & Smits, 2005) show that, in spite of migration and a radical change in the power relations between ethnic groups, the prevalence of intermarriage stayed fundamentally the same before and after the transition and into the times of transformation, except for a very short period of high tension. In particular, increased ethnic consciousness did not result in less intermarriage between Latvians and Russians; rather, the rates increased among Russian women, owing to selective outmigration by their group and because of increased opportunities for them to integrate into the new society.

Value Orientations

According to Inglehart (1977, 1997), experiences with economic hardship during the first two decades of life represent a legacy that determines whether one leans toward the materialist or the postmaterialist pole of value orientations. Thus, if scarcity characterized one's early life, materialist orientations, such as striving for security, are dominant. In contrast, the human development hypothesis expects value orientations to change as a function of life achievements, and in this regard life transitions during adulthood offer an avenue to new orientations. Higher education and status attainment in one's work and family are candidates for instilling a more liberal orientation.

In their comparative study of Hong Kong and Guangzhou in China, Ting and Chiu (2000) found evidence for an integrative view because different birth cohorts as well as differences in adult status attainments played a role. As expected, owing to the gap in economic development between the two regions, a higher share of the 21- to 60-year-olds in Guangzhou expressed a materialist orientation (that is, they chose income over respectability, power, qualification, training, serving the public, and contributions to society when asked to rank the social standing of an occupation). The birth cohort effect was also more important in Guangzhou than in Hong Kong in that the younger cohorts from Guangzhou were more materialistic, reflecting the recent rapid social and economic change in this region. In contrast, education played a stronger role in Hong Kong, but none of the adult experiences that was assessed replaced the effect of birth cohorts. Thus, although value orientations may be malleable across the lifespan, early experiences seem to be important in their own right.

Concerning adolescents, Cen and Li (2006) conclude their review of research over the past two decades by asserting that the collectivist values in Chinese adolescents have largely been replaced by the notions of individual benefit, financial success, and self-realization. When asked about their biggest wishes for the next 5 years, 39% of the Beijing college students studied by Yang and Yan (1997, cited in Cen & Li, 2006) gave career success, 21% named achievement in studies, and 18% cited the ability to earn big money. Good health, an ideal companion, and family harmony were hardly mentioned by any student! The apparent shift from collectivist to individualist values can partly be explained by the openness of Chinese young people to foreign cultures and languages. For instance, a study by Wu (2002, cited in Cen & Li, 2006), conducted against the backdrop of China's imminent entry into the World Trade Organization, found that some 80% of adolescents and young adults had learned a foreign language, read foreign books, magazines, or newspapers at least occasionally, and disagreed with the idea that exchanges with foreign cultures must be rejected in order to protect the relics of traditional Chinese culture.

Coming back to the European situation, Reitzle and Silbereisen (2000a) compared same-age samples in East and West Germany 5 years apart during the postunification period of transformation and found a stronger tendency toward the Western value profile among youths in the East as compared to older age groups. More specifically, for the 1991 cohort the authors found that participants in the East endorsed collectivist values, such as family safety, politeness, or respect for tradition, more strongly, whereas those from the West more strongly endorsed individualist values such as freedom and social power. These differences were attenuated in the 1996 cohort, suggesting some convergence. This effect was particularly strong among younger participants who had not yet completed their transition to adulthood by the time of German unification and who were still in the process of identity formation when major societal changes took place.

Exo Context

Next we refer to the tremendous effects of the political and economic transformation on the exo contexts that potentially affect people's lives and development. Examples are the measures to restore the quality of life in polluted areas, the deindustrialization of entire regions, the change in population density in rural areas, the labor migration within countries, the increase in commercialization for consumption and leisure, and many more such changes in the physical and social environment. It seems obvious that such changes should result in changes in people's behaviors, and thus the exo contexts can be seen as vehicles of social change.

In our own research (Pinquart, Silbereisen, & Körner, 2009), we found that the economic prosperity of the political-administrative regions where people live had a particularly strong effect on the relationship between well-being and the extent to which there were new demands relating to globalization pressures on work and family. Overall, this effect was negative, as one might have expected. Those who lived in economically challenged regions, however, seemingly suffered less in their well-being, even when confronted with the same amount of negative experiences concerning employment uncertainty and instability in the family. According to our interpretation, this finding reflected people's comparing themselves to others who fared even worse. As a matter of fact, in the regions affected worst by unemployment and with the highest need for welfare payments, the relationship between well-being and the level of demands was virtually nil, whereas in better-off regions it was clearly negative. Interestingly, the relationship between engagement with demands and well-being was in the opposite direction. Those living in prosperous regions showed a more positive association with well-being than those in economically challenged ones, probably owing to the presence of more positive role models of how to be active in overcoming the mismatch between new claims and accustomed ways of behavior vis-à-vis the transformation challenges.

Our comparison of regions in terms of their economic prosperity was guided by its relevance to our conception of transformation demands. Both the contextual and the individual measures reflected the same phenomena. In general, research attempting to demonstrate the role of contexts in individual adaptation has often had difficulty finding strong empirical evidence because of certain ambiguity about the appropriate measurement level of the context (see Leventhal & Brooks-Gunn, 2000; Picket & Pearl, 2001).

Although not directly related to political change in our understanding, an exceptional study by Axinn and Yabiku (2001) on Nepal is of considerable interest because it introduced features relevant for the macro–micro linkage in more general terms. The researchers investigated changes in neighborhoods that were the result of macro changes in the economy and the spread of new ideas in a remote area of Nepal. As, owing to economic development, the physical distance to employment opportunities, schools, and health services became dramatically reduced, a shift in daily activities took place from concentrating on the family to heightened attendance or participation at places and in institutions outside the home. The consequences for family functions, such as socialization and recreation, were manifold, including opening up to ideational influences and a decline in family integration.

Obviously, family integration is of relevance beyond the specific example. According to Yabiku, Axinn, and Thornton (1999), it entails various organizational aspects of the family, such as activities within the home, interactions with the extended family, and supportive exchanges within the family. These aspects may be changed by some experiences rooted in societal transformation. While the higher unemployment risk for women after the transition may have increased opportunities for integration activities, other experiences, such as intensified work stress, may have had the opposite result. At any rate, research showed a strong relationship between family integration and the grown-ups' self-esteem many years later. This relationship is probably attributable to earlier perceived increase in opportunities to believe that one is needed, that others are interested in oneself, and that one belongs to a strong network. In addition, better family integration may have an indirect effect by promoting more emotional and ideational aspects of parenting.

Meso Context

The meso context is understood as representing the intersection of other micro contexts. We use the example of the changes in social networks following the decline of the communist-era command economy. That development brought an end to the systemic shortages in consumer goods and in pressures for conformity. People in the former East Germany had a relatively small social network of others they knew well and could trust, and they often befriended people who could provide goods in short supply from the informal economy. As Völker and Flap (1995) reported, the transition of the political system after 1989 revealed the malleability of these social networks. In terms of size, during the earliest years after unification social networks tended to become somewhat smaller, density decreased (as one no longer needed to be cautious when discussing sensitive ideological matters), as did heterogeneity in terms of occupations and social strata, owing to a reduction in dependency on the informal economy. Attributing all this to the system change alone, however, would be misleading. According to Nauck and Schwenk (2001), who also had comparative data from West Germany, a similar reduction in network size occurred in the West. Kinship ties became more important at the expense of members outside the family. However, this development was also probably not a particular reaction to unification but rather more a reflection of attempts to cope with the deregulation of the welfare system, aimed at reducing the rising costs attributable to demographic changes. The close family system is a rather steady and tested barrier against such strains from social change in general.

Network analyses on urban samples in China also demonstrated the linkage between structural changes in the economy and personal networks on the meso level. As reported by Ruan and collaborators (Ruan, Freeman, Dai, Pan, & Zhang, 1997), over a period of just 7 years the old pattern of a network mainly composed of co-workers and kin changed quite dramatically to include a much higher share of friends and others outside of work and family. This trend reflected the declining need to rely on the benefits and supports provided by state-run industry as well as increased risks for unemployment in *all* sectors of the economy. However, kinship is no substitute for "weak" ties from outside that help an individual to take advantage of the new economic and social opportunities. Compared to the German data, during the earliest transformation years, reliance on the family appeared to be weaker and the new relationships found outside of work and the family stronger. Interestingly enough, in spite of the political differences between the situation in Germany and China, after the early 1990s the overall network size declined somewhat in both countries—in Germany in favor of family ties and in China in favor of new instrumental relationships outside the family—with both reflecting the changed contingencies of life.

Micro Context

The family represents one of the most central developmental contexts for children and adolescents (Trommsdorf, 2006). Studies on economic hardship during the Great Depression of the 1920s–1930s (Elder, 1974) and the farm crisis of the 1980s (Conger & Elder, 1994) provide evidence for the mediating role of parents' mood and behaviors between economic hardship and the socioemotional development of children. Liker and Elder (1983), for instance, demonstrated that pressures from economic hardship and marital conflict were related to each other via the emotional instability of the father. Other reports provide evidence that emotional distress, marital conflict, and disrupted parenting are the key family variables with which to understand the negative psychosocial outcomes of social change on offspring (e.g., Conger et al., 1992; Conger, Jewbury-Conger, Matthews, & Elder, 1999).

Noack, Hofer, Kracke, and Klein-Allermann (1995) found similar results in the case of German unification. There, changes of perceived uncertainty in society negatively affected the quality of family relations, which in turn had negative effects on the psychosocial adaptation of the family members. The outcomes investigated included adolescents' externalizing tendencies, somatic health, consumption of alcohol and nicotine, and sociopolitical intolerance. However, these effects may be moderated by causal attribution. Forkel and Silbereisen (2001), for instance, provided some evidence that appraising the negative effects of social change as beyond one's control, or as systemic failure in the course of German unification, may attenuate the effect of economic hardship on parental mood.

When it directly affects their daily lives, people seem to react rather quickly to changed opportunities resulting from the political and economic transformation. We know from research on the "value of children" that with economic development a shift takes place—the importance of children's economic role for their parents' life declines, and the psychological role for joy and fulfillment increases. Kăgitcibaşi (2005; Kăgitcibaşi & Ataca, 2005) interpreted the same trends, observed over 30 years in Turkey, as suggesting the emergence of a mindset characterized by psychological interdependence where, in spite of economic improvements, psychological relatedness prevails over autonomy as the goal of parenting. In Kăgitcibaşi's view, this predisposition is characteristic of societies with a collectivist tradition that undergo rapid social change. The economic development permits a growing sense of independence between generations within families, but the psychological interdependence remains unchanged because of its strong roots in the culture and its ultimate compatibility with the new lifestyles of a more affluent society.

In the past, differences in the balance between the importance ascribed to autonomy and relatedness were often seen as a more or less static cultural difference. With Kăgitcibaşi and others, it became clear that this balance may change rather swiftly in response to various forms of economic and political change. The transition from a command economy to a market economy in China is a case in point. Recent research shows that young Chinese mothers place almost equal importance on autonomy and relatedness, and they see both as equally related to the promotion of achievements (Tamis-LeMonda et al., 2008). This pattern is different from the traditional *guanxi*, that is, the Chinese belief that personal needs can be better satisfied by having established social connections, which itself seems partly to be an adaptation to the past shortage economy. This understanding of relationships is also in decline in business and personal transactions across urban China (Guthrie, 2006).

As Chen and Chen (2010) report, parental support of children's autonomy can quickly gain in importance if the pace of social change requires rapid adjustment to the new social reality. However, a comparison of Chinese parents in 1998 and 2002 revealed a significantly higher endorsement of autonomy support in mothers but not in fathers and a significantly lower endorsement of power-assertive parenting strategies in both mothers and fathers. There are similar findings that relate to a decline in the traditional appreciation accorded to shy and inhibited behaviors in Chinese children— since under the new economic opportunities such behaviors impede self-expression and active exploration (Chang, 2003; Chang et al., 2005; Hart et al., 2000). Chinese parents may therefore have suddenly realized that children need to attain the competencies associated with autonomy and independence to function adequately under the new economic rule in China, and they may therefore have adapted their parenting goals and practices accordingly (Liu et al., 2005). Similar conclusions may be drawn from a study of South Korean mothers by Cheah and Park (2006).

Effects on Individual Adjustment

In this section we address the case of the child or adolescent in a changing society from complementary perspectives. We begin with studies on how the societal transitions were perceived by those affected. This emphasis represents the demands part of our model depicted in Figure 13.1 and is the important starting point for adaptive behavior at the individual level (Pinquart & Silbereisen, 2004; Tomasik & Silbereisen, 2009).

Perceptions of Social and Economic Change

Several studies were performed to investigate the perception of social change in different countries, and all conclude that individuals are usually ambivalent about social and political change, especially if it happens very quickly. In early1990, a few months before German unification, more than two-thirds of the youths in West and East Germany surveyed stated that they would prefer a *gradual* growing together of the two former parts of the country (Behnken et al., 1991). In another study following reunification, a similar proportion of respondents indicated that they believed German unification had been accomplished too rapidly (Deutsches Jugendinstitut, 1992). Macek and colleagues (1998) asked Bulgarian, Czech, and Hungarian adolescents about their perceptions regarding the economy and the local community. The results showed that many youths were not positive about the changes occurring in their countries and disliked the increasing economic disparities. Further, a study conducted in Shanghai in 1994 (as cited by Cen & Li, 2006) found that about 40% of the Chinese adolescents interviewed endorsed the statement that "today there are some things making it so that people don't know what is right or wrong and don't know how to deal with it [*sic*]" (p. 161).

Subjective uncertainty thus seems to be a common response to societies in transition. However, individuals differ in their perceptions of social change as a function of the political context and the sociodemographic niche in which they live (Tomasik & Silbereisen, 2009). In a study conducted in Germany a few years after the country's unification, Noack, Kracke, Wild, and Hofer (2001) reported that perceived uncertainty was higher in the East as compared to the West, reflecting the more profound social change in the formerly socialist part of the country. Plichtová and Erös (1997) compared a sample of younger and older adults from Slovakia and Hungary and found that the younger adults felt a greater sense of agency than the older age group in planning their future. This finding might indicate that younger adults perceive social change as less threatening, probably because they are less tied to commitments concerning work and family that certainly reduce the freedom to engage in new opportunities (Elder et al., 1994; Van Snippenburg & Hendriks Vettehen, 1992).

The experience of social change may also differ as a function of gender. Studies showed that girls experienced economic decline, economic disparities, or political conflict more often than boys (Deutsches Jugendinstitut, 1992; Macek et al., 1998). Such gender effects are also known to be operative in more stable societies, but they appear to be particularly elevated in countries undergoing transition (Grob, Little, Wanner, Wearing, & Euronet, 1996). We also have some evidence that people with higher education are more positive about social change as compared to those with lower educational attainment (Malmberg & Trempala, 1997; Plichtová & Erös, 1997). Education seems to have a strong effect on social mobility, income, and status (Titma & Tuma, 2005; Titma et al., 2007); so, those who are better educated probably endure fewer costs and enjoy more benefits from social change over time.

Adjustment of Developmental Timetables

In the study by Noack and colleagues (2001), the perception of uncertainty was the key variable in understanding how social change affects individuals. This notion is also prominent in more recent psychological (Tomasik & Silbereisen, 2009) and sociological research (Hofäcker et al., 2010; Jeffrey & McDowell, 2004). Shifting the timing of major biographical transitions can be seen as an adaptive response to contextual constraints on individuals' developmental aspirations as a result of heightened economic and job-related uncertainties (Bynner, 2001; Furlong & Cartmel, 1997; Reitzle, 2006; Wyn & White, 2000). Social change, though, is not likely to affect all biographical transitions alike. Silbereisen and Wiesner (2000) have demonstrated that German unification affected only transitions that were closely related to social institutions that underwent significant change. So, for instance, the timing of the earliest vocational preferences changed in East German adolescents—but not the timing of their first romantic involvement.

Cohort differences in developmental timetables can be explained by the experience of what we call the demands of social change. Reitzle and Silbereisen (2000b) examined the timing of the transition from school to work and financial self-support, and they demonstrated that a large share of interindividual variance in timing was related to strains rooted in German unification, such as periods of unemployment and attendance at professional retraining courses offered by the state in the East. In other words, the coupling between the change of social structure and the revision of individual developmental goals could be explained by individual experiences in the very proximal developmental contexts of young people, exactly as predicted by Bronfenbrenner (1985).

Social Change and Psychosocial Adjustment

Based on a classification proposed by Evans (1994), Grob and colleagues (1996) argue that the most prominent antecedents of psychosocial adjustment in childhood and adolescence comprise a stable cultural and social context in terms of a person–environment–fit (Bronfenbrenner, 1985), the sound accomplishment of normative and age-specific developmental tasks (Havighurst, 1948), meaningful life goals that require a positive future perspective (Brunstein, 1993; Emmons, 1992), and a sense of personal control in important life domains (Bandura, 1995; Seligmann, 1975). Social change can affect all these factors in a positive or negative way, either by providing new opportunities or new constraints for these antecedents.

Against this conceptual backdrop, Grob and colleagues (1996) compared the subjective well-being of adolescents from contexts experiencing rapid social change (eastern Europe) with adolescents from more stable contexts (western Europe and the United States). They found that adolescents from the Eastern countries reported lower positive attitudes and lower self-esteem as compared to their Western counterparts. This finding may be attributable to the fact that rapid political change, combined with economic turmoil in the East, made it difficult to maintain a positive future perspective and long-term life goals, which in turn negatively influenced subjective well-being.

Various other studies tried to demonstrate the effects of large-scale social and political change on individual psychosocial adjustment, although studies on children, adolescents, or families are rather rare. Taimalu, Lahikainen, Korhonen, and Kraav (2007) focused on children and investigated their self-reported fears as an indicator of well-being. The authors compared 6-year-olds, from Finland and Estonia in 1993 and 2003, and found an increase in self-reported fears in both countries. However, this increase was much stronger for the Estonian sample. The authors conclude that this finding may reflect increased television viewing by these children, who remain unattended more often due to the work stress of the parents.

Although fear is usually a functional emotion, excessive fears can inhibit and disturb growth (Craske, 1997), evoke various psychosomatic disorders (Valkenburg, 2004), and become socially incapacitating (Rutter & Rutter, 1993). The results reported by Taimalu and colleagues (2007) are thus giving cause for concern. In the same vein, epidemiological data on alcohol use and abuse of teenagers in eastern European countries are worrisome. Okulicz-Kozaryn and Borucka (2008), for instance, report data from Poland comparing five cohorts of 15-year-old students. In general, they found a decrease in abstainers and light drinkers and an increase in heavy drinkers. Significantly, a distinct cluster of students who drank alcohol "in order to get drunk" appeared during the early 1990s—parallel to the political changes in the country. The authors suggest that deregulated advertising and a higher availability of alcohol together with a change in adolescents' values were responsible for the changes in their drinking patterns.

Conclusion

Taking all the concepts and results reported as a whole, the scope of research on socioemotional behavior and development that explicitly references political and economic transitions appears to be rather limited. Most studies in the field dealt with adulthood, and these were dominated by research on age-typical achievements and psychological well-being. Despite these limitations, we see a growing body of literature analyzing transitions from one political or economic order to another. Together with sociologists (e.g., Nee & Matthews, 1986), we argue that it is necessary to consider the actions of key economic and social actors as prominent explanations for attendant institutional change and societal transformation. Certainly much more research exists on phenomena, such as unemployment or economic hardship, that coexist with social change. However, studying potential manifestations without addressing the larger framework of social change can be misleading, because it ignores the reciprocal interactions between the different levels of developmental contexts.

At the core is a radical change in people's macro context, followed by cascaded effects on the various more proximal contexts, from exo to micro. Ultimately, it confronts individuals with demands to which they are not accustomed and that require serious efforts for their mastery. The resulting psychosocial outcomes have the potential—although this aspect was almost never studied thus far in a psychological format—to influence changes on the societal level for better or worse. Seen from an interdisciplinary perspective, dealing with demands represents the "transformational mechanism" Hedström and Swedberg (1996) had in mind when they explain how social structures change through the actions of the individuals affected. Thus, beyond its immediate effects on psychological insights about the role of changing ecological contexts in adaptation and development, psychological research on political transitions and transformations also helps to establish better links with the social sciences.

People often misjudge the comprehensiveness and pace of social change. Given our model, it should be clear that the cascading events and processes from macro to micro take time—often more years than one would expect. A comparison with the pace of acculturation among immigrants is telling. For the necessities of everyday life, adaptation is quickly accomplished, whereas it may take more than a generation for *values* to change (Kăgitcibaşi & Ataca, 2005). From this perspective, the rapid pace of changes in parental goals for childrearing reported by Chen and Chen (2010) is impressive. While the pace of social change is often overestimated, the continuity in spite of change is often underestimated. For instance, Melvin Kohn's research comparing stable societies with societies in transition revealed that the relationship between social stratification and personality remained surprisingly stable, as did the mediating role of work-related experiences, such as the complexity of work (e.g., Kohn, 2006). Since this conclusion also applied to urban Chinese samples and because work experiences tend to be translated into values of child socialization, the basic goals of parenting should not have changed dramatically, as far as the appreciation of autonomy is concerned. However, autonomy can come in diverse versions, as Kăgitcibaşi (2005) has shown.

The design of studies addressing social change and its role on the individual level is a challenge in itself. A common approach used to discover change at the structural level is to compare samples of individuals gathered at different periods of the process of social change. Such studies are legitimate, but they often share the conceptual weakness that interindividual differences in exposure to political and economic change are only addressed implicitly, at best. However, according to our framework, actual assessments are crucial, and the dimensions addressed need to be informed by the nature of societal changes. This happens only very rarely. Furthermore, almost all of the research on political transitions and transformations we have discussed thus far is nonexperimental and relies on covariation among variables, sometimes including longitudinal assessments. The advantage is the obvious ecological relevance and interdisciplinary nature of the research. Moreover, in some cases, there was a clear theoretical rationale delineating the pathways between the macro level and individual adaptation and development. Nevertheless, as with all nonexperimental data, concerns remain that the covariation pattern between demands rooted in the transition and transformation, on the one hand, and levels of adaptation, on the other, may be attributable to processes other than those claimed in the conceptual model.

Although it would be difficult or unethical to change the fabric of a society for the purpose of improved causative analyses, nevertheless there is a whole strand of experimental research on the role of economic hardship in children's development—and economic hardship is certainly often involved in the types of social change addressed here. A case in point is randomized control trials on means to improve parenting and child adjustment by providing employment and income to poor families. As Huston (2005) reports, increased income but not employment per se indeed had an impact on various measures of children's adjustment, such as school achievement. Rather than being mediated by improved parenting (McLoyd, 1998), it was the fact that the offspring received qualitatively better child care and opportunities for out-of-school experiences. Overall this change offered more structured activities and the kinds of experiences known to be the most relevant of developmentally instigative leisure activities (Larson, 2000).

Research on social change addressed in this chapter not only has implications for individual adaptation and development, but it but also gives further insights into the processes by which distal economic and social conditions influence the development of children and adolescents (and vice versa). The latter effect is obviously relevant for a better scientific understanding of the pathways linking macro with micro contexts and the resulting individual behavior. Moreover, such knowledge is also helpful in the systematic design of social policies aimed at supporting children, adolescents, and their families in negotiating social change. Research providing insights into the mediating processes between macro and micro levels can identify conditions in the causal chain that can be changed efficiently through interventions.

References

Aneshensel, C. S. (1992). Social stress: Theory and research. *Annual Review of Sociology, 18*, 15–38.

Axinn, W. G., & Yabiku, S. T. (2001). Social change, the social organization of families, and fertility limitation. *American Journal of Sociology, 106*, 1219–1261.

Bandura, A. (1995). *Self-efficacy: The exercise of control*. New York: Freeman.

Behnken, I., Günther, C., Kabat vel Job, O., Keiser, S., Karig, U., Krüger, H. H. et al. (1991). *Schülerstudie '90. Jugendliche im Prozeß der Vereinigung* [Pupil study '90. Adolescents in the process of unification]. Weinheim, Germany: Juventa.

Bronfenbrenner, U. (1985). Ecology of the family as a context for human development: Research perspectives. *Developmental Psychology, 22*, 723–742.

Brunstein, J. C. (1993). Personal goals and subjective well-being: A longitudinal study. *Journal of Personality and Social Psychology, 65*, 1061–1070.

Bynner, J. (2001). British youth transitions in comparative perspective. *Journal of Youth Studies, 4*, 5–23.

Caldwell, J. C. (2004). Social upheaval and fertility decline. *Journal of Family History, 29*, 382–406.

Cen, G., & Li, D. (2006). Social transformation and values conflict among youth in contemporary China. In C. Daiute, Z. F. Beykont, C. Higson-Smith, & L. Nucci (Eds.), *International perspectives on youth conflict and development* (pp. 156–170). New York: Oxford University Press.

Chang, L. (2003). Variable effects on children's aggression, social withdrawal, and prosocial leadership as functions of teacher beliefs and behaviors. *Child Development, 74*, 538–548.

Chang, L., Lei, L., Li, K. K., Liu, H., Guo, B, Wang, Y., et al. (2005). Peer acceptance and self-perceptions of verbal and behavioural aggression and withdrawal. *International Journal of Behavioral Development, 29*, 49–57.

Cheah, C. S. L., & Park, S.-Y. (2006). South Korean mothers' beliefs regarding aggression and social withdrawal in preschoolers. *Early Childhood Research Quarterly, 21*, 61–75.

Chen, X., & Chen, H. (2010). Children's socioemotional functioning and adjustment in the changing Chinese society. In R. K. Silbereisen & X. Chen (Eds.), *Social change and human development: Concepts and results* (pp. 209–226). London: Sage.

Cohen, S., & Wills, T. A. (1985). Stress, social support, and the buffering hypothesis. *Psychological Bulletin, 98*, 310–357.

Conger, R. D., Conger, K. J., Elder, G. H., Jr., Lorenz, F. O., Simons, R. L., & Whitbeck, L. B. (1992). A family process model of economic hardship and adjustment of early adolescent boys. *Child Development, 63*, 526–541.

Conger, R. D., & Elder, G. H., Jr. (Eds.). (1994). *Families in troubled times: Adapting to change in rural America*. New York: Aldine de Gruyter.

Conger, R. D., Jewsbury-Conger, K., Matthews, L. S., & Elder, G. H., Jr. (1999). Pathways of economic influence on adolescent adjustment. *American Journal of Community Psychology, 27*, 519–541.

Craske, M. G. (1997). Fear and anxiety in children and adolescents. *Bulletin of the Menninger Clinic, 61*, 14–36.

Deutsches Jugendinstitut (Ed.). (1992). *Schüler an der Schwelle zur deutschen Einheit: Politische und persönliche Orientierung in Ost und West* [Pupils at the cusp of German unity: Political and personal orientation in East and West]. Opladen, Germany: Leske+Budrich.

Dreher, A. (2006). Does globalization affect growth?: Evidence from a new Index of Globalization. *Applied Economics, 38*, 1091–1110.

Elder, G. H., Jr. (1974). *Children of the Great Depression*. Chicago: University of Chicago Press.

Elder, G. H., Jr., Shanahan, M. J., & Clipp, E. C. (1994). When war comes to men's lives: Life-course patterns in family, work, and health. *Psychology and Aging, 9*, 5–16.

Emmons, R. A. (1992). Abstract versus concrete goals: Personal striving level, physical illness, and psychological well-being. *Journal of Personality and Social Psychology, 62*, 292–300.

Esping-Andersen, G. (1990). *The three worlds of welfare capitalism*. Princeton, NJ: Princeton University Press.

Evans, D. R. (1994). Enhancing quality of life in the population at large. *Social Indicators Research, 33*, 47–88.

Fenwick, R., & Tausig, M. (1994). The macroeconomic context of job stress. *Journal of Health and Social Behavior, 35,* 266–282.

Forkel, I., & Silbereisen, R. K. (2001). Family economic hardship and depressed mood among young adolescents from former East and West Germany. *American Behavioral Scientist, 44,* 1955–1971.

Fuller, L. (2000). Socialism and the transition in East and Central Europe. *Annual Review of Sociology, 26,* 585–609.

Furlong, A., & Cartmel, F. (1997). *Young people and social change: Individualisation and risk in late modernity.* Buckingham, UK: Open University Press.

Grob, A., Little, T. D., Wanner, B., Wearing, A. J., & Euronet (1996). Adolescents' well-being and perceived control across 14 sociocultural contexts. *Journal of Personality and Social Psychology, 71,* 785–795.

Guthrie, D. (2006). *China and globalization: The social, economic, and political transformation of Chinese society.* London: Routledge.

Hart, C. H., Yang, C., Nelson, L. J., Robinson, C. C., Olson, J. A., Nelson, D. A., et al. (2000). Peer acceptance in early childhood and subtypes of socially withdrawn behaviour in China, Russia and the United States. *International Journal of Behavioral Development, 24,* 73–81.

Havighurst, R. J. (1948). *Developmental tasks and education.* New York: McKay.

Heckhausen, J. (1999). *Developmental regulation in adulthood: Age-normative and sociostructural constraints as adaptive challenges.* New York: Cambridge University Press.

Hedström, P., & Swedberg, R. (1996). Social mechanism. *Acta Sociologica, 39,* 281–308.

Hofäcker, D., Buchholz, S., & Blossfeld, H.-P. (2010). Globalization, institutional filters and changing life course: Patterns in modern societies: A summary of the results from the GLOBALIFE-project. In R. K. Silbereisen & X. Chen (Eds.), *Social change and human development: Concepts and results* (pp. 101–124). London: Sage.

Huston, A. C. (2005). The effects of welfare reform and poverty policies on children and families. In D. B. Pillemer & S. H. White (Eds.), *Developmental psychology and social change* (pp. 83–103). New York: Cambridge University Press.

Inglehart, R. (1977). *The silent revolution: Changing values and political styles among Western publics.* Princeton, NJ: Princeton University Press.

Inglehart, R. (1997). *Modernization and postmodernization: Cultural, economic and political change in 43 societies.* Princeton, NJ: Princeton University Press.

Jeffrey, C., & McDowell, L. (2004). Youth in a comparative perspective: Global change, local lives. *Youth and Society, 36,* 131–142.

Jerusalem, M., & Mittag, W. (1995). Self-efficacy in stressful life transitions. In A. Bandura (Ed.), *Self-efficacy in changing societies* (pp. 177–201). New York: Cambridge University Press.

Kăgitcibaşi, C. (2005). Autonomy and relatedness in cultural context. Implications for self and family. *Journal of Cross-Cultural Psychology, 36,* 403–422.

Kăgitcibaşi, C., & Ataca, B. (2005). Value of children and family change: A three-decade portrait from Turkey. *Applied Psychology: An International Review,* 54, 317–337.

Kohn, M. L. (2006). *Change and stability: A cross-national analysis of social structure and personality.* Boulder, CO: Paradigm.

Kunovich, R. M., & Deitelbaum, C. (2004). Ethnic conflict, group polarization and gender attitudes in Croatia. *Journal of Marriage and Family, 66,* 1089–1107.

Larson, R. (2000). Toward a psychology of positive youth development. *American Psychologist, 55,* 170–183.

Lazarus, R. S., & Folkman, S. (1984). *Stress, appraisal and coping.* New York: Springer.

Lerner, R. M., & Busch-Rossnagel, N. (1981). Individuals as producers of their development: Conceptual and empirical bases. In R. M. Lerner & N. A. Busch-Rossnagel (Eds.), *Individuals as producers of their development: A life-span perspective* (pp.1–36). New York: Academic Press.

Leventhal, T., & Brooks-Gunn, J. (2000). The neighborhoods they live in: The effects of neighborhood residence on child and adolescent outcomes. *Psychological Bulletin, 126,* 309–337.

Liker, J. K., & Elder, G. H., Jr. (1983). Economic hardship and marital relations in the 1930s. *American Sociological Review, 48,* 343–359.

Liu, M., Chen, X., Rubin, K. H., Zheng, S., Cui, L., Li, D., et al. (2005). Autonomy- vs. connectedness-oriented parenting behaviors in Chinese and Canadian mothers. *International Journal of Behavioral Development, 29,* 489–495.

Macek, P., Flanagan, C., Gallay, L., Kostron, L., Botcheva, L., & Csapo, B. (1998). Postcommunist societies in times of transition: Perceptions of change among adolescents in central and eastern Europe. *Journal of Social Issues, 54,* 547–561.

Malmberg, L.-E., & Trempala, J. (1997). Anticipated transition to adulthood: The effect of educational track, gender, and self-evaluation on Finnish and Polish adolescents' future orientation. *Journal of Youth and Adolescence, 26,* 517–537.

Matutinovic, I. (1988). Quality of life in transition countries: Central East Europe with special reference to Croatia. *Social Indicators Research, 43,* 97–119.

McLoyd, V. C. (1998). Socioeconomic disadvantage and child development. *American Psychologist, 53,* 185–204.

Monden, C., & Smits, J. (2005). Ethnic intermarriage in times of social change: The case of Latvia. *Demography, 42,* 323–345.

Nauck, B., & Schwenk, O. G. (2001). Did societal transformation destroy the social networks of families in East Germany? *American Behavioral Scientist, 44,* 1864–1878.

Noack, P., Hofer, M., Kracke, B., & Klein-Allermann, E. (1995). Adolescents and their parents in East and West Germany facing social change. In P. Noack, M. Hofer, & J. Youniss (Eds.), *Psychological responses to social change* (pp. 129–148). Berlin: Walter de Gruyter.

Noack, P., Kracke, B., Wild, E., & Hofer, M. (2001). Subjectve experiences of social change in East and West Germany: Analyses of the perceptions of adolescents and their parents. *American Behavioral Scientist, 44,* 1798–1817.

Nee, V., & Matthews, R. (1996). Market transition and societal transformation in reforming state socialism. *Annual Review of Sociology, 22,* 401–435.

Okulicz-Kozaryn, K., & Borucka, A. (2008). Warsaw adolescent alchohol use in a period of social change in Poland: Cluster analyses of five consecutive surveys, 1998 to 2004. *Addictive Behaviors, 33,* 439–450.

Picket, K. E., & Pearl, M. (2001). Multilevel analyses of neighbourhood socioeconomic context and health outcomes: A critical review. *Journal of Epidemiology and Community Health, 55,* 111–122.

Pillemer, D. B., & White, S. H. (Eds.). (2005). *Developmental psychology and social change.* New York: Cambridge University Press.

Pinquart, M., Juang, L. P., & Silbereisen, R. K. (2004). The role of self-efficacy, academic abilities, and parental education in the change in career decisions of adolescents facing German unification. *Journal of Career Development, 31,* 125–142.

Pinquart, M., & Silbereisen, R. K. (2004). Human development in times of social change: Theoretical considerations and research needs. *International Journal of Behavioral Development, 28,* 289–298.

Pinquart, M., Silbereisen, R. K., & Juang, L. P. (2004a). Moderating effects of adolescents' self-efficacy beliefs on psychological responses to social change. *Journal of Adolescent Research, 19,* 340–359.

Pinquart, M., Silbereisen, R. K., & Juang, L. P. (2004b). Changes in psychosocial distress among East German adolescents facing German unification: The role of commitment to the old system and of self-efficacy beliefs. *Youth and Society, 36,* 77–101.

Pinquart, M., Silbereisen, R. K., & Körner, A. (2009). Do associations between perceived social change, coping, and psychological well-being vary by regional economic conditions?: Evidence from Germany. *European Psychologist, 14,* 207–219.

Plichtová, J., & Erös, F. (1997). The significance of political and economic change in two generations of Slovaks and Hungarians. *Journal of Community and Applied Social Psychology, 7,* 89–101.

Reitzle, M. (2006). The connections between adulthood transitions and the self-perception of being adult in the changing contexts of East and West Germany. *European Psychologist, 11,* 25–28.

Reitzle, M., & Silbereisen, R. K. (2000a). Adapting to social change: Adolescents' values in Eastern and Western Germany. In J. Bynner & R. K. Silbereisen (Eds.), *Adversity and challenge in life in the New Germany and England* (pp. 123–152). Basingstoke, UK: Macmillan.

Reitzle, M., & Silbereisen, R. K. (2000b). The timing of adolescents' school-to-work transition in the course of social change: The example of German unification. *Swiss Journal of Psychology, 59,* 240–255.

Ritter, G. A. (2006). *Der Preis der deutschen Einheit: Die Wiedervereinigung und die Krise des Sozialstaates* [The price of German unity: Reunification and the crisis of the welfare state]. München, Germany: Beck.

Ruan, D., Freeman, L. C., Dai, X., Pan, Y., & Zhang, W. (1997). On the changing structure of social networks in urban China. *Social Networks, 19*, 75–89.

Rutter, M., & Rutter, M. (1993). *Developing minds: Challenge and continuity across the life span.* London: Penguin Books.

Schmitz, M. (1995). *Wendestre?: Die psychosozialen Kosten der deutschen Einheit* [Reunification stress: Psychosocial costs of German unity]. Berlin: Rowohlt.

Schneider, N. F. (1994). *Familie und private Lebensführung in West- und Ostdeutschland: Eine vergleichende Analyse des Familienlebens 1970–1992* [Family and private lifestyle in West and East Germany: A comparative analysis of family life, 1970–1992]. Stuttgart, Germany: Enke.

Seligman, M. E. P. (1975). *Helplessness.* San Francisco: Freeman.

Silbereisen, R. K., & Chen, X. (Eds.). (2010). *Social change and human development: Concepts and results.* London: Sage.

Silbereisen, R. K., Eyferth, K., & Rudinger, G. (Eds.). (1986). *Development as action in context: Problem behavior and normal youth development.* New York: Springer.

Silbereisen, R. K., & Pinquart, M. (Eds.). (2008). *Individuum und sozialer Wandel: Eine Studie zu Anforderungen, psychosozialen Ressourcen und individueller Bewältigung* [Individual and social change: A study of demands, psychosocial resources, and individual coping]. Weinheim, Germany: Juventa.

Silbereisen, R. K., & Wiesner, M. (2000). Cohort change in adolescent developmental timetables after German unification: Trends and possible reasons. In J. Heckhausen (Ed.), *Motivational psychology of human development: Developing motivation and motivating development* (pp. 271–284). Amsterdam: Elsevier.

Taimalu, M., Lahikainen, A. R., Korhonen, P., & Kraav, I. (2007). Self-reported fears as indicators of young children's well-being in societal change: A cross-cultural perspective. *Social Indicators Research, 80*, 51–78.

Tamis-LeMonda, C. S., Way, N., Hughes, D, Yoshikawa, H., Kalman, R. K., & Niwa, E. Y. (2008). Parents' goals for children: The dynamic coexistence of individualism and collectivism in cultures and individuals. *Social Development, 17*, 183–209.

Thoits, P. (1995). Stress, coping, and social support processes: Where are we, what next? *Journal of Health and Social Behavior, Extra Issue,* 53–79.

Ting, K. F., & Chiu, C. C. H. (2000). Materialistic values in Hong Kong and Guangzhou: A comparative analysis of two Chinese societies. *Sociological Spectrum, 20*, 15–40.

Titma, M., & Trapido, D. (2002). Prediction of success in post-communist societies: Evidence from Latvia and Estonia. *Society and Economy, 24*, 297–331.

Titma, M., & Tuma, N. B. (2005). Human agency in the transition from communism. In K. W. Schaie & G. H. Elder Jr. (Eds.), *Historical influences on lives and aging* (pp. 108–143). New York: Springer.

Titma, M., Tuma, N. B., & Roots, A. (2007). Adolescent agency and adult economic success in a transitional society. *International Journal of Psychology, 42*, 102–109.

Tomasik, M. J., & Silbereisen, R. K. (2009). Demands of social change as a function of the political context, institutional filters, and psychosocial resources. *Social Indicators Research, 94*, 13–28.

Tomasik, M. J., Silbereisen, R. K., & Heckhausen, J. (2010). Is it adaptive to disengage from demands of social change? Adjustment to developmental barriers in opportunity-deprived regions. *Motivation and Emotion, 34*, 384–398.

Tuma, N. B., Titma, M., & Murakas, R. (2002). Transitional economies and income inequality: The case of Estonia. In B. J. Weinert (Ed.), *Transition to democracy in Eastern Europe and Russia: Impact on politics, economy and culture* (pp. 111–140). Westport, CT: Praeger.

Trommsdorff, G. (2006). Parent–child relations over the life-span: A cross-cultural perspective. In K. Rubin (Ed.), *Parenting beliefs, behaviors, and parent–child relations* (pp. 143–183). New York: Psychology Press.

Valkenburg, P. M. (2004). *Children's responses to the screen: A media psychological approach*. Mahwah, NJ: Erlbaum.

Van Snippenburg, L. B., & Hendriks Vettehen, P. G. J. (1992). Dutch youth in transition to adulthood: Differential changes in their political and sociocultural values since the 1970s. *Journal of Youth and Adolescence, 21*, 573–591.

Völker, B., & Flap, H. (1995). The effects of institutional transformation on personal networks: East Germany, four years later. *Netherlands Journal of Social Sciences, 31*, 87–110.

Wheaton, B. (1980). The sociogenesis of psychological disorder: An attributional theory. *Journal of Health and Social Behavior, 21*, 100–124.

Wu, Y. (2002). The openness and awareness of Shanghai's youth under the background of China's WTO entry. In J. Yin (Ed.), *2002 report on Shanghai society* (pp. 305–334). Shanghai: Shanghai Academy of Social Science Press.

Wyn, J., & White, R. (2000). Negotiating social change: The paradox of youth. *Youth and Society, 32*, 165–183.

Yabiku, S. T., Axinn, W. G., & Thornton, A. (1999). Family integration and children's self-esteem. *American Journal of Sociology, 104*, 1494–1524.

Yang, D., & Yan, K. (1997). (Eds.). *Research on values among university students in China in the contemporary era*. Shanghai: Shanghai Education Press.

Zhou, X., & Moen, P. (2001). Explaining life chances in China's economic transformation: A life course approach. *Social Science Research, 30*, 552–577.

Index